Progress in Inflammation Research

Series Editor

Prof. Dr. Michael J. Parnham
Senior Scientific Advisor
PLIVA dd
Prilaz baruna Filipovica 25
10000 Zagreb
Croatia

Advisory Board

Forthcoming titles:

Antirheumatic Therapy: Actions and Outcomes,
R.O. Day, D.E. Furst, P.L. van Riel, B. Bresnihan (Editors), 2004
Antibiotics as Anti-inflammatory and Immunomodulatory Agents,
B.K. Rubin, J. Tamaoki (Editors), 2004
Bone Morphogenetic Proteins: Bone Regeneration and Beyond,
S. Vukicevic, K.T. Sampath (Editors), 2004

(Already published titles see last page.)

Cancer and Inflammation

Douglas W. Morgan
Ulf J. Forssmann
Marian T. Nakada

Editors

Springer Basel AG

Editors

Douglas W. Morgan
TAP Pharmaceuticals
675 North Field Dr.
Lake Forest, IL 60045
USA

Ulf J. Forssmann
IPF PharmaCeuticals
Feodor-Lynen-Strasse 31
30625 Hannover
Germany

Marian T. Nakada
Oncology Research
Centocor
200 Great Valley Parkway
Malvern, PA 19355
USA

A CIP catalogue record for this book is available from the Library of Congress, Washington D.C., USA

Bibliographic information published by Die Deutsche Bibliothek
Die Deutsche Bibliothek lists this publication in the Deutsche Nationalbibliografie;
detailed bibliographic data is available in the internet at http://dnb.ddb.de

ISBN 978-3-7643-6592-9 ISBN 978-3-0348-7861-6 (eBook)
DOI 10.1007/978-3-0348-7861-6

Originally published by Birkhäuser Verlag, Basel - Boston - Berlin in 2004

Cover design: Markus Etterich, Basel
Cover illustration: CD68-positive macrophages (red) are observed in close proximity to CD31-positive endothelial cells (black) using double immunohistochemical techniques in a representative area of a human colon carcinoma. All nuclei (blue) have been counterstained with hematoxylin. Mags are as follows: 40× objective, total mag 600×, if use a bar size of 1.5 cm, then bar = 25 microns. We like to thank Danielle Lawrence and Dr. Michael R. D'Andrea of Johnson & Johnson Pharmaceutical Research & Development, Spring House, PA, for their contribution of this micrograph.

ISBN 978-3-7643-6592-9

9 8 7 6 5 4 3 2 1

www.birkhasuer-science.com

Contents

List of contributors vii

Preface ix

Jong H. Nam and Sreekant Murthy
Chronic inflammation and cancer in various organ systems 1

Michael T. Lotze and Ronald B. Herberman
Cancer as a chronic inflammatory disease: role of immunotherapy 21

Frances R. Balkwill
Inflammatory chemokines: their role in tumor growth and progression 53

Karin E. de Visser and Lisa M. Coussens
Inflammation and matrix metalloproteinases: implications for cancer development 71

Li Yan, Xiao-yu R. Song, Marian T. Nakada
Interplay between inflammation and tumor angiogenesis 99

Barbara Fingleton and Howard C. Crawford
Apoptotic responses common to cancer and inflammation 123

John P. Lynch and Gary R. Lichtenstein
Cyclooxygenase activity in gastrointestinal cancer development and progression: prospects as a therapeutic target 147

Christoph A. Maurer and Katharina M. Kessler
Effects of COX-2 inhibitors in colorectal cancer 177

Michael T. Lotze
Inflammation, necrosis, and cancer 189

Index 197

List of contributors

Frances R. Balkwill, Cancer Research UK, Translational Oncology Laboratory, Barts and The London Queen Mary's Medical School, Charterhouse Square, London EC1M 6BQ, UK; e-mail: frances.balkwill@cancer.org.uk

Lisa M. Coussens, Cancer Research Institute, Department of Pathology and Comprehensive Cancer Center, University of California, San Francisco 2340 Sutter St., San Francisco, CA 94143, USA; e-mail: coussens@cc.ucsf.edu

Howard C. Crawford, Dept. of Pharmacological Sciences, SUNY, Stony Brook, NY 11794, USA; e-mail: crawford@pharm.sunysb.edu

Barbara Fingleton, Dept. of Cancer Biology, Vanderbilt University Medical Center, Nashville TN 37232-6840, USA; e-mail: barbara.fingleton@vanderbilt.edu

Ronald B. Herberman, Hillman Cancer Center, University of Pittsburgh Cancer Institute and Centers, 5115 Centre Drive, Pittsburgh, PA 15323, USA; e-mail: herbermanrb@upmc.edu

Katharina M. Kessler, Surgical Clinic, Hospital of Liestal (affiliated hospital to the University of Basel), Rheinstrasse 26, 4410 Liestal, Switzerland; e-mail: katharina.kessler@ksli.ch

Gary R. Lichtenstein, Hospital of the University of Pennsylvania, Division of Gastroenterology/3rd fl Ravdin, 39th and Spruce Streets, Philadelphia, PA 19104, USA; e-mail: grl@mail.med.upenn.edu

Michael T. Lotze, Translational Research, Molecular Medicine Institute, University of Pittsburgh School of Medicine, 300 Technology Drive, Pittsburgh, PA 15219, USA; e-mail: lotzemt@upmc.edu

John P. Lynch, Division of Gastroenterology/660 CRB, Department of Medicine, University of Pennsylvania, 415 Curie Blvd., Philadelphia, PA 19104, USA; e-mail: lynchj@mail.med.upenn.edu

Christoph A. Maurer, Surgical Clinic, Hospital of Liestal (affiliated hospital to the University of Basel), Rheinstrasse 26, 4410 Liestal, Switzerland; e-mail: christoph.maurer@ksli.ch

Sreekant Murthy, Division of Gastroenterology and Hepatology, Drexel University College of Medicine, Drexel University, 245 N 15th Street, Philadelphia, PA 19102-1192, USA; e-mail: s.murthy@drexel.edu

Marian T. Nakada, Centocor, Inc, 200 Great Valley Parkway, Malvern, PA 19355, USA; e-mail: mnakada@cntus.jnj.com

Jong H. Nam, Division of Gastroenterology and Hepatology, Drexel University College of Medicine, Drexel University, 245 N 15th Street, Philadelphia, PA 19102-1192, USA

Yiao-yu R. Song, Centocor, Inc, 200 Great Valley Parkway, Malvern, PA 19355, USA

Karin E. de Visser, Cancer Research Institute, University of California, San Francisco, 2340 Sutter St., San Francisco, CA 94143, USA; e-mail: kdevisser@cc.ucsf.edu

Li Yan, Centocor, Inc, 200 Great Valley Parkway, Malvern, PA 19355, USA

Preface

This book provides a practical appreciation for the many biochemical and cellular mechanisms shared by cancer and inflammatory processes. It also explores the hypothesis that cancer and chronic inflammation are causally linked. It is written to scientists and physicians alike interested in biomedical research. Relatively few texts are available that truly integrate these two fields in spite of the many common underlying mechanisms. Few would dispute that there are common points in the two pathologies, but research on these areas has evolved to a large extent into groups working almost independently. Perhaps this is due to the differences in the overall clinical presentations that, historically, have spawned separate areas of research efforts. A closer look at both is taken by this book and reveals how interrelated the two are. It is hoped that this approach will stimulate more integration of knowledge, thinking and activity to benefit advancement of both areas.

To this end and as a part of the ongoing series *Progress in Inflammation Research*, edited by M. Parnham, we have assembled a collection of manuscripts that explore the links between cancer and inflammation. These manuscripts were written by prominent researchers working in both basic and clinical aspects of these fields and who represent the current critical thinking in the area. This is by no means intended to be exhaustive but primarily to broaden the reader's knowledge of this emerging area by means of collecting some of the current scholarly work.

For content we included areas where investigation of the interrelationship between the fields has received significant attention and that illustrates the integration already taking place. Areas covered include cytokines, proliferation, apoptosis, immunity, matrix metalloproteinases, cyclooxygenase and angiogenesis. We also included clinical studies in gastrointestinal diseases where hypotheses linking the diseases are being tested.

While our collection is really only a tip-of-the-iceberg view of a potentially whole new field, we hope that such coverage will help stimulate efforts to further our understanding fundamentally and to ultimately bring new therapeutics.

April 2004

Douglas W. Morgan
Ulf J. Forssmann
Marian T. Nakada

Chronic inflammation and cancer in various organ systems

Jong H. Nam and Sreekant Murthy

Division of Gastroenterology and Hepatology, Drexel University College of Medicine, Drexel University, 245 N 15th Street, Philadelphia, PA 19102-1192, USA

Introduction

Cancer is one of the leading causes of mortality and morbidity worldwide. The Global Burden of Disease Study estimated that, in 1990, 6 million out of 50.5 million deaths worldwide (12%) were attributable to cancer [1]. Among the top 30 causes of deaths worldwide that year, lung cancer, stomach cancer, liver cancer, colorectal cancer, esophageal cancer, and breast cancer ranked 10th, 14th, 22nd, 24th, 26th and 29th, respectively. In 1999, as per the World Health Organization mortality data, 23% of the total deaths in the United States occurred from cancer [2]. The United Kingdom and Japan reported similar rates at 24% and 30%, respectively. Mortality data from other countries are available at the World Health Organization website (http://www.who.int/en).

Interestingly, cancer is a disease that has strong links to chronic inflammation. There are many cancers that develop in the background of chronic inflammation, and some of these are listed in Table 1. Although the mechanisms have not been elucidated, it is hypothesized that reactive oxygen and nitrogen species produced by inflammatory cells cause DNA damage and cell mutation. These inflammatory cells also secrete various cytokines and chemokines, some of which are known to function as regulators of tumor growth, tumor metastasis, and angiogenesis [3]. Moreover, inflammation is known to cause upregulation of the enzyme cyclooxygenase type 2 (COX-2), and there is accumulating evidence that COX-2 upregulation plays an important role in neoplastic progression [4].

Associating chronic inflammation with cancer is really not a novel concept. In 1863, Virchow [5] wrote about leukocytes being present in neoplastic tissues. Later, he hypothesized that cancers originated from sites of chronic inflammation. In 1986, Dvorak [6] described how wound healing and tumor stoma formation share many important properties, referring to tumors as "wounds that fail to heal". It has since become more widely accepted that chronic inflammation provides a favorable environment for cancer to form and grow. In this chapter, we identify those cancers that have strong associations with inflammation, and discuss their epidemiology and the evidence that links their origin to inflammation.

Cancer and Inflammation, edited by Douglas W. Morgan, Ulf J. Forssmann and Marian T. Nakada

Table 1 - Chronic inflammation and associated cancer

Inflammatory condition/stimulus	Associated cancer
Schistosomiasis	Bladder cancer
H. pylori-induced gastritis	Gastric adenocarcinoma and MALT lymphoma
Hepatitis C virus infection	Hepatocellular carcinoma
Inflammatory bowel disease	Colon cancer
Reflux esophagitis/Barrett's esophagus	Esophageal adenocarcinoma
Asbestosis	Mesothelioma
Chronic pancreatitis	Pancreatic adenocarcinoma
Hepatitis B virus infection*	Hepatocellular carcinoma
Human papilloma virus infection*	Cervical cancer
Human herpes simplex virus type 8*	Kaposi's sarcoma

MALT, mucosa-associated lymphoid tissue.
**Inflammatory states where integration of the viral genome into the host genome is believed to be the principal cause of carcinogenesis rather than inflammation itself.*

Heliobacter pylori chronic gastritis and gastric adenocarcinoma

In recent years, it has become clear that the most important factor responsible for development of gastric cancer is *H. pylori* gastritis. *H. pylori* is a curved Gram-negative organism that infects roughly 50% of the world's population, more so in developing countries [7]. It is most commonly acquired in childhood, and once acquired, the organism persists on the gastric epithelium and causes chronic gastritis in essentially all those infected [8]. A small proportion of these persons go on to develop clinically significant diseases, such as gastric cancer and peptic ulcer disease. The World Health Organization has recognized this link and has declared *H. pylori* a class I carcinogen [9].

Gastric cancer is now the third most common cancer worldwide, and the second leading cause of cancer mortality [10]. This remains true despite the sharp decline in both the incidence and mortality observed in the second half of the 20th century [11, 12]. It was estimated that there were more than 870 000 deaths from gastric cancer in the year 2000, which accounted for about 12% of cancer deaths [13]. Gastric cancer also varies in incidence by geography. The highest rates are seen in the Far East, in countries such as Japan, China, and Korea, while the lowest rates are seen in North America, Western Europe, and Australia [14].

There are several lines of evidence to support the link between gastric cancer and *H. pylori* infection. The first real epidemiological evidence came from a study by

Parsonnet et al. [15], who performed a case-control study to compare the *H. pylori* serology status of 186 patients with gastric cancer to those of matched controls. They reported that significantly more gastric cancer patients had seropositivity to *H. pylori* than did the matched controls (84% *versus* 61%). The Eurogast group [16] conducted a study where 17 populations from 13 countries were involved, and confirmed that there was clearly a significant relationship between *H. pylori* prevalence and both gastric cancer incidence and mortality. There was approximately a 6-fold increase in risk of cancer in populations with 100% infection compared with populations with no infection. Other studies have reported similar conclusions [17–19]. Furthermore, there are even studies that have shown that the fall in gastric cancer incidence has paralleled the fall in *H. pylori* prevalence [20, 21].

Prospective studies, however, provide the strongest support for the link. Parsonnet and Forman [22] analyzed data from three prospective studies and reported that the risk of gastric cancer following *H. pylori* infection increased almost 9-fold after 15 years or more of *H. pylori* infection. Other meta-analyses of prospective studies have confirmed this association, reporting 2–3-fold increased risk in those chronically infected with *H. pylori* [23, 24]. Even more powerful evidence is available from a study by Uemura et al. [25]. In this study, 1526 patients with known *H. pylori* serology status were followed over an 8-year period. Of the 1246 patients who were *H. pylori*-positive, 36 (2.9%) eventually developed gastric cancer, whereas of the 280 patients who were *H. pylori* negative, none did. Uemura et al. [26] also studied the effect of *H. pylori* eradication in gastric cancer recurrence. They reported that no recurrent cancer occurred in those who had successful eradication of the organism.

Heliobacter pylori infection and gastric mucosa-associated lymphoid tissue (MALT) lymphomas

In 1983, Isaacson and Wright [27] first introduced the term MALT lymphoma to characterize primary low-grade B-cell lymphomas in the stomach and small bowel. A more recent term put forth by the World Health Organization is "extranodal marginal zone B-cell lymphoma of mucosa-associated lymphoid tissue". Nevertheless, the gastric form of this lymphoma is still most commonly referred to as gastric MALT lymphoma.

Overall, gastric lymphomas account for only about 3–6% of all gastric malignancies [28]. Its association with *H. pylori* infection, as in gastric adenocarcinomas, has also clearly been established. First of all, evidence suggests that *H. pylori* can be found in most cases of gastric MALT lymphomas. Wotherspoon et al. [29], for example, examined 110 cases of gastric MALT lymphomas and found *H. pylori* infection in 101 of them (92%). Moreover, *H. pylori*-infected patients appear to be at increased risk of developing gastric lymphomas. Parsonnet et al. [30] collected and stored serum from 230 593 subjects who were followed for a median of 14 years, at which time 33 patients developed gastric lymphomas. They noted that patients with gastric lymphomas were 6.3 times more likely than matched controls to have seropositivity to *H. pylori*. The prevalence of MALT lymphoma also appears to parallel that of *H. pylori* infection. In northern Italy, for example, where *H. pylori* prevalence is 87%, there is an extraordinarily high incidence of primary gastric lymphomas (13 times that of the UK) [31].

More direct evidence comes from clinical studies in which *H. pylori* was eradicated and the effect on the disease noted. In 1993, Wotherspoon et al. [32] reported regression of gastric MALT lymphoma in five of their six patients who were treated for and successfully eradicated *H. pylori*. Another study reported complete regression of low-grade MALT lymphoma for 16 months following *H. pylori* eradication, with subsequent relapse of the lymphoma following re-infection with the organism [33]. Other studies have reported similar findings [34, 35]. Studies in Mongolian gerbils lend further support to this notion [36].

The mechanism *via* which MALT lymphomas arise from chronic *H. pylori* infection is unclear. Interestingly, normal stomach is considered to be devoid of organized lymphoid tissue. Hence, acquisition of MALT is probably the first step toward carcinogenesis, and infection by *H. pylori* appears to trigger this. *H. pylori* is known to stimulate T-cells in very non-specific ways and, as such, *H. pylori* has often been referred to as a "super-antigen". This is in contrast to the normal antigen-recognition process that takes place between T-cell receptors and specific antigens. In the midst of non-specific T-cell activation, interleukin-2 (IL-2) is secreted and B-cells are stimulated, and when a single B-cell clone takes over and propagates, lymphoma can develop. Moreover, neutrophilic involvement during inflammation produces oxygen free radicals, which can damage DNA and help acquire genetic abnormalities [37].

Hepatitis C and hepatocellular carcinoma (HCC)

Hepatitis C virus (HCV) is an etiological agent that is linked to chronic hepatitis, cirrhosis, and HCC. In the United States it is the most common indication for liver transplant [38]. The worldwide prevalence of HCV seropositivity is about 3% (170 million people), although large variations do exist by geography [39,40]. Seroprevalence in North America, for example, is 0.4–1.8%, while that in North Africa is 9.6–13.6% [41]. In the United States, a national survey of non-institutionalized persons during 1988 through 1994 revealed a seroprevalence of 1.8%, among which 74% had detectable viral RNA levels [42]. This translates to 3.9 million Americans having antibody to HCV, and 2.7 million having persistent viremia. The US Surgeon General declared HCV a "silent epidemic" as of July 2000.

In the US and Australia, most HCV infections occur in persons aged 30–40, suggesting that the peak of HCV incidence has been relatively recent. In other countries, such as Japan, most HCV infections occur in much older persons, suggesting the peak of incidence was in the distant past (i.e. World War II). In other regions, such as North Africa, HCV occurs across all ages, reflecting ongoing high risk of HCV acquisition.

The most striking aspect of HCV infection is that once acquired, the virus will persist in 60–85% of infected persons, despite vigorous humoral and cellular host immune responses [43]. The precise mechanism of this viral persistence is unknown, but it appears that the quasispecies nature of HCV (genetic heterogeneity) is an important contributing factor. Once acquired, the virus causes chronic hepatitis in most persons, although with varying degrees of severity. Over the next 5–20 years, fibrosis of the liver will occur and a proportion of these persons will eventually develop cirrhosis. It is in this setting of chronic hepatic inflammation and fibrosis that HCC is known to emerge.

HCC is one of the most common solid tumors worldwide, with about 0.5–1 million cases occurring per year [44]. It is the 5th most common cancer in men and 9th in women. The age-adjusted incidence varies by geography, but worldwide it is 14.67 for men and 4.92 for women [45]. The lowest rates occur in developed countries, such as North America and Europe, where the primary etiologic agent is the hepatitis B virus (HBV). The highest rates, on the other hand, occur in east Asia and sub-Saharan Africa, and HCV is the primary agent here. HCC is also a cancer with very high mortality. In fact, the mortality rate of HCC closely approximates the incidence rate because there is a rapid death rate after diagnosis in most cases. In certain countries, such as those in sub-Saharan Africa and Far East, including China, Hong Kong, Taiwan, Korea, Vietnam, and Cambodia, HCC is one of the most frequent causes of death [46].

It is also clear that the global patterns of HCC are changing. HCC incidence rates in many developed areas, such as North America, Europe, and Japan, have clearly increased. In the United States, for example, HCC incidence has increased from 1.4 per 100 000 during 1976–1980 to 3.0 per 100 000 during 1996–1998, a 2-fold increase [47]. It has been pointed out that these figures likely underestimate the true incidence by 20–30%, since they represent only HCC confirmed by histopathological examinations [48]. Not surprisingly, the mortality rate due to HCC has increased also. According to vital US statistics, the overall age-adjusted mortality rate for HCC increased from 1.8 per 100 000 during 1979–1983 to 3.1 per 100 000 during 1994–1998 [44].

The strongest support for the link between HCV and HCC comes from epidemiologic studies where HCV was identified as a clear risk factor for HCC. In a recent meta-analysis of 21 case-control studies, for example, the risk of HCC was 17-fold among HCV-infected patients compared with HCV-negative controls [49]. Several prospective studies have confirmed the increased risk of HCC in HCV-infected cohorts [50, 51].

The precise mechanism by which chronic HCV causes HCC is unknown. Unlike the hepatitis B virus, whose DNA genome integrates itself into the host cell's genome,

HCV probably initiates carcinogenesis *via* chronic inflammation and fibrosis generation. This notion would be supported by the observation that virtually all HCV-related HCCs arise in a setting of chronic inflammation and cirrhosis [60]. Once cirrhosis is established, the annual risk of HCC is estimated to be 1–4% [52, 53].

Inflammatory bowel disease (IBD) and colorectal cancer (CRC)

IBD is a group of disorders where the gastrointestinal tract undergoes chronic or relapsing idiopathic immune activation and inflammation. Crohn's disease and ulcerative colitis are the two major forms of IBD, and lymphocytic colitis and collagenous colitis are the much less common types. Crohn's disease is characterized by chronic inflammation involving any region of the gastrointestinal tract, from mouth to anus. The inflammation is often transmural, meaning that it can affect the entire wall of the gut from mucosa to serosa. The affected areas also tend to occur in discontinuous regions along the gut, often described as "skipped lesions". Numerous extraintestinal manifestations may exist, such as arthralgias, skins lesions, and ocular diseases. Ulcerative colitis shares many similar features with Crohn's disease. In fact, it is sometimes difficult to distinguish the two diseases clinically. Nevertheless, ulcerative colitis and Crohn's disease are distinct syndromes with important differences. Ulcerative colitis always involves the rectum, with variable involvement proximally into the colon. In contrast to Crohn's disease, the affected areas are superficial (involving mucosa and submucosa) and continuous. Like Crohn's disease, though, there are similar extraintestinal manifestations of the disease.

Defining the precise epidemiology of IBD has been a challenge for various reasons. Because there are no gold-standard criteria for diagnosis of IBD, certain diseases, such as infectious colitis, have often been misclassified as IBD. Sometimes it is also difficult to differentiate between Crohn's disease and ulcerative colitis clinically, and hence reassignment of diagnosis is not uncommon, occurring in as much as 10% of cases in the first 2 years of diagnosis [54]. Then there is also that tendency for studies from large referral centers to underestimate the true incidence in the general population [55]. Despite these challenges, however, there are ample data to suggest that IBD affects numerous individuals in many parts of the world, particularly in North America and Europe, and that its incidence is rising rapidly in areas such as east Asia where rates have been historically low. In North America, the incidence rates of Crohn's disease and ulcerative colitis are in the range of 3.1–14.6 and 2.2–14.3 cases per 100 000, respectively [55]. In Europe, the rates are in the range of 0.7–9.8 and 1.5–20.3 cases per 100 000, respectively [55]. In Australia and New Zealand, the incidence rates have been low to moderate, ranging from 1.75–2.1 per 100 000 [55]. As mentioned previously, east Asian countries have much lower incidence rates of IBD than those of Western countries. Japan, for example, has reported incidence rates between 0.08 and 0.5 per 100 000 [56, 57].

These areas, however, are also experiencing rapid rises in IBD incidence. Korea, for example, has reported a 10-fold increase in incidence of ulcerative colitis since the mid 1980s [58]. South America and Africa still report the lowest incidence of IBD, with the exception of South Africa, where the rate among the white population is about 2.6 per 100 000 [59].

Increased risk of CRC is one of the most frightening aspects of IBD. This increased risk has been recognized since the 1930s, and many epidemiologic studies have since confirmed it. In ulcerative colitis, there is about a 20–30-fold higher risk of developing CRC than in the general population [60]. In fact, CRC is responsible for about one out of six deaths in ulcerative colitis [61]. It is rare to develop cancer when the duration of disease is less than 8 years, but thereafter the incidence accumulates at 0.5–1% per year [62]. Recently, a meta-analysis was performed to estimate the overall risk of CRC in ulcerative colitis by decade [63]. A total of 116 published studies were analyzed, and the cumulative incidences were 2% by 10 years of disease, 8% by 20 years, and 18% by 30 years. The overall prevalence of CRC in all ulcerative colitis patients was 3.7%. The risk of cancer in IBD patients is more likely related to the duration and extent of disease than the age of onset [64, 65]. The risk is clearly most increased in patients with pancolitis, whereas it is only minimally increased in left-sided colitis and not increased in proctitis [62].

The increased risk of CRC is being increasingly recognized in Crohn's disease as well. The estimated risk, however, varies as widely as in ulcerative colitis. Patients with Crohn's disease have a higher percentage of right-sided lesions, perhaps reflecting the tendency for right-sided Crohn's colitis in patients with ileocolitis [66]. Most studies based on hospital data report standardized incidence ratios between 1.0 and 4.3, but also as high as 26.6 [61, 67–69, 71, 72]. Population-based studies report ratios between 1.36 and 2.64 [70–73]. When Crohn's disease involves the colon, the risk of CRC appears to be similar to that of ulcerative colitis. One hospital-based study reported that cumulative incidence rates for extensive Crohn's disease and ulcerative colitis were 8% at 22 years and 7% at 20 years, respectively [67]. Another study reported slightly higher rates, at 12% and 13% at 20 years [74].

Inflammation-associated colon cancer has also been observed in many natural and experimental models of colitis. Cotton top tamarins develop colitis-associated colon cancer in a captive environment [75]. Although colon cancer is not observed in mice, certain genetically engineered mice such as interleukin-10 and G-1 knockouts [76, 77] develop colitis-associated adenocarcinoma.

In addition to genetically engineered mice, several studies have reported the occurance of dysplasia and cancers in mice, rats, and hamsters when they are fed dextran sulfate sodium solutions. A recent study [78] has also shown that colitis acts as a promoter of cancer in mice with multiple intestinal neoplasia (MIN model of cancer), which has a single germline mutatation of the adenomatous polyposis coli. These animal studies further confirm that inflammation could be a precursor for the development of colon cancer in animals as well.

Reflux esophagitis, Barrett's esophagus, and esophageal adenocarcinoma

Reflux esophagitis results from mucosal injury caused by gastric contents refluxing abnormally into the esophagus. It is difficult to ascertain the exact prevalence of esophagitis in gastroesophageal reflux disease (GERD), but available studies suggest that between 48% and 79% of GERD patients have esophagitis [79,80]. Given that GERD is a highly prevalent condition, particularly in North America and Europe, significant numbers of people will suffer from reflux esophagitis.

Barrett's esophagus is an acquired premalignant condition that arises from a setting of GERD and chronic esophagitis. It essentially describes a metaplastic change in the esophageal epithelium from the normal squamous epithelium to the specialized intestinal epithelium containing columnar cells and goblet cells. The incidence of Barrett's esophagus has increased markedly since the 1970s in the United States, mostly in the white male population. The prevalence in the general population is currently estimated to be about 1% [81, 82], but this may be an underestimate. A study from Olmsted County, Minnesota, suggested that for every known case of Barrett's esophagus, 20 additional cases go unrecognized [83].

Barrett's esophagus would be of no importance were it not for its well-recognized association with esophageal adenocarcinoma. As with Barrett's esophagus, the incidence of esophageal adenocarcinoma has also been increasing rapidly in many parts of the world, mainly North America and Europe. In fact, esophageal adenocarcinoma is the fastest rising malignancy among white men in the United States, with an annual increase of 4–10% since the 1970s [84, 85]. Whereas it accounted for less than 15% of all esophageal cancers in white men in the mid-1970s, it now accounts for over half of them [86]. Similar reports have come from other countries. Denmark, for example, experienced an increase in incidence 8-fold from 1970 to 1990 [87].

There are several lines of evidence to link GERD with Barrett's esophagus and esophageal adenocarcionoma. First of all, GERD patients are much more likely to have Barrett's esophagus than the general population. For example, Barrett's esophagus is reported to occur in about 1% of unselected patients undergoing endoscopies, but in about 6–12% of GERD patients [88]. The duration and severity of GERD symptoms also appear to influence the risk of developing Barrett's esophagus. Lieberman et al. [89] reported that compared to patients with reflux symptoms for less than 1 year, patients with GERD symptoms for 1–5 years were three times more likely to have Barrett's esophagus. Those with symptoms for more than 10 years were even more likely to have Barrett's – 6.4 times. Patients with Barrett's esophagus also have more severe GERD by objective criteria. Singh et al. [90] determined that Barrett's patients had a higher percentage of acid exposure ($pH < 4$) and lower pressure in the lower esophageal sphincter (LES) than non-Barrett's patients with GERD. There was also a strong correlation between degree of acid exposure and length of Barrett's segment. Oberg et al. [91] performed esophageal motility and

24-h pH monitoring in 556 patients undergoing endoscopy for symptoms suggestive of GERD, and similarly reported that the extent of Barrett's correlated strongly with the degree of esophageal acid exposure and duration of symptoms, and inversely with lower esophageal sphincter pressure.

The severity of GERD appears to influence the risk of not only Barrett's, but esophageal adenocarcionoma as well. Lagergren et al. [92] performed a large population-based case-control study in Sweden involving 189 patients with esophageal adenocarcinoma, and reported that patients with recurrent symptoms of reflux were 7.7 times more likely to have esophageal adenocarcinoma than those without GERD. The more frequent, severe, and extended the symptoms of reflux were, the greater the risk of cancer. In fact, the risk was increased to 43.5 times in patients with long-standing and severe reflux disease. Others have confirmed this [93].

Chronic pancreatitis and pancreatic adenocarcinoma

Pancreatic cancer is a relatively rare tumor. In the United States, for example, the number of new cases diagnosed per year is about 28 000 [94]. The disease is rare before age 45, but rises in incidence sharply thereafter. Pancreatic cancer is also a disease with extreme high mortality. Of the 28 000 persons diagnosed every year, only 10–20% have resectable disease, and 83% will die within 12 months of diagnosis [95, 96]. Appropriately, this cancer has been ranked fourth as a cause of cancer-related deaths in the United States, despite the relatively low incidence.

It is known that chronic pancreatitis is a risk factor for the development of pancreatic adenocarcinoma. Initial studies linking chronic pancreatitis to pancreatic cancer emerged in the 1980s, when two small case-control studies reported an increased yet non-significant number of pancreatic cancers among patients with chronic pancreatitis [97, 98]. Three additional studies emerged in the early 1990s that reported similar observations [99–101]. Lowenfels et al. [102] conducted the most convincing study; they recruited and followed 2015 patients with chronic pancreatitis enrolled from various centers around the world. They identified 56 patients who developed pancreatic cancer, and their analysis showed that at 10 years after diagnosis of chronic pancreatitis, the cumulative risk of pancreatic cancer was 1.8%. At 20 years, the risk increased to 4.0%. Similarly, Talamini et al. [103] followed 715 cases of chronic pancreatitis for a median of 10 years, and compared the incidence of pancreatic cancer with that of the general population. They noticed a significant increase in the incidence of pancreatic cancer in the chronic pancreatitis group (standardized incidence ratio = 18.5).

The highest risk of pancreatic cancer is seen in hereditary pancreatitis, a rare autosomal dominant disorder involving mutation of the trypsinogen gene. These patients present with pancreatitis at an early age (< 20 years), followed by a chronic relapsing pattern of disease. Lowenfels et al. [102] gathered medical records of

246 patients with presumed hereditary pancreatitis to assess the strength of association between pancreatitis and pancreatic cancer. They found that these patients had a 53-fold increased risk of pancreatic cancer, and that the cumulative risk by age 70 years was 40%.

Schistosomiasis and bladder cancer

Schistosomiasis, also known as bilharziasis, is a widespread endemic disease found most commonly in agricultural communities, particularly those that are dependent on irrigation to support their agriculture. The etiological agent is a fluke, a kind of parasitic worm that has complex life cycle involving fresh-water snails as intermediate hosts. Initially, fresh water becomes infected from contaminated urine or stool. Here, the eggs hatch, and if water snails are present, the parasites grow and develop in them. The snails eventually release large numbers of larvae into the water, which penetrate through the skin of unsuspecting hosts swimming in contaminated water. Within several weeks, the worms produce eggs that are passed into the urine or stool.

It is estimated that more than 200 million people are infected with these flukes worldwide [104]. *Schistosoma haematobium*, is one species of schistosome that is endemic to the Nile River valley in Egypt and other parts of Africa, and this species has been strongly linked to squamous cell carcinoma of the bladder. The exact mechanism by which the parasite causes bladder cancer is unknown, but it is thought that chronic inflammation may be an important culprit. The mechanical irritation caused by egg deposits in the bladder wall cause chronic inflammation, and in this setting activated macrophages generate reactive oxygen radicals that damage DNA and mutate cells.

There is strong epidemiologic evidence to support the relationship between schistosomiasis and bladder cancer. In countries where schistosomiasis is endemic, bladder cancer often tops the list in terms of cancer incidence and mortality. In Egypt, for example, bladder cancer ranks first among all types of cancer in men, and second only to breast cancer in women [104]. In one report, of the 11 626 cancer cases reported between 1970 and 1974, 27.6% were due to bladder cancers associated with schistosomiasis [105]. The same study reported that among the 2500 new cases of cancer reported to the Cairo Cancer Institute every year, about 27% were bladder cancers associated with schistosomiasis. Reports from other countries such as Iraq, Malawi, Zambia, and Kuwait, where schistosomiasis is also endemic, have reported similar findings [106, 107]. These figures are in clear contrast to those found in countries free of schistosomiasis, where bladder cancer ranks only 5th to 14th in incidence [108]. The association between *S. haematobium* and bladder cancer has also been confirmed in experimental models of schistosomiasis [109, 110].

Asbestosis and mesothelioma

Asbestos refers to a naturally occurring group of fibers that have flexible and fire-resistant properties. They are often used in industry to make heat insulation and fire resistance products. Although these fibers are typically combined with binding agents, some fibers are released into the air inadvertently and inhaled by workers. Naturally, some of the heaviest exposures occur in settings of building demolition and renovation. Workers in textile, insulation, and automobile brake-repair industries are also at increased risk of exposure to airborne asbestos. It is estimated that a total of 1.3 million workers are at significant risk of exposure to asbestos in the United States.

Asbestosis is a serious disease of the lung caused by inhalation of asbestos. It is characterized by a gradual scarring of the lung parenchyma, which eventually leads to inefficient oxygen exchange and subsequently to dyspnea, weakness, and weight loss. The mechanism by which asbestos causes these changes is probably *via* chronic irritation and inflammation. The body will attempt to clear the fibers *via* mucociliary actions and macrophages, but some fibers manage to migrate distally into the parenchyma and cause on-going inflammation and eventual fibrosis.

One of the most frightening complications of asbestosis is the occurrence of mesothelioma, a rare tumor of the pleura. Mesotheliomas can be benign or malignant, but as most are malignant they are routinely referred to as just mesotheliomas. Several observations support the link between asbestos and mesothelioma. In 1960, Wagner et al. [111] first demonstrated clearly that among South African miners occupational and environmental exposure to crocidolite was associated with deaths from malignant mesothelioma 30–40 years later. Selikoff et al. [112] similarly reported later that an association between asbestos exposure and mesothelioma existed among a group of pipe fitters. Since then, many similar observations have been reported from around the world. It is now clear that about 80% of malignant mesotheliomas, at least in the Western world, are associated with asbestos exposure. The latency period is also very prolonged. In a review of 1690 mesothelioma cases, 99% of cases occurred more than 15 years after asbestos exposure, but none occurred less than 10 years from exposure [113].

Malignant mesothelioma is still a relatively rare tumor, although it is continuing to grow in incidence. The precise incidence is difficult to estimate because the disease has been frequently coded as lung cancer in the past. Nevertheless, the available data allow estimation of the incidence of newly diagnosed mesothelioma in US males to be in the range of 2000–3000 cases per year [114, 115]. Interestingly, because of its association with work-related asbestos exposure, mesothelioma is more frequently seen in men than in women. The incidence is expected to continue to rise well into the next century, reflecting the 8 million workers who were exposed to asbestos in the past (before governmental regulations) and the long latency period to its developement. It is predicted that the annual death rate from malignant mesothelioma will continue to rise annually at least until the year 2020. Currently, mesothelioma leads to some 10 000 worldwide deaths annually [116].

The exact mechanism *via* which asbestos fibers cause mesothelioma is unclear. As mentioned previously, when asbestos fibers are inhaled, macrophages will attempt to phagocytose them and mucocililary actions will help to clear them. The inhaled fibers that are not cleared by these mechanisms migrate distally through the endothelial lining and into the interstitial tissues. Here they accumulate in the lower third of the lungs and penetrate the visceral pleura. It is here that asbestos can induce DNA damage and mutations by direct physical interaction and/or by indirect action of superoxides and free radicals produced by macrophages.

Summary

There is convincing evidence that inflammation plays an important role in the neoplastic progression of many types of cancer. It is generally agreed that inflammation provides an ideal setting for carcinogenesis because inflammatory cells, growth factors, and genotoxic agents work in concert to potentiate and promote neoplastic progression. Much evidence comes from epidemiologic studies and animal studies where the links between certain chronic inflammatory conditions and cancers have been clearly established. Probably the strongest evidence, however, comes from studies that have assessed cancer risk among long-term users of aspirin and non-steroidal anti-inflammatory drugs. It is clear from these studies that these drugs have chemopreventive effects, reducing the incidence of certain cancers, such as esophageal cancer [117], gastric cancer [118], colorectal cancer [119–121], lung cancer [122], bladder cancer [123], and breast cancer [124]. Celecoxib, a COX-2 inhibitor, for example, has been shown in a double-blind placebo-controlled study to significantly reduce colorectal polyp burden in familial adenomatous polyposis [125]. Aspirin has also been shown to reduce the number of adenomatous polyps in patients with histories of both colorectal polyps and colorectal cancer [126, 127]. The putative role by which inflammation promotes tumor growth, angiogenesis, and metastasis are subjects of intense investigation and are discussed in subsequent chapters of this book.

References

1 Murray CJL, Lopez AD (1997) Mortality by cause for eight regions of the world: Global Burden of Disease Study. *Lancet* 349: 1269–1276
2 http://www-depdb.iarc.fr/who/menu.htm
3 Coussens LM, Werb Z (2002) Inflammation and cancer. *Nature* 420: 860–867

4 O'Byrne KJ, Dalgleish AG (2001) Chronic immune activation and inflammation as the cause of malignancy. *Br J Cancer* 85: 473–483
5 Balkwill F, Mantovani A (2001) Inflammation and cancer: back to Virchow? *Lancet* 357: 539–545
6 Dvorak HF (1986) Tumors: wounds that do not heal. Similarities between tumor stroma generation and wound healing. *N Engl J Med* 315: 1650–1659
7 Williams MP, Pounder RE (1999) *Helicobacter pylori*: From the benign to the malignant. *Am J Gastroenterol* 94 (Suppl): S11–S16
8 Kuipers EJ, Uyterlinde AM, Pena AS, Roosendaal R, Pals G, Nelis GF, Festen HP, Meuwissen SG (1995) Long-term sequelae of *Helicobacter pylori* gastritis. *Lancet* 345: 1525–1528
9 International Agency for Research on Cancer Schistosomes, liver flukes and *Helicobacter pylori* (1994) *IARC monographs on the evaluation of carcinogenic risks to humans*, Vol. 61. International Agency for Research on Cancer, Lyon
10 Parkin DM, Bray FI, Devesa SS (2001) Cancer burden in the year 2000. The global picture. *Eur J Cancer* 37: S4–S66
11 Howson CP, Hiyama T, Wynder EL (1986) The decline of gastric cancer: epidemiology of an unplanned triumph. *Epidemiol Rev* 8:1–27
12 Kelley JR, Duggan JM (2003) Gastric cancer epidemiology and risk factors. *J Clin Epidemiol* 56: 1–9
13 Parkin DM, Pisani P, Ferlay J (1993) Estimates of the worldwide incidence of eighteen major cancers in 1985. *Int J Cancer* 54: 594–606
14 Kelley JR, Duggan JM (2003) Gastric cancer epidemiology and risk factors. [Review]. *J Clin Epidemiol* 56: 1–9
15 Parsonnet J, Friedman GD, Vandersteen DP, Chang Y, Vogelman JH, Orentreich N, Sibley RK (1991) *Helicobacter pylori* infection and the risk of gastric carcinoma. *N Engl J Med* 325: 1127–1131
16 The Eurogast Study Group (1993) An international association between *Helicobacter pylori* infection and gastric cancer. *Lancet* 341: 1359–1362
17 Sipponen P, Kosunen TU, Valle J, Riihela M, Seppala K (1992) *Helicobacter pylori* infection and chronic gastritis in gastric cancer. *J Clin Pathol* 45: 319–323
18 Kikuchi O, Wada T, Nakajima T, Nishi T, Kobayashi O, Konishi T, Inaba Y (1995) Serum anti-*Helicobacter pylori* antibody and gastric carcinoma among young adults. *Cancer* 75: 2789–2793
19 Asaka M, Kimura T, Kato M, Kudo M, Miki K, Ogoshi K, Kato T, Tatsuta M, Graham DY (1994) Possible role of *Helicobacter pylori* infection in early gastric cancer development. *Cancer* 73: 2691–2694
20 Banatvala N, Mayo K, Megraud F, Jennings R, Deeks JJ, Feldman RA (1993) The cohort effect and *Helicobacter pylori*. *J Infect Dis* 168: 219–221
21 Webb PM, Forman D (1995) *Helicobacter pylori* as a risk factor for cancer. *Baillieres Clin Gastroenterol* 9: 563–582

22 Parsonnet J, Forman D (2004) *Helicobacter pylori* and gastric cancer. *JAMA* 291: 187–194
23 Danesh J (1999) *Helicobacter pylori* and gastric cancer; systematic review of epidemiological studies. *Aliment Pharmacol Ther* 13: 851–856
24 Eslick GD, Lim LL, Byles JE, Xia HH, Talley NJ (1999) Association of *Helicobacter pylori* infection with gastric carcinoma: a meta-analysis. *Am J Gastroenterol* 94: 2373–2379
25 Uemura N, Okamoto S, Yamamoto S, Matsumura N, Yamaguchi S, Yamakido M, Taniyama K, Sasaki N, Schlemper RJ (2001) *Helicobacter pylori* infection and the development of gastric cancer. *N Engl J Med* 345: 784–789
26 Uemura N, Mukai T, Okamoto S, Yamaguchi S, Mashiba H, Taniyama K, Sasaki N, Haruma K, Sumi K, Kajiyama G (1997) Effect of *Helicobacter pylori* eradication on subsequent development of cancer after endoscopic resection of early gastric cancer. *Cancer Epidemiol Biomarkers Prev* 6: 639–642
27 Isaacson P, Wright DH (1983) Malignant lymphoma of mucosa-associated lymphoid tissue. A distinctive type of B cell lymphoma. *Cancer* 52: 1410–1416
28 Morgner A, Bayerdörffer E, Neubauer A, Stolte M (2000) Malignant tumors of the stomach. Gastric mucosa-associated lymphoid tissue lymphoma and *Helicobacter pylori*. *Gastroenterol Clin North Am* 29: 593–607
29 Wotherspoon AC, Ortiz Hidalgo C, Falzon MR, Isaacson PG (1991) *Helicobacter pylori*-associated gastritis and primary B cell gastric lymphoma. *Lancet* 338: 1175–1176
30 Parsonnet J, Hansen S, Rodriguez L, Gelb AB, Warnke RA, Jellum E, Orentreich N, Vogelman JH, Friedman GD (1994) *Helicobacter pylori* infection and gastric lymphoma. *N Engl J Med* 330: 1267–1271
31 Doglioni C, Wotherspoon AC, Moschini A, De Boni M, Isaacson PG (1992) High incidence of primary gastric lymphoma in northeastern Italy. *Lancet* 339: 834–835
32 Wotherspoon AC, Doglioni C, Diss TC, Pan L, Moschini A, De Boni M, Isaacson PG (1993) Regression of primary low-grade B cell gastric lymphoma of mucosa-associated lymphoid tissue type after eradication of *Helicobacter pylori*. *Lancet* 342: 575–577
33 Cammarota G, Montalto M, Tursiet A, Vecchio FM, Fedeli G, Gasbarrini G (1995) *Helicobacter pylori* reinfection and rapid relapse of low-grade B-cell gastric. *Lancet* 345: 192
34 Bayerdorffer E, Neubauer A, Rudolph B, Thiede C, Lehn N, Eidt S, Stolte M (1995) Regression of primary gastric lymphoma of mucosa-associated lymphoid tissue type after cure of *Helicobacter pylori* infection. *Lancet* 345: 1591–1594
35 Morgner A, Miehlke S, Fischbach W, Schmitt W, Muller-Hermelink H, Greiner A, Thiede C, Schetelig J, Neubauer A, Stolte M et al (2001) Complete remission of primary high-grade B-cell gastric lymphoma after cure of *Helicobacter pylori* infection. *J Clin Oncol* 19: 2041–2048
36 Morgner A, Lehn N, Andersen LP, Thiede C, Bennedsen M, Trebesius K, Neubauer B, Neubauer A, Stolte M, Bayerdorffer E (2000) *Helicobacter heilmannii*-associated pri-

mary gastric low-grade MALT lymphoma: complete remission after curing the infection. *Gastroenterology* 118: 821–828
37 Du MQ (2002) Gastric MALT lymphoma: from aetiology to treatment. *Lancet Oncol* 3: 97–104
38 Seaberg EC, Belle SH, Beringer KC, Schivins JL, Detre KM (1999) Liver transplantation in the United States from 1987–1998: Updated results from the Pitt-UNOS liver transplant registry. In: JM Cecka, PI Terasaki (eds): *Clinical transplants 1998*. UCLA Tissue Typing Laboratory, Los Angeles, 17–37
39 Wasley A, Alter MJ (2000) Epidemiology of hepatitis C: geographic differences and temporal trends. *Semin Liver Dis* 20: 1–16
40 World Health Organization (1999) Global surveillance and control of hepatitis C. Report of a WHO Consultation organized in collaboration with the Viral Hepatitis Prevention Board, Antwerp, Belgium. *J Viral Hepat* 6: 35–47
41 Wasley A, Alter MJ (2000) Epidemiology of hepatitis C: Geographic differences and temporal trends. *Semin Liver Dis* 20: 1–16
42 Alter MJ, Kruszon-Moran D, Nainan OV, McQuillan GM, Gao F, Moyer LA, Kaslow RA et al (1999) The prevalence of hepatitis C virus infection in the United States, 1988 through 1994. *N Engl J Med* 341: 556–562
43 Yen T, Keeffe EB, Ahmed A (2003) The epidemiology of hepatitis C virus infection. *J Clin Gastroenterol* 36: 47–53
44 El-Serag HB (2002) Hepatocellular carcinoma: an epidemiologic view. *J Clin Gastroenterol* 35: S72–S78
45 Bosch FX, Ribes J, Borras J (1999) Epidemiology of primary liver cancer. *Semin Liver Dis* 19: 271–286
46 El-Serag HB (2001) Global epidemiology of hepatocellular carcinoma. *Clin Liver Dis* 5: 87–107
47 El-Serag HB, Mason AC (1999) Rising incidence of hepatocellular carcinoma in the United States. *N Engl J Med* 340: 745–750
48 El-Serag HB (2002) Hepatocellular carcinoma and hepatitis C in the United States. *Hepatology* 36 (5, Suppl 1): S74–S83
49 Donato F, Boffetta P, Puoti M (1998) A meta-analysis of epidemiological studies on the combined effect of hepatitis B and C virus infections in causing hepatocellular carcinoma. *Int J Cancer* 75: 347–354
50 Di Bisceglie AM, Goodman ZD, Ishak KG, Hoofnagle JH, Melpolder JJ, Alter HJ (1991) Long-term clinical and histopathological follow-up of posttransfusion hepatitis. *Hepatology* 14: 969–974
51 Ikeda K, Saitoh S, Koida I, Arase Y, Tsubota A, Chayama K, Kumada H, Kawanishi M (1993) A multivariate analysis of risk factors for hepatocellular carcinogenesis. *Hepatology* 18: 47–53
52 Colombo M (1999) Hepatitis C virus and hepatocellular carcinoma. *Baillieres Best Pract Res Clin Gastroenterol* 13: 519–528

53 Di Bisceglie AM (1997) Hepatitis C and hepatocellular carcinoma. *Hepatology* 26: 34S–38S
54 Moum B, Ekbom A, Vatn MH, Aadland E, Sauar J, Lygren I, Schulz T, Stray N, Fausa O (1997) Inflammatory bowel disease: re-evaluation of the diagnosis in a prospective population based study in south eastern Norway. *Gut* 40: 328–332
55 Loftus EV, Sandborn WJ (2002) Epidemiology of inflammatory bowel disease. *Gastroenterol Clin North Am* 31: 1–20
56 Morita N, Toki S, Hirohashi T, Minoda T, Ogawa K, Kono S, Tamakoshi A, Ohno Y, Sawada T, Muto T (1995) Incidence and prevalence of inflammatory bowel disease in japan: nationwide epidemiological survey during the year 1991. *J Gastroenterol* 30 (Suppl 8): 1–4
57 Yoshida Y, Murata Y (1990) Inflammatory bowel disease in Japan: studies of epidemiology and etiopathogenesis. *Med Clin North Am* 74: 67–90
58 Yang SK, Hong WS, Min YI, Kim HY, Yoo JH, Rhee PL, Rhee JC, Chang DK, Song IS, Jung SA et al (2000) Incidence of and prevalence of ulcerative colitis in the Songpa-Kangdong District, Seoul, Korea, 1986–1997. *J Gastroenterol Hepatol* 15: 1037–1042
59 Wright JP, Froggatt J, O'Keefe EA, Ackerman S, Watermeyer S, Louw J, Adams G, Girdwood AH, Burns DG, Marks IN (1986) The epidemiology of inflammatory bowel disease in Cape Town 1980–1984. *S Afr Med J* 70: 10–15
60 Levin B (1992) Inflammatory bowel disease and colon cancer. *Cancer* 70: 1313–1316
61 Gyde S, Prior P, Dew NJ, Saunders V, Waterhouse JA, Allan RN (1982) Mortality in ulcerative colitis. *Gastroenterology* 83: 36–43
62 Sharan R, Schoen RE (2002) Cancer in inflammatory bowel disease: An evidence-based analysis and guide for physicians and patients. *Gastroenterol Clin North Am* 31: 237–254
63 Eaden JA, Abrams KR, Mayberry JF (2001) The risk of colorectal cancer in ulcerative colitis: a meta-analysis. *Gut* 48: 526–535
64 Sugita A, Sachar DB, Bodian C, Ribeiro MB, Aufses AH, Greenstein AJ (1991) Colorectal cancer in ulcerative colitis. Influence of anatomical extent and age at onset on colitis-cancer interval. *Gut* 32: 167–169
65 Markowitz J, McKinely M, Kahn E, Stiel L, Rosa J, Grancher K, Daum F (1997) Endoscopic screening for dysplasia and mucosal aneuploidy in adolescents and young adults with childhood onset colitis. *Am J Gastroenterol* 92: 2001–2006
66 Bansal P, Sonnenberg A (1996) Risk for colorectalcoancer in inflammatory bowel disease. *Am J Gastroenterol* 91: 44–48
67 Gillen CD, Walmsley RS, Prior P, Andrews HA, Allan RN (1994) Ulcerative colitis and Crohn's disease: A comparison of the colorectal cancer risk in extensive colitis. *Gut* 35: 1590–1592
68 Munkholm P, Langholz E, Davidsen M, Binder V (1993) Intestinal cancer risk and mortality in patients with Crohn's disease. *Gastroenterology* 105: 1716–1723
69 Weedon DD, Shorter RG, Ilstrup DM, Huizenga KA, Taylor WF (1973) Crohn's disease and cancer. *N Engl J Med* 289: 1099–1103

70 Bernstein CN, Blanchard JF, Kliewer E, Wajda A (2001) Cancer risk in patients with inflammatory bowel disease: A population-based study. *Cancer* 91: 854–862
71 Ekbom A, Helmick C, Zack M, Adami HO (1990) Increased risk of large-bowel cancer in Crohn's disease with colonic involvement. *Lancet* 336: 357–359
72 Fireman Z, Grossman A, Lilos P, Hacohen D, Bar Meir S, Rozen P, Gilat T (1989) Intestinal cancer in patients with Crohn's disease: A population study in central Israel. *Scand J Gastroenterol* 24: 346–350
73 Gallop JH, Phillips SF, Melton III LJ, Zinsmeister AR. (1988) Epidemiologic aspects of Crohn's disease: A population-based study in Olmsted County, Minnesota, 1943–1982. *Gut* 29: 49–56
74 Friedman S, Rubin PH, Bodian C, Goldstein E, Harpaz N, Present DH (2001) Screening and surveillance colonoscopy in chronic Crohn's colitis. *Gastroenterology* 120: 820–826
75 Johnson RD, Ausmn LM, Sehggal PK, King NW Jr (1996) A prospective study of the epidemiology of colitis and colon cancer in cotton top tamarins (*Sanguinas oedipus*). *Gastroenterology* 110: 102–115
76 Berg DJ, Davidson N, Kuhn R, Muller W, Mennon S, Holland DG, Thompson-Snipes L, Leach MW, Rennick D (1995) Enterocolitis and colon cancer in interleukin 10 deficient mice are associated with abnormal cytokine production and CD 4^+ TH-1 like responses. *J Clin Invest* 98: 1010–1020
77 Rudolph U, Finegold MJ, Ridge SS, Harriman GR, Srinivasan Y, Brabert P, Goyley G, Bradley A, Birnbaumer L (1995) Ulcerative colitis and adenocarcinoma of a colon in G alpha 1-2 deficient mice. *Nat Genet* 10: 143–150
78 Cooper HS, Everley L, Chang WC, Pfeiffer G, Lee B, Murthy S, Clapper ML (2001) The role of mutant Apc in the development of dysplasia and cancer in the mouse model of dextran sulfate sodium-induced colitis. *Gastroenterology* 121: 1407–1416
79 DeMeester TR, Wang CI, Wernly JA, Pellegrini CA, Little G, Klementschitsch P, Bermudez G, Johnson LF, Skinner DB (1980) Technique, indications, and clinical use of 24-hour esophageal pH monitoring. *J Thorac Cardiovasc Surg* 79: 656–670
80 Johnsson F, Joelsson B, Gudmundsson K, Freiff L (1987) Symptoms and endoscopic findings in the diagnosis of gastroesophageal reflux disease. *Scand J Gastroenterol* 22: 714–718
81 Cameron AJ, Zinsmeister AR, Ballard DJ, Carney JA (1990) Prevalence of columnar-lined (Barrett's) esophagus: Comparison of population-based clinical and autopsy findings. *Gastroenterology* 99: 918–922
82 Spechler SJ, Zeroogian JM, Antonioli DA, Wang HH, Goyal RK (1994) Prevalence of metaplasia at the gastro-esophageal junction. *Lancet* 344: 1533–1536
83 Cameron AJ, Zinsmeister AR, Ballard DJ, Carney JA (1990) Prevalence of columnar-lined (Barrett's esophagus). *Gastroenterology* 99: 918–922
84 Blot WJ, Devesa SS, Kneller RW, Fraumeni JF Jr (1991) Rising incidence of adenocarcinoma of the esophagus and gastric cardia. *JAMA* 265: 1287–1289
85 Bollschweiler E, Wolfgarten E, Gutschow C, Holscher AH (2001) Demographic varia-

tions in the rising incidence of esophageal adenocarcinoma in white males. *Cancer* 92: 549–555
86 Devesa SS, Blot WJ, Fraumeni JF Jr (1998) Changing patterns in the incidence of esophageal and gastric carcinoma in the United States. *Cancer* 83: 2049–2053
87 Bytzer P, Christensen PB, Damkier P, Vinding K, Seersholm N (1999) Adenocarcinoma of the esophagus and Barrett's esophagus: a population-based study. *Am J Gastroenterol* 94: 86–91
88 Falk GW (2002) Barrett's esophagus. *Gastroenterology* 122: 1569–1591
89 Lieberman DA, Oehlke M, Helfand M (1997) Risk factors for Barrett's esophagus in community-based practice. *Am J Gastroenterol* 92: 1293–1297
90 Singh P, Taylor RH, Colin-Jones DG (1994) Esophageal motor dysfunction and acid exposure in reflux esophagitis are more severe if Barrett's metaplasia is present. *Am J Gastroenterol* 89: 349–356
91 Oberg S, DeMeester TR, Peters JH, Hagen JA, Nigro JJ, DeMeester SR, Theisen J, Campos GM, Crookes PF (1999) The extent of Barrett's esophagus depends on the status of the lower esophageal sphincter and the degree of esophageal acid exposure. *J Thorac Cardiovasc Surg* 117: 572–580
92 Lagergren J, Bergström R, Lindgren A, Nyrén O (1999) Symptomatic gastroesophageal reflux disease as a risk factor for esophageal adenocarcinoma. *N Engl J Med* 340: 825–831
93 Farrow DC, Vaughan TL, Sweeney C, Gammon MD, Chow WH, Risch HA, Stanford JL, Hantsen PD, Mayne ST, Schoenberg JB et al (2000) Gastroesophageal reflux disease, use of H2 receptor antagonists and risk of esophageal and gastric cancer. *Cancer Causes Control* 11: 231–238
94 Lowenfels AB, Maisonneuve P (2002) Epidemiologic and etiologic factors of pancreatic cancer. *Hematol Oncol Clin of North Am* 16: 1–16
95 Greenlee RT, Murray T, Bolden S, Wingo PA (2000) Cancer statistics 2000. *CA Cancer J Clin* 50: 7–33
96 Ries LAG, Eisner MP, Kosary CL, Hankey BF, Miller BA, Clegg L, Mariotto A, Feuer EJ, Edwards BK (2000) Seer Cancer Statistics Review, 1973–1996. National Cancer Institute, Bethesda, MD
97 Gold EB, Gordis L, Diener MD, Seltser R, Boitnott JK, Bynum TE, Seltser R, Boitnott JK, Bynum TE, Hutcheon DF (1985) Diet and other risk factors for cancer of the pancreas. *Cancer* 55: 460–467
98 Mack TM, Yu MC, Hanisch R, Henderson BE (1986) Pancreas cancer and smoking, beverage consumption and past medical history. *J Natl Cancer Inst* 76: 49–60
99 Farrow DC, Davis S (1990) Risk of pancreatic cancer in relation to medical history and use of tobacco, alcohol and coffee. *Int J Cancer* 45: 816–820
100 Jain M, Howe GR, St Louis P, Miller AB (1991) Coffee and alcohol as determinants of risk of pancreatic cancer: a case-control study from Toronto. *Int J Cancer* 47: 384–389
101 Kalapothaki V, Tzonou A, Hsieh CC, Toupadaki N, Trichopoulos D (1993) Tobacco,

ethanol, coffee, pancreatitis, diabetes mellitus, and cholelithiasis as risk factors for pancreatic carcinoma. *Cancer Causes Control* 4: 1433–1437
102 Lowenfels AB, Maisonneuve P, Cavallini G, Ammann RW, Lankisch PG, Andersen JR, Ammann RW, Lankisch PG, Andersen JR, Dimagno EP et al (1993) Pancreatitis and the risk of pancreatic cancer. International Pancreatitis Study Group. *N Engl J Med* 328: 1433–1447
103 Talamini G, Falconi M, Bassi C, Sartori N, Salvia R, Caldiron E, Frulloni L, Di Francesco V, Vaona B, Bovo P et al (1999) Incidence of cancer in the course of chronic pancreatitis. *Am J Gastroenterol* 94: 1253–1260
104 Mostafa MH, Sheweita A, O'Connor PJ (1999) Relationship between schistosomiasis and bladder cancer. *Clin Microbiol Rev* 12: 97–111
105 El-Sebai I (1977) Parasites in the etiology of cacaner; bilharziasis and bladder cancer. *CA Cancer J Clin* 27: 100–106
106 Al-Shukri SM, Alwan H, Nayef M, Rahman AA (1987) Bilharziasis in malignant tumors of the urinary bladder. *Br J Urol* 59: 59–62
107 Elem B, Purohit R (1983) Carcinoma of urinary bladder in Zambia: a quantitative estimate of *Schistosoma haematobium* infection. *Br J Urol* 55: 275–278
108 Lucas SB (1982) Squamous cell carcinoma of the bladder and Schistosomiasis. *East Afr Med J* 59: 345–351
109 El-Sebai I (1977) Parasites in the etiology of cancer; bilharziasis and bladder cancer. *CA Cancer J Clin* 27: 100–106
110 Kuntz RE, Cheever AW, Myers BJ (1972) Proliferative lesions of the urinary bladder of non-human primates infected with *Schistosoma haematobium*. *J Natl Cancer Inst* 48: 223–235
111 Wagner JC, Sleggs EA, Marchand P (1960) Diffuse pleural mesothelioma and asbestos in the North Western Cape Province. *Br J Ind Med* 17: 260–270
112 Selikoff IJ, Churg J, Hammond EC (1964) Asbestos exposure and neoplasia. *JAMA* 188: 22–26
113 Lanphear BP, Buncher CR (1992) Latent period for malignant mesothelioma of occupational origin. *J Occupat Med* 34: 718–721
114 Enterline PE, Henderson VL (1987) Geographic patterns for female pleural mesothelioma deaths for 50 states. *J Natl Cancer Inst* 79: 31–37
115 Walker AM, Loughlin JE, Freidlander ER, et al (1983) Projections of asbestos-related disease 1980–2009. *J Occupat Med* 25: 409–425
116 Peto J, Hodgson JT, Mathews FE, Jones JR (1995) Continuing increase in mesothelioma mortality in Britain. *Lancet* 345: 535–539
117 Funkhouser EM, Sharp GB (1995) Aspirin and reduced risk of esophageal carcinoma. Cancer 76: 1116–1169
118 Aker K, Ekstsrom AM, Signorello LB, Hansson LE, Nyren O (2001) Aspirin and risk of gastric cancer: a population based case-control studying Sweden. *Br J Cancer* 84: 965–968

119 Giovannucci E, Eagan KM, Hunter DJ, Stampfer MJ, Colditz GA, Willet WC, Speizer FE (1995) Aspirin and risk of colorectal cancer in women. *N Engl J Med* 333: 609–614
120 Giovannucci E, Rimm EG, Stampfer MJ, Colditz GA, Ascherio A, Willett WC (1994) Aspirin use and the risk of colorectal cancer and adenoma in male health professionals. *Ann Intern Med* 121: 241–246
121 Thun MJ, Namboodiri MM, Dealth CW Jr (1991) Aspirin use and reduced risk of fatal colon cancer. *N Engl J Med* 325: 1593–1596
122 Schreinemachers DM, Everson RB (1994) Aspirin use and lung, colon, and breast cancer incidence in a prospective study. *Epidemiology* 5: 138–146
123 Castelao JE, Yuan JM, Gago-Dominguez M, Yu MC, Ross RK (2000) Non-steroidal anti-inflammatory drugs and bladder cancer prevention. *Br J Cancer* 82: 1364–1369
124 Harris RE, Kasbari S, Farrar WB (1999) Prospective study of nonsteroidal anti-inflammatory drugs and breast cancer. *Oncol Rep* 6: 71–73
125 Steinbach G, Lynch PM, Phillips RKS, Wallace MH, Hawk E, Gordon GB, Wakabayashi N, Saunders B, Shen Y, Fujimura T (2000) The effect of celecoxib, a cylooxygenase-2 inhibitor, in familial adenomatous polyposis. *N Engl J Med* 342: 1946–1952
126 Sandler RS, Halabi S, Baron JA, Budinger S, Paskett E, Keresztes R, Petrelli N, Pipas JM, Karp DD, Loprinzi CL et al (2003) A randomized trial of aspirin to prevent colorectal adenomas in patients with previous colorectal cancer. *N Engl J Med* 348: 883–890
127 Baron JA, Cole BF, Sandler RS, Haile RW, Ahnen D, Bresalier R, Mckeown-Eyssen G, Summers RW, Rothstein R, Burke CA et al (2003) A randomized trial of aspirin to prevent colorectal adenomas. *N Engl J Med* 348: 891–899

Cancer as a chronic inflammatory disease: role of immunotherapy

Michael T. Lotze[1] *and Ronald B. Herberman*[2]

[1]Molecular Medicine Institute, University of Pittsburgh School of Medicine, 300 Technology Drive, Pittsburgh, PA 15219, USA; [2]University of Pittsburgh Cancer Institute and Centers, 5115 Centre Drive, Pittsburgh, PA 15232, USA

Introduction

Cancer is fundamentally the end stage of many chronic inflammatory diseases, representing a state of continuous angiogenic and stromagenic support for the established neoplasm [1, 2]. Indeed, a substantial literature now exists to support the notion that cancer in adults arises most often in the setting of chronic inflammation [3]. Efforts to arrest and diminish tumor growth applied late in the setting of metastatic disease, at a time when the host and the tumor have established their *folie à deux*, are regrettably largely ineffective. The absence of suitable biomarkers and surrogates of response likewise limit application of biologic therapies early in disease. Many of these markers are of tissue remodeling and inflammation associated with the neoplastic state [4–11]. New findings about the interactions of natural killer (NK) cells and dendritic cells (DCs) [12–32] in the initiation of the inflammatory response as well as secondary responses suggest their critical role in immunity and potential utility as immunotherapies or the use of cytokine or cytokine gene therapy designed to elicit/activate them. Although the period following resection of the primary tumor is most often a period of seeming quiescence, we now recognize that considerable changes including continued genomic instability and immunologic alterations in the host and tumor target molecules are occurring. Having a means to identify suitable biomarkers and surrogates of tumor during this nominally quiescent period is one of great need so that novel agents might be applied at a time when they are most likely to modify the biology of the tumor. Promising new approaches applying proteomics, genomics [33–36], and cellomics (imaging cytometric) [37–41] strategies may make this possible.

Cancer and Inflammation, edited by Douglas W. Morgan, Ulf J. Forssmann and Marian T. Nakada

Chronic inflammation leads to cancer: an unusual situation of pediatric neoplasms

Cancer arises as a consequence of mutations in genes regulating cell growth or cell death. Although acute inflammation (Fig. 1) is most often associated with control of a pathogen and resultant long term T-cell memory, chronic inflammation is the result of persistent inflammatory stimuli. In adults, with the incidence increasing with age, tumors arise following years of chronic inflammation in the setting of intact immunity [2, 3, 5, 7–9, 11, 42–58]. Such chronic inflammatory pre-cancerous states are associated with a number of chronic viral infections (hepatitis B virus, hepatitis C virus, human papillomavirus, and Epstein-Barr virus, etc.), bacterial infections (*Helicobacter pylori*), toxins (arsenic, asbestos, smoking), hormonal cycling of breast or uterine tissues, or repetitive chemical or physical irritation (esophagitis, solar irradiation). T cells, recruited to the site, mediate rounds of stromal and epithelial destruction. When identified within the established tumor later, or infiltrating the precancerous lesions, they are often found to be anergic or suppressive. Progression of a tumor occurs once mutations limit apoptosis, permitting necrotic cell death, and subsequent reconstituting growth have occurred. In children, many of the targeted mutations in growth-controlling genes occur while the immune system is still in a nominal immature state, resulting in so-called immunologic “ignorance” [59–61]. Although many reports document the presence of NK cells, T cells and DCs within adult neoplasms, only a paucity of reports on Hodgkin’s disease [62–65] and leukemia [59, 66] in children make similar claims. Indeed our own recent unpublished observations suggest that, unlike their adult counterparts, there are almost no inflammatory cells within the tumor prior to or even after cancer chemotherapy (Fig. 2).

Stress response: cancer as stressed cells

During inflammation, mediators including tumor necrosis factor α (TNFα) and interferon γ (INFγ) promote arrest in cell growth, processing of endogenous proteins in epithelial and stromal cells, expression of processed peptides in the context of MHC Class I and Class II molecules and, particularly in epithelial cells, expression of cell surface “stress molecules” including MHC class I chain-like genes A and B (MICA/B) [67–75] and Letal [76]. MHC molecules presented as peptides are targets for activated memory effector and regulatory T cells. MICA/B and presumably other virally induced molecules such as Letal are targets for natural killer G2D (NKG2D)-expressing NK cells. Recently, it has been suggested that MICA/B can be expressed on IFNα stimulated DCs allowing engagement and activation of NK cells as well [77]. Similarly Letal has been shown to promote T-cell survival and enhance substrate uptake, even in the presence of nominal apoptosis-inducing stimuli including

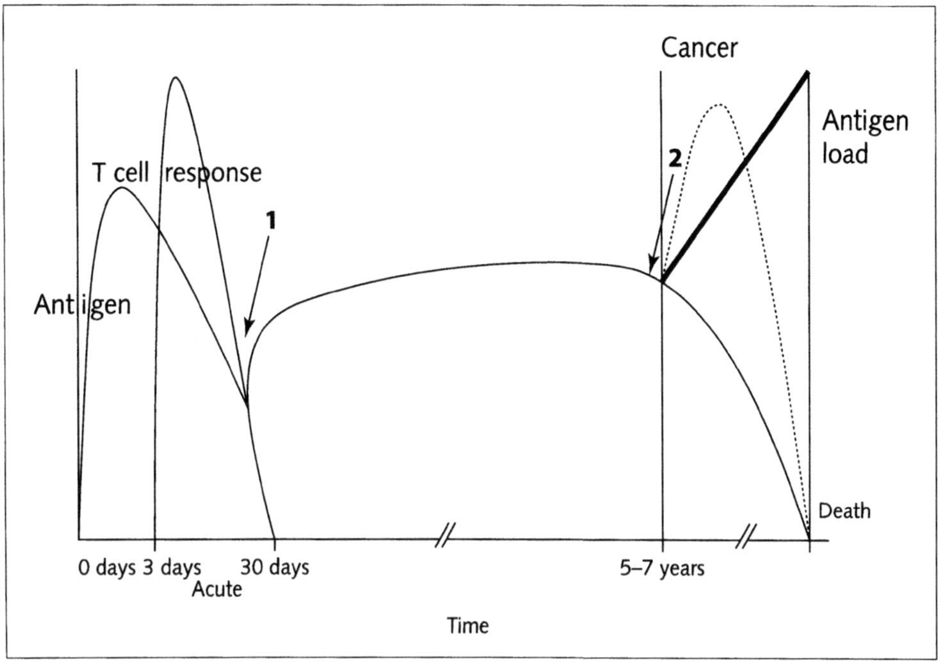

Figure 1
Chronic inflammation and cancer.
In the setting of viral or bacterial infections, or other inflammatory signals, typically an acute inflammatory response is associated with a rapid rise in antigen over the first few days followed by an emergent T-cell response (which we now recognize as balanced between effectors and suppressors of immunity). With persistence of antigen or inflammatory signals, a chronic inflammatory state ensues (↑1) which is associated with cyclical increases in antigen, triggering a renewed inflammatory response and T-cell immigration, and attempts to limit or wall off the focus. In sites characterized by diminution of antigen and waning of inflammation, renewed danger/damage or injury signals recruits NK cells and NK cells/T cells into the site to launch another round of inflammation with delivery of antigen to DCs, release of chemokines and cytokines limiting local stromal and epithelial proliferation, and enabling the recruitment of additional inflammatory cells. The consequence of this is another round of T-cell immigrants, including both effectors and balanced regulatory cells including $CD4^+CD25^+$ cells, limiting the pathogen and ultimately allowing healing and epithelial and stromal proliferation to repair the local damage. Following rounds of inflammation, epithelial death and proliferation, sufficient mutational events ensue, particularly in the background of a genetically susceptible individual, to enable the expansion of a malignant clone (↑2) imbued with the ability to expand with a concomitant diminution in specific and global immunity, ultimately eventuating in death. Our goals with biologic therapy are to reinitiate an "acute inflammatory" response to the tumor (shown by dotted line), with the ability of new T cells emergent and capable of limiting the growth of the malignant clone.

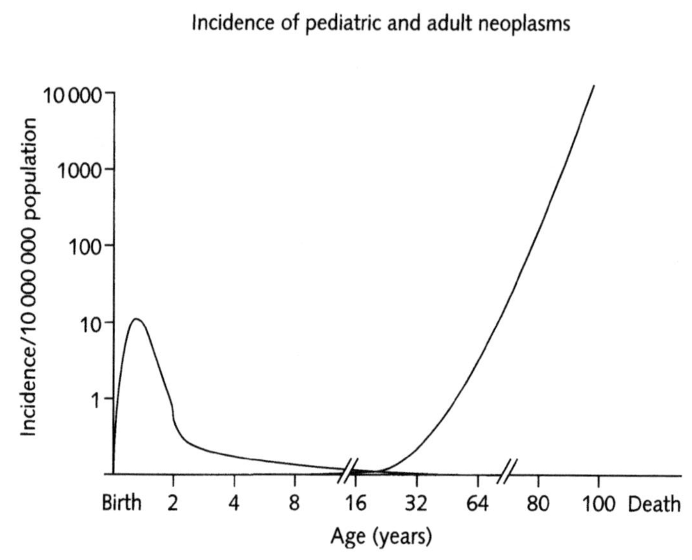

Figure 2
Two major etiologies for cancer.
Pediatric neoplasms arise embryologically during rapid expansion of the cell mass during early fetal development with either acquired or hereditary mutations affecting genes regulating cell contact, cell growth, and cell death. Most of these tumors indeed are successfully eradicated by aggressive combination chemotherapy although rare variants of rhabdomyosarcoma, osteosarcoma, Wilm's tumor, and gliomas continue to be identified through adult life, albeit at low incidence. This is presumably because of a lower growth fraction than those presenting earlier in life. Hematologic neoplasms, melanoma, and aggressive colorectal cancers are observed as early as the teenage years and a progressive increase in frequency of epithelial neoplasms. A preponderance of adult neoplasms (shown in the ascending curve > 16 years) takes place as a result of years of chronic inflammation, hormonal cycling, exposure to toxins, and accumulation of mutations, often with facilitatory hereditary genetic alterations. This results in tumors with low responsiveness to chemotherapeutics associated with inflammatory infiltrates. Biologic therapies have little role in the treatment of pediatric neoplasms but are being increasingly pursued and applied in the setting of adult neoplasms with modest success.

chemotherapeutic agents. It is likely that the consequence of chronic inflammation is the destruction of epithelial and stromal elements resulting in renewed proliferation of these cells during the healing phase. Necrotic cell death, as a stimulator of inflammation, and apoptosis as the preferred type of antigen to launch an immune response [78–83], may be distinguished by a variety of specialized cell-surface molecular receptors for heat-shock proteins (Hsps) [84] and the molecule HMGB-1, as this is released by necrotic but not apoptotic cells. During inflammatory responses inducing both apoptosis and necrosis of premalignant and malignant cells, the cells with altered genes promoting cell growth and limiting cell death are selected for in the setting of inflammation. In addition, those cells which lose expression of individual MHC molecules or antigens that they present are also powerfully selected for in the tumor microenvironment. Loss of tumor antigen expression during and subsequent to effective immunotherapy has now been well documented, particularly in the setting of melanoma [85–95]. Other molecules released by necrotic cells are likely to play an important role and include uric acid [96], Hsp70 [67, 97–100], and ATP [101] among others.

Signals 1–5

Although substantial information has been attained about the signals (Tab. 1) eliciting the adaptive immune response mediated by T cells, the classic Bretscher and Cohn model [102] of two signals published over 30 years ago does not adequately define the biological activity taking place. Although we recognize that MHC/peptide or Signal 1 and the provision of costimulation, Signal 2, are requisite to driving naïve T cells, it was not until the last decade that it became apparent that this was the unique set of signals provided by DCs to either immunize or tolerize. Furthermore, Janeway [103] suggested that there needed to be a so-called Signal 0. This was initially believed to be derived as signals coming directly from bacteria, viruses, or other forms of injury or "danger" which prompted the initiation of the immune response. We now recognize that these signals largely drive Toll-like receptors on macrophages recruiting acutely polymorphonuclear leukocytes, NK cells, and DCs to the site. Subsequently Signal 3, reflecting the nature of the environmental stimuli provides a polarizing signal, initiating the Th1 or Th2 type of response [104–112] and Signal 4, the selective imprinting by DCs of the site from which the inflammatory focus derived [113–115], enabling the appropriate T cells to migrate more selectively to the appropriate site. At some point after continued inflammation, signals associated with healing, containment, or persistence of chronic inflammation are found (Signal 5) [116–126]. As noted above, cancer often arises in the setting of chronic viral infections, toxins, or irritation and several states of chronic inflammation. Interfering with this complex process using conventional vaccination strategies and recapitulating individual Signals 1–4 is believed to be unlikely to succeed because of the established chronic inflammatory state mediated by nominal Signal 5 factors such as transforming growth factor β (TGFβ) [118, 127, 128], nitric oxide [129–133], interleukin-10 (IL-10) [121, 123, 134–140], prostanoids [110, 112, 141–143], and others. These latter signals limit the ability to launch an acute inflam-

Table 1 - Signals/messages in immunity

	Class	Examples	Origin	Effectors
Signal 0	Danger	TLR1–13, IFNα, HMGB 1, Hsp, CD1+	Mφ	Polys, NK cells
Signal 1	Antigen	MHC / peptide	DCs	NK cells, NKT
Signal 2	Costimulation	CD80, CD86	DCs, NK cells	T cells
Signal 3	Polarization	Cytokines, IL-4, -10, -12	DCs, NK cells, NKT	T cells
Signal 4	Localization	Integrins; chemokine receptors	DCs	T cells
Signal 5	Termination, continuation, healing	PGE_2, TGFβ, IL-10, CTLA4	T cells, NK cells, DCs	T cells

HMBG 1, high mobility group B 1; Mφ, macrophage; polys, polymorphonuclear leukocytes; NKT, natural killer/T cells; IL, interleukin; TGFβ, transforming growth factor β; PGE_2, prostaglandin E_2

matory response. One of our central hypotheses is that inducing an acute inflammatory response with the adoptive transfer of NK cells and DCs (Fig. 3) will allow induction of a new T-cell response. Data coming from several centers now including our own [12–32, 144] suggest that this NK cell–DC interaction plays a primary role in polarizing the DCs and enhancing IL-12 and possibly IL-23 production.

IFNγ and IL-10 as pivotal cytokines in the inflammatory/tumor response: induction by cytokine therapies

A set of cytokines promoting an inflammatory response has now been tested clinically. These include IL-1 [145], IL-2 [146 147], IL-3 (PIXY-321), IL-4 [87, 148–150], IL-6 [151–157], IL-7 [158], IL-11 [159–164], IL-12 [165–169], IL-18 [170–175], IFNs α, β, and γ [176–178], the colony-stimulating factors M-CSF, GM-CSF, G-CSF [179–183], and erythropoietin [184–188], as well as TNFα [99, 189–191]. Interestingly, few of these have shown substantial enough activity for one to be enthusiastic about their application as therapeutic agents (Tab. 2). In large part this is due to the fact that soon after administration, counter-regulatory factors, including the IFNγ-inducible suppressor of signalling 1 (SOCS1) and SOCS3 feedback inhibitor [192–199], limit signaling through these molecules' Janus kinase/signal transduction and activators of transcription (JAK/STAT) signaling pathways,

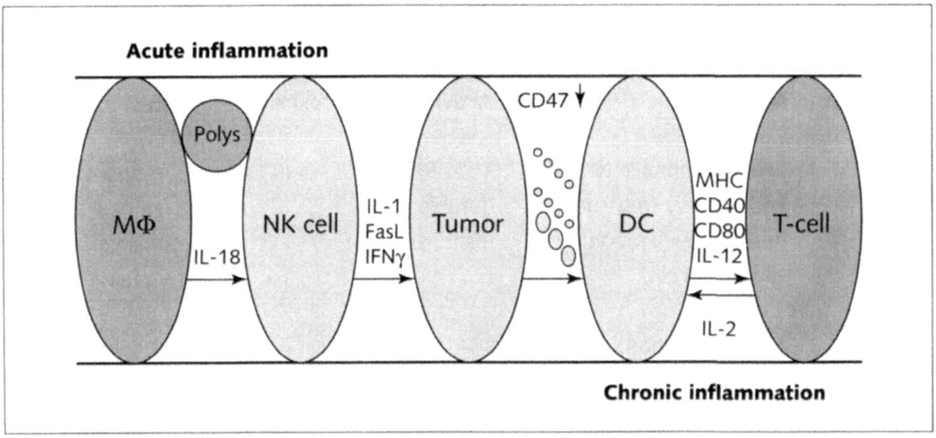

Figure 3
Coordinate delivery of NK cells and DCs to enhance the anti-cancer response.
Acute inflammation is induced in response to early signals of danger, damage, or injury; typically these are necrotic cell death, signaled by the release of heat shock proteins or HMGB 1, bacterial products including lipopolysaccharide and CpG (cytidine/guanine without methylation) containing single-stranded DNA, double-stranded RNA, etc. Tissue macrophages and immature dendritic cells, stimulated by these events typically produce cytokines and chemokines that trigger endothelial activation, ingestion of lysed cells, and recruitment of additional inflammatory cells including polymorphonuclear leucocytes and NK cells. These cells respond appropriately to environmental stimuli ingesting and/or lysing bacteria and stressed cells expressing molecules such as MICA/B. Release of monokines including IL-18 following its cleavage by caspase 1 allows promotion of a cellular immune response and enhances NK production of IFNγ, expression of Fas ligand (FasL) and release of other inflammatory mediators. Lysis of tumor cells allows release of apoptotic bodies, which are captured and further processed by dendritic cells. These in turn interact with memory effector and regulatory T cells recruited to the inflammatory site within 24–48 h. Retention of these cells within the acute and in some situations the chronic inflammatory site allows persistence of inflammation during periods of cell necrosis and apoptosis. When T cells are not appropriately retained or recruited, TNF is released by NK cells prompting traffic of DCs to the regional lymph nodes to recruit additional T cells capable of recognizing antigen. The reinitation of acute inflammation in the setting of cancer progression and the chronic inflammatory response represents a strategy targeting the late signal 5's within the tumor including immunosuppressive TGFβ, prostaglandin E_2, and IL-10.

which continues with subsequent administration. IL-10 is also induced within the tissues and plasma which limits the ability of new dendritic cells to provide critical costimulatory molecules in the tissues. It is perhaps surprising, given the increasing-

Table 2 - Cytokine therapy of cancer

Cytokine	Mechanism	Activity	Toxicity	Status
IL-2	Expand/enhance NK cells and delivery to tissues; promote generation of specific T cells	15% RR; durable responses	++++	FDA approved; stage IV renal cell cancer and melanoma
IFNα	↑DC maturation; antigen presentation by tumor; antiproliferative; antiangiogenic	10–15% RR; some durable	++	FDA approved; stage III melanoma, hairy cell leukemia, lymphoma
GM-CSF	DC activation; survival	↓Recurrence; responses as gene therapy	+	In Phase III
IL-12	Th1 shift; IFNγ inducer; antiangiogenic	Modest in lower, tolerable doses	++	Phase I and II; combinations with IL-2, IFN
IL-18	IFNγ inducer; Fas-dependent	Early response in melanoma	??	Phase I

FDA, US Food and Drug Administration; RR, relative response; GM-CSF, granulocyte-macrophage colony-stimulating factor

ly sophisticated understanding of cytokine networks and regulatory pathways that any responses were observed at all!

DC/NK cell cross-talk and DC/T-cell cross-talk are mediated in part by IL-1 family members

We have previously shown *in vitro* that the anti-tumor effects of recombinant IL-18 delivered in murine tumor models can be mimicked with coculture of DCs, NK cells, tumor, T cells, and IL-18, leading to the generation of tumor-specific T cells [170–175, 200–203]. There are now at least 10 distinct IL-1 family members. The biologic role of many of these cytokines is unclear; however, in murine models IL-

1α, IL-1β, IL-18, and IL-1F7 promote an effective anti-tumor response when used as genetic constructs. We are exploring whether the IL-1 homologues, including IL-1α, IL-1β, IL-1RA, IL-1F5, IL-1H4 (IL-1F7), and IL-1F9, mediate similar or dissimilar effects [204–208]. Whether IL-12 production is enhanced in an IFNγ-dependent manner in such cultures, generating successful development of specific T cells in NK cells and DCs cultured with tumor, is as yet unknown. The role of the IL-1 family members in cooperation with TNF family members in initiation of the adaptive immune response to cancer when applied locally is largely unexplored. An important question will be to test these premises *in vivo* in patients with melanoma. (We plan to assess this in an innovative clinical protocol assessing local tumor response in patients with multiple cutaneous melanoma metastases.) Although DC-based immunizations are effective in inducing cytotoxic T-lymphocyte (CTL) responses against cancer cells, clinical responses are rarely observed. Similarly, adoptively transferred T cells are effective only in limited types of cancer. We hypothesize that chronic inflammation, which clearly precedes progression of cancer in many cases and is present in the tumor microenvironment after the change into invasive malignant disease has occurred, is suppressive for anti-cancer effector cells; thus, the need to reinitiate acute inflammation seems a plausable interventive approach. In this respect, we are turning our studies into combination cellular therapy, and we propose that direct application of NK cells and DCs in the tumor microenvironment will create an acute inflammatory focus in the tumor, and promote the development of an effective anti-tumor immune response [17, 20, 209, 210].

The use of cellular therapy in cancer

Requirements for immune control of cancer include the need to attain T cells capable of migrating across endothelial barriers, surviving at the tumor site, and mediating a prolonged memory response [15, 87, 211–219]. Multiple studies in murine models predict that the induction and delivery of therapeutic T cells mediates important anti-tumor effects. A number of studies, particularly in the setting of patients with melanoma have now demonstrated that adoptive transfer of such cells mediates anti-tumor effects. Substantial host modification is required including the use of cytotoxic agents to "open space" for the adoptively transferred cells or to inhibit nominal suppressor T cells. An alternative strategy, and one which we are promoting, is the notion that the chronic inflammatory response to cancer is already mediated endogenously by T cells and DCs, and furthermore that the T cells found within tumors are ineffective and, with expansion, of limited utility. Our fundamental premise, based on an integration of the available insights into tumor biology, is that delivery of NK cells and DCs directly into the tumor will coordinately elicit new tumor-specific effector cells, driving the acute inflammatory response with Th1-promoting DC1s matured with NK cells *in vitro* or *in vivo*. Nonspecific strategies using bacterial injection such as bacille Calmette-Guérin (BCG) or *Corynebacterium parvum* have had limited application as have the application of immunostimulatory antibodies such as anti-CD3. More promising has been the application of antibodies such as those to CTLA4 to limit the negative inflammatory signal provided by resident regulatory cells with tissues and secondary nodal sites [220, 221].

The use of T cells to treat cancer in murine tumor models and application to humans arose in the 1970s. NK cells were also identified as critical effectors *in vitro* and in some *in vivo* systems with continued interest in their application today [15, 222–231]. In the late 1970s through the mid-1980s, so-called lymphokine-activated killer cells (LAKs) derived from IL-2-activated T cells and NK cells in the peripheral blood were generated in the presence of IL-2. They were administered systemically with high doses of IL-2 to patients with a variety of cancers including glioma, colorectal cancer, melanoma, and renal cell cancer. This treatment was associated with substantial toxicity and randomized, prospective trials showed comparable anti-tumor activity of the combination of LAKs and IL-2 to IL-2 alone. This prompted much of the current use of modified fibroblasts and antigen-pulsed or engineered DCs to deliver cytokines into the tumor microenvironment. At this point over 1000 individuals have been treated with DCs with only modest anti-tumor effects, especially in clinical trials in melanoma. We would propose that many of the DCs applied have not been suitably polarized or designed to deliver IL-12/IL-18 or other cytokines sufficiently [168, 232–247]. Many of the cytokines which mediate the cross-talk between immune cells are produced by DCs, and thus termed "dendrikines". They are not alone and are quite complex with microarray assays now revealing substantial complexity of the network of cytokines playing both synergistic and antagonistic roles in the tumor environment (Fig. 4). Rather than introducing single cytokines, we believe it is more plausible to deliver multiple cytokines produced following the coordinate interaction of DCs and NK cells, with the expectation that efficient adaptive immune responses will ensue, overcoming the polarized and only partially effective adaptive immune response identified in the cancer patient. Indeed, evidence that there is immune suppression in the peripheral blood of patients with cancer has continued to be provided by our group [248–251] as well as others.

Hypothetical impact of inducing an acute inflammatory response to cancer with NK cells and DCs

Although DC-based immunizations are effective in inducing CTL-responses against cancer cells, clinical responses are rarely observed. Similarly, adoptively transferred T cells are effective only in limited types of cancer. We hypothesize that chronic inflammation, which clearly precedes progression of cancer in many cases and is present in the tumor microenvironment after the change into invasive malignant dis-

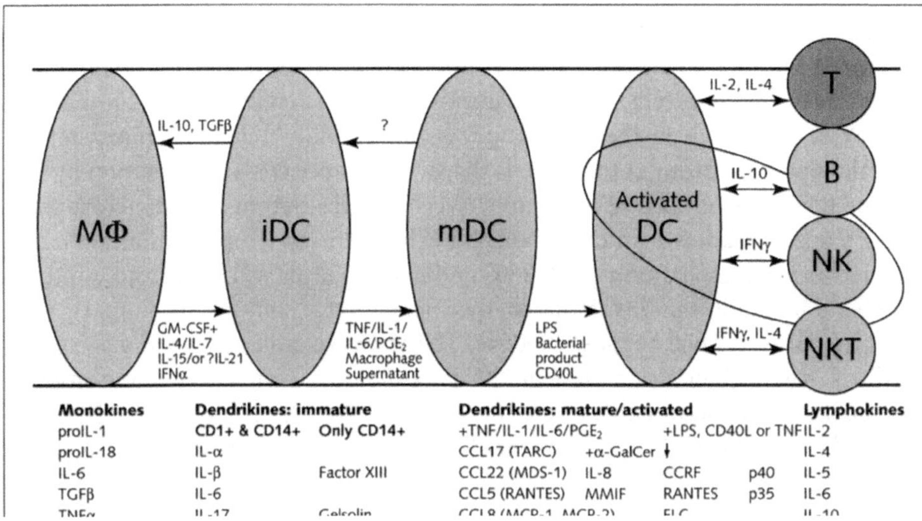

Figure 4

NK cells/DCs promote an adaptive immune response.

Our current understanding of early events in antigen uptake and processing by myeloid cells involves uptake of antigen by macrophages in the tissues and its complete degradation. When immune stimuli promote more of an immature dendritc cell pattern, antigen is processed and then protected from further degradation by association with Class I and Class II molecules. Transformation to mature dendritic cells by factors released by NK cells or bacterial products allows lymphatic entry and traffic to secondary nodal sites where interaction with resident B cells and T cells, as well as postulated NK cells and NK cells/T cells presenting antigen and other information derived in the tumor microenvironment, to enable initiation of the adaptive immune response, linking these cells with the innate immune response. Interestingly the cross-talk of inflammatory mediators is substantial and differs during different phases of the immune response. Coordinate interaction of the monokine or dendrikines and chemokines and their respective receptors enables the next set of interactions to occur. The fine interaction of the adaptive immune response with each other and innate inflammatory cells is mediated by a series of lymphokines, equally complex in their biology. LPS, lipopolysaccharide; GM-CSF, granulocyte-macrophage colony-stimulating factor; mCSF, monocyte colony-stimulating factor; iDC, immature DC; mDC, mature DC.

ease has occurred, is suppressive for anti-cancer effector cells. This supports the need to reinitiate acute inflammation. In this respect, we are turning our studies to combination cellular therapy. We propose that direct application of NK cells and DCs in the tumor microenvironment will create an acute inflammatory focus in the tumor, and promote the development of an effective anti-tumor immune response [17, 20, 209, 210]. We hypothesize that NK cells will enhance DC function and vaccine efficacy in driving the expansion of tumor-reactive T cells that may be recruited into the tumor microenvironment and mediate tumoricidal effects. We also hypothesize that NK cells delivered intra-tumorally, particularly in combination with DCs, will result in the apoptotic (*via* Fas ligand, TNF, and granzyme) and necrotic (perforin) death of tumor cells that will enhance cross-presentation by DCs and the development of new anti-tumor T cells. In this setting inflammatory mediators, tissue-breakdown products, and both inflammatory and non-inflammatory cells such as endothelial cells [252–255] and macrophages will be delivered into the peripheral blood. It is in this setting that we imagine that some of the biomarker and surrogate measures will be most effective. The ability to either suppress macrophage products which limit the nature of the inflammatory response in the setting of chronic infection and/or enhance the NK cell/DCs interactions promoting IL-1 family members and/or IL-12 family member production by DC's seems like a plausible strategy to enhance new T cell reactivity.

Future immunotherapeutic strategies

The twin premises of weak antigens and lack of immune responses which were the operative paradigms of the last 50 years have now been subjected to a major test. As such, interestingly, the current stage of evolution of immunotherapies for cancer is in a bit of a quandary. We have come through a period where cancer was thought to have little in the way of antigenic targets, being largely derived from normal cells with little in the way of an immune response. We now recognize that the immune response to tumor is well established in most tumors and that modifying immunity will require earlier application of novel agents and their evaluation in the setting when suitable biomarkers and surrogates can be tested.

The notion of weak antigens

Many of the tissue-specific targets can be recognized by antibodies or T cells. Furthermore, the genomic instability of cancer is capable of generating a plethora of targets for immune recognition. The identification and testing of these targets as immunogens has arguably engaged the major efforts of tumor immuologists for the last decade, with the notion that induction of an inflammatory response was relatively straightforward. The paucity of clinically important responses, arguably in the most advanced settings of disease, has not confirmed these hopes or expectations of focusing on the afferent limb of the immune response.

The notion of immunologic quiescence

The other major sentiment has been that the tumor was quiescent immunologically. Pro-inflammatory stimuli including BCG and C. *parvum*, and administration of IFNα, IL-2, TNF, IL-12, and IL-18 were driven by mouse models of acute inflammation, resulting in enhanced afferent stimuli for an immune response. Although occasional responses, especially in what we now recognize as immunologically responsive neoplasms, melanoma, renal cell carcinoma, and lymphoma, were observed, clear delineation of the mechanisms for this response or predicting response have been slow in coming. Indeed, with the exception of most childhood neoplasms, tumors arising later in life are the end result, in most instances, of a complex interplay of immune cells and host stromal and epithelial cells. Tumors arise in the setting of chronic inflammation and the prognosis for individuals with virtually every tumor type is tied to the level of inflammatory cells – NK cells, T cells, and DCs – found within it. As such the tumor is not seen as a silent, immunologically quiescent manifestation of genes gone awry but rather the genetic alterations are seen as Darwinian consequences of inflammation-mediated destruction and selection.

Paradigmatic shifts focus on anti-inflammatory strategies prior to tumorigenesis and pro-infammatory effector strategies following establishment of a neoplastic clone

So, the immunotherapies of the future for most adult neoplasms will focus on the earliest and most amenable to change. This will include identifying and eliminating the causes of chronic inflammation or limiting the chronic inflammation. An example of this type of therapy will be the paradigmatic application [6, 50, 57, 256-258] of cyclooxygenase 1 and 2 inhibitors in the setting of polyps arising in the colon, hysterectomy, or conization for women with advanced cervical intraepithelial neoplasia, and the widespread immunization of individuals for Hepatitis B. More problematic is the treatment of a patient with an established malignant neoplasm. Most thoughtful individuals would agree that earlier application of immunotherapy will be more effective, when applied in the adjuvant postoperative or neoadjuvant preoperative period following resection of a neoplasm. We favor strategies focusing on the efferent limb of the immune response, enabling delivery of activated NK cells and DCs to promote not only better tumor eradication by recruited and newly elicited T-effector cells, but the elimination of regulatory T cells, and the drive for new T cells accompanying host tumor destruction. The best exemplar of this strategy has been the application of adjuvant IFNα in the setting of melanoma, the direct delivery of LAKs or DCs into established neoplasms, and the administration of antibodies to cytotoxic T lymphocyte antigen 4 (CTLA4) to block some of the function of regulatory T cells. Understanding the signals involved in generation of the chronic inflammatory response and focusing on those most amenable to therapeutic intervention will likely be the beginnings of a more sound and rational oncologic armamentarium.

Identification of blood biomarkers and surrogates of cancer and the host response

We have now embarked on a discovery strategy designed to identify means to apply earlier therapies in the clinic, perhaps during the adjuvant or neoadjuvant period. The earlier application of therapies before the tumor–host interaction is so disordered to preclude correction. We believe it will be necessary to test some of the novel strategies suggested above in the setting where blood surrogates are validated and useful to guide therapy [259–261].

References

1 Sallusto F, Lanzavecchia A (1999) Mobilizing dendritic cells for tolerance, priming, and chronic inflammation. *J Exp Med* 189: 611–614

2 Lotze MT (1997) Future directions for recombinant interleukin-2 in cancer: a chronic inflammatory disorder *Cancer J Sci Am* 3: S106–S108

3 Coussens LM, Werb Z (2002) Inflammation and cancer. *Nature* 420: 860–867

4 Solakidi S, Dessypris A, Stathopoulos GP, Androulakis G, Sekeris CE (2004) Tumour-associated trypsin inhibitor, carcinoembryonic antigen and acute-phase reactant proteins CRP and alpha1-antitrypsin in patients with gastrointestinal malignancies. *Clin Biochem* 37: 56–60

5 Senthil K, Aranganathan S, Nalini N (2004) Evidence of oxidative stress in the circulation of ovarian cancer patients. *Clin Chim Acta* 339: 27–32

6 Phipps RP, Ryan E, Bernstein SH (2004) Inhibition of cyclooxygenase-2: a new targeted therapy for B-cell lymphoma? *Leuk Res* 28: 109–111

7 Melillo G (2004) HIF-1: A target for cancer, ischemia and inflammation – too good to be true? *Cell Cycle* 3: 154–155

8 Dranoff G (2004) Cytokines in cancer pathogenesis and cancer therapy. *Nat Rev Cancer* 4: 11–22

9 Baek HY, Lim JW, Kim H, Kim JM, Kim JS, Jung HC, Kim KH (2004) Oxidative stress-

related proteome changes in *Helicobacter pylori*-infected human gastric mucosa. *Biochem J* 379: 291–299

10 Ucur A, Palanduz S, Cefle K et al (2003) Sister chromatid exchange and mitotic index in patients with cirrhosis related to hepatitis B and C viruses and in chronic carriers. *Hepatogastroenterology* 50: 2137–2140

11 Wang TC, Goldenring JR (2002) Inflammation intersection: gp130 balances gut irritation and stomach cancer. *Nat Med* 8: 1080–1082

12 Munster DJ, MacDonald KP, Kato M, Hart DJ (2004) Human T lymphoblasts and activated dendritic cells in the allogeneic mixed leukocyte reaction are susceptible to NK cell-mediated anti-CD83-dependent cytotoxicity. *Int Immunol* 16: 33–42

13 Hayakawa Y, Screpanti V, Yagita H et al (2004) NK Cell TRAIL eliminates immature dendritic cells *in vivo* and limits dendritic cell vaccination efficacy. *J Immunol* 172: 123–129

14 Albright JW, Bream JH, Bere EW, Young HA, Winkler-Pickett R, Ortaldo JR (2004) Aging of innate immunity: functional comparisons of NK/LAK cells obtained from bulk cultures of young and aged mouse spleen cells in high concentrations of interleukin-2. *Exp Gerontol* 39: 73–82

15 Vakkila J, Lotze MT (2003) Cellular therapy of cancer. *Blood Therap Med* 3: 84–90

16 Tourkova IL, Yamabe K, Chatta G, Shurin GV, Shurin MR (2003) NK cells mediate Flt3 ligand-induced protection of dendritic cell precursors *in vivo* from the inhibition by prostate carcinoma in the murine bone marrow metastasis model. *J Immunother* 26: 468–472

17 Strbo N, Oizumi S, Sotosek-Tokmadzic V, Podack ER (2003) Perforin is required for innate and adaptive immunity induced by heat shock protein gp96. *Immunity* 18: 381–390

18 Moretta L, Ferlazzo G, Mingari MC, Melioli G, Moretta A (2003) Human natural killer cell function and their interactions with dendritic cells. *Vaccine* 21: S38–S42

19 Mailliard RB, Son YI, Redlinger R et al (2003) Dendritic cells mediate NK cell help for Th1 and CTL responses: two-signal requirement for the induction of NK cell helper function. *J Immunol* 171: 2366–2373

20 Valteau-Couanet D, Leboulaire C, Maincent K et al (2002) Dendritic cells for NK/LAK activation: rationale for multicellular immunotherapy in neuroblastoma patients. *Blood* 100: 2554–2561

21 Ferlazzo G, Morandi B, D'Agostino A et al (2003) The interaction between NK cells and dendritic cells in bacterial infections results in rapid induction of NK cell activation and in the lysis of uninfected dendritic cells. *Eur J Immunol* 33: 306–313

22 Heusel JW, Ballas ZK (2003) Natural killer cells: emerging concepts in immunity to infection and implications for assessment of immunodeficiency. *Curr Opin Pediatr* 15: 586–593

23 Poggi A, Carosio R, Spaggiari GM et al (2002) NK cell activation by dendritic cells is dependent on LFA-1-mediated induction of calcium-calmodulin kinase II: inhibition by HIV-1 Tat C-terminal domain. *J Immunol* 168: 95–101

24 Gerosa F, Baldani-Guerra B, Nisii C, Marchesini V, Carra G, Trinchieri G (2002) Reciprocal activating interaction between natural killer cells and dendritic cells. *J Exp Med* 195: 327–333
25 Fujii S, Shimizu K, Kronenberg M, Steinman RM (2002) Prolonged IFN-gamma-producing NKT response induced with alpha-galactosylceramide-loaded DCs. *Nat Immunol* 3: 867–374
26 Fernandez NC, Flament C, Crepineau F, Angevin E, Vivier E, Zitvogel L (2002) Dendritic cells (DC) promote natural killer (NK) cell functions: dynamics of the human DC/NK cell cross talk. *Eur Cytokine Netw* 13: 17–27
27 Ferlazzo G, Tsang ML, Moretta L, Melioli G, Steinman RM, Munz C (2002) Human dendritic cells activate resting natural killer (NK) cells and are recognized *via* the NKp30 receptor by activated NK cells. *J Exp Med* 195: 343–351
28 Engering A, Van Vliet SJ, Geijtenbeek TB, Van Kooyk Y (2002) Subset of DC-SIGN(+) dendritic cells in human blood transmits HIV-1 to T lymphocytes. *Blood* 100: 1780–1786
29 Coudert JD, Coureau C, Guery JC (2002) Preventing NK cell activation by donor dendritic cells enhances allospecific CD4 T cell priming and promotes Th type 2 responses to transplantation antigens. *J Immunol* 169: 2979–2987
30 Wilson JL, Heffler LC, Charo J, Scheynius A, Bejarano MT, Ljunggren HG (1999) Targeting of human dendritic cells by autologous NK cells. *J Immunol* 163: 6365–6370
31 Fernandez NC, Lozier A, Flament C et al (1999) Dendritic cells directly trigger NK cell functions: cross-talk relevant in innate anti-tumor immune responses *in vivo*. *Nat Med* 5: 405–11
32 Shah PD, Gilbertson SM, Rowley DA (1985) Dendritic cells that have interacted with antigen are targets for natural killer cells. *J Exp Med* 162: 625–636
33 Unwin RD, Knowles MA, Selby PJ, Banks RE (1999) Urological malignancies and the proteomic-genomic interface. *Electrophoresis* 20: 3629–3637
34 Lotze MT, Kost TA (2002) Viruses as gene delivery vectors: application to gene function, target validation, and assay development. *Cancer Gene Ther* 9: 692–699
35 Omenn GS (2002) Genetic advances will influence the practice of medicine: examples from cancer research and care of cancer patients. *Gen Med* 4: 15S–20S
36 Espina V, Dettloff KA, Cowherd S, Petricoin ERE, Liotta LA (2004) Use of proteomic analysis to monitor responses to biological therapies. *Expert Opin Biol Ther* 4: 83–93
37 Dow AI, Shafer SA, Kirkwood JM, Mascari RA, Waggoner AS (1996) Automatic multiparameter fluorescence imaging for determining lymphocyte phenotype and activation status in melanoma tissue sections. *Cytometry* 25: 71–81
38 Vakkila J, DeMarco RM, Lotze MT (2004) Rapid assessment of blood-derived dendritic cell activation by imaging cytometry. *J Immunol Methods; in press*
39 Stephens DJ, Allan VJ (2003) Light microscopy techniques for live cell imaging. *Science* 300: 82–86
40 Waggoner A, Taylor L, Seadler A, Dunlay T (1996) Multiparameter fluorescence imaging microscopy: reagents and instruments. *Hum Pathol* 27: 494–502

41 Galbraith W, Wagner MC, Chao J et al (1991) Imaging cytometry by multiparameter fluorescence. *Cytometry* 12: 579–596
42 Pasquinelli C, Bhavani K, Chisari FV (1992) Multiple oncogenes and tumor suppressor genes are structurally and functionally intact during hepatocarcinogenesis in hepatitis B virus transgenic mice. *Cancer Res* 52: 2823–2829
43 Vitolo D, Zerbe T, Kanbour A, Dahl C, Herberman RB, Whiteside TL (1992) Expression of mRNA for cytokines in tumor-infiltrating mononuclear cells in ovarian adenocarcinoma and invasive breast cancer. *Int J Cancer* 51: 573–580
44 Brentnall TA, Crispin DA, Bronner MP et al (1996) Microsatellite instability in nonneoplastic mucosa from patients with chronic ulcerative colitis. *Cancer Res* 56: 1237–1240
45 Jankowski JA, Harrison RF, Perry I, Balkwill F, Tselepis C (2000) Barrett's metaplasia. *Lancet* 356: 2079–2085
46 Balkwill F, Mantovani A (2000) Inflammation and cancer: back to Virchow? *Lancet* 357: 539–545
47 Coussens LM, Tinkle CL, Hanahan D, Werb Z (2000) MMP-9 supplied by bone marrow-derived cells contributes to skin carcinogenesis. *Cell* 103: 481–490
48 Fitzpatrick FA (2001) Inflammation, carcinogenesis and cancer. *Int Immunopharmacol* 1: 1651–1667
49 Gasche C, Chang CL, Rhees J, Goel A, Boland CR (2001) Oxidative stress increases frameshift mutations in human colorectal cancer cells. *Cancer Res* 61: 7444–7448
50 O'Byrne KJ, Dalgleish AG (2001) Chronic immune activation and inflammation as the cause of malignancy. *Br J Cancer* 85: 473–483
51 O'Byrne KJ, Dalgleish AG (2001) Infection and cancer. *Lancet* 358: 156
52 Brigati C, Noonan DM, Albini A, Benelli R (2002) Tumors and inflammatory infiltrates: friends or foes? *Clin Exp Metastasis* 19: 247–258
53 Caine GJ, Stonelake PS, Lip GY, Kehoe ST (2002) The hypercoagulable state of malignancy: pathogenesis and current debate. *Neoplasia* 4: 465–473
54 Shacter E, Weitzman SA (2002) Chronic inflammation and cancer. *Oncology (Huntingt)* 16: 217–226, 229; discussion 230–232
55 Guo HH, Loeb LA (2003) Tumbling down a different pathway to genetic instability. *J Clin Invest* 112: 1793–1795
56 Hahm KB, Song YJ, Oh TY et al (2003) Chemoprevention of *Helicobacter pylori*-associated gastric carcinogenesis in a mouse model: is it possible? *J Biochem Mol Biol* 36: 82–94
57 Ruegg C, Zaric J, Stupp R (2003) Non steroidal anti-inflammatory drugs and COX-2 inhibitors as anti-cancer therapeutics: hypes, hopes and reality. *Ann Med* 35: 476–487
58 Lucia MS, Torkko KC (2004) Inflammation as a Target for Prostate Cancer Chemoprevention: Pathological and Laboratory Rationale. *J Urol* 171: S30–S35
59 Pollock BH, Jenson HB, Leach CT et al (2003) Risk factors for pediatric human immunodeficiency virus-related malignancy. *JAMA* 289: 2393–2399
60 Kline NE, Sevier N (2003) Solid tumors in children. *J Pediatr Nurs* 18: 96–102

61 Vakkila J, Vettenranta K, Sariola H, Saarinen-Pihkala UM (2001) Poor yield of dendritic cell precursors from untreated pediatric cancer. *J Hematother Stem Cell Res* 10: 787–793
62 Bohlen H, Kessler M, Sextro M, Diehl V, Tesch H (2000) Poor clinical outcome of patients with Hodgkin's disease and elevated interleukin-10 serum levels. Clinical significance of interleukin-10 serum levels for Hodgkin's disease. *Ann Hematol* 79: 110–113
63 Viviani S, Notti P, Bonfante V, Verderio P, Valagussa P, Bonadonna G (2000) Elevated pretreatment serum levels of Il-10 are associated with a poor prognosis in Hodgkin's disease, the milan cancer institute experience. *Med Oncol* 17: 59–63
64 Ortac R, Aktas S, Diniz G, Erbay A, Vergin C (2002) Prognostic role of natural killer cells in pediatric mixed cellularity and nodular sclerosing Hodgkin's disease. *Anal Quant Cytol Histol* 24: 249–253
65 Smith RS, Chen Q, Hudson MM et al (2003) Prognostic factors for children with Hodgkin's disease treated with combined-modality therapy. *J Clin Oncol* 21: 2026–2033
66 Adler A, Albo V, Blatt J, Whiteside TL, Herberman RB (1989) Interleukin-2 induction of lymphokine-activated killer (LAK) activity in the peripheral blood and bone marrow of acute leukemia patients: II. Feasibility of LAK generation in children with active disease and in remission. *Blood* 74: 1690–1697
67 Groh V, Bahram S, Bauer S, Herman A, Beauchamp M, Spies T (1996) Cell stress-regulated human major histocompatibility complex class I gene expressed in gastrointestinal epithelium. *Proc Natl Acad Sci USA* 93: 12445–12450
68 Orchard TR, Dhar A, Simmons JD, Vaughan R, Welsh KI, Jewell DP (2001) MHC class I chain-like gene A (MICA) and its associations with inflammatory bowel disease and peripheral arthropathy. *Clin Exp Immunol* 126: 437–440
69 Groh V, Wu J, Yee C, Spies T (2002) Tumour-derived soluble MIC ligands impair expression of NKG2D and T-cell activation. *Nature* 419: 734–738
70 Lopez-Vazquez A, Rodrigo L, Fuentes D et al (2002) MHC class I chain related gene A (MICA) modulates the development of coeliac disease in patients with the high risk heterodimer DQA1*0501/DQB1*0201. *Gut* 50: 336–340
71 Pende D, Rivera P, Marcenaro S et al (2002) Major histocompatibility complex class I-related chain A and UL16-binding protein expression on tumor cell lines of different histotypes: analysis of tumor susceptibility to NKG2D-dependent natural killer cell cytotoxicity. *Cancer Res* 62: 6178–6186
72 Salih HR, Rammensee HG, Steinle A (2002) Cutting edge: down-regulation of MICA on human tumors by proteolytic shedding. *J Immunol* 169: 4098–4102
73 Maccalli C, Pende D, Castelli C, Mingari MC, Robbins PF, Parmiani G (2003) NKG2D engagement of colorectal cancer-specific T cells strengthens TCR-mediated antigen stimulation and elicits TCR independent anti-tumor activity. *Eur J Immunol* 33: 2033–2043
74 Qi J, Zhang J, Zhang S, Cui L, He W (2003) Immobilized MICA could expand human Vdelta1 gammadelta T cells *in vitro* that displayed major histocompatibility complex

class I chain-related A-dependent cytotoxicity to human epithelial carcinomas. *Scand J Immunol* 58: 211–220
75 Beal RK, Powers C, Wigley P, Barrow PA, Smith AL (2004) Temporal dynamics of the cellular, humoral and cytokine responses in chickens during primary and secondary infection with *Salmonella enterica* serovar *Typhimurium*. *Avian Pathol* 33: 25–33
76 Conejo-Garcia JR, Benencia F, Courreges MC et al (2003) Letal, A tumor-associated NKG2D immunoreceptor ligand, induces activation and expansion of effector immune cells. *Cancer Biol Ther* 2: 446–451
77 Jinushi M, Takehara T, Kanto T et al (2003) Critical role of MHC class I-related chain A and B expression on IFN-alpha-stimulated dendritic cells in NK cell activation: impairment in chronic hepatitis C virus infection. *J Immunol* 170: 1249–1256
78 Vujanovic NL, Nagashima S, Herberman RB, Whiteside TL (1996) Nonsecretory apoptotic killing by human NK cells. *J Immunol* 157: 1117–1126
79 Gallucci S, Lolkema M, Matzinger P (1999) Natural adjuvants: endogenous activators of dendritic cells. *Nat Med* 5: 1249–1255
80 Vanderheyde N, Aksoy E, Amraoui Z, Vandenabeele P, Goldman M, Willems F (2001) Tumoricidal activity of monocyte-derived dendritic cells: evidence for a caspase-8-dependent, Fas-associated death domain-independent mechanism. *J Immunol* 167: 3565–3569
81 Friedman EJ (2002) Immune modulation by ionizing radiation and its implications for cancer immunotherapy. *Curr Pharm Res* 8: 1765–1780
82 Reddy SM, Hsiao KH, Abernethy VE et al (2002) Phagocytosis of apoptotic cells by macrophages induces novel signaling events leading to cytokine-independent survival and inhibition of proliferation: activation of Akt and inhibition of extracellular signal-regulated kinases 1 and 2. *J Immunol* 169: 702–713
83 Scheffer SR, Nave H, Korangy F et al (2003) Apoptotic, but not necrotic, tumor cell vaccines induce a potent immune response *in vivo*. *Int J Cancer* 103: 205–211
84 Hanahan D, Lanzavecchia A, Mihich E (2003) Fourteenth annual pezcoller symposium: the novel dichotomy of immune interactions with tumors. *Cancer Res* 63: 3005–3008
85 Herberman RB (1973) *In vivo* and *in vitro* assays of cellular immunity to human tumor antigens. *Fed Proc* 32: 160–164
86 Herberman RB, Campbell DA, Jr., Oldham RK et al (1976) Immunogenicity of tumor antigens. *Ann NY Acad Sci* 276: 26–44
87 Lotze MT, Custer MC, Bolton ES, Wiebke EA, Kawakami Y, Rosenberg SA (1990) Mechanisms of immunologic antitumor therapy: lessons from the laboratory and clinical applications. *Hum Immunol* 28: 198–207
88 Tratkiewicz JA, Szer J (1990) Loss of natural killer activity as an indicator of relapse in acute leukaemia. *Clin Exp Immunol* 80: 241–246
89 Salerno C, Crepaldi T, Savoia P, Richiardi P (1990) Expression of HLA class I antigens in human tumors and their involvement in tumor growth. *Ric Clin Lab* 20: 85–93
90 Fountain JW, Karayiorgou M, Ernstoff MS et al (1992) Homozygous deletions within

human chromosome band 9p21 in melanoma. *Proc Natl Acad Sci USA* 89: 10557–10561

91 Restifo NP, Kawakami Y, Marincola F et al (1993) Molecular mechanisms used by tumors to escape immune recognition: immunogenetherapy and the cell biology of major histocompatibility complex class I. *J Immunother* 14: 182–190

92 Maeurer MJ, Gollin SM, Storkus WJ et al (1996) Tumor escape from immune recognition: loss of HLA-A2 melanoma cell surface expression is associated with a complex rearrangement of the short arm of chromosome 6. Clin *Cancer Res* 2: 641–652

93 Restifo NP, Marincola FM, Kawakami Y, Taubenberger J, Yannelli JR, Rosenberg SA (1996) Loss of functional beta 2-microglobulin in metastatic melanomas from five patients receiving immunotherapy. *J Natl Cancer Inst* 88: 100–108

94 Cormier JN, Hijazi YM, Abati A et al (1998) Heterogeneous expression of melanoma-associated antigens and HLA-A2 in metastatic melanoma *in vivo*. *Int J Cancer* 75: 517–524

95 Rosenberg SA, Yang JC, White DE, Steinberg SM (1998) Durability of complete responses in patients with metastatic cancer treated with high-dose interleukin-2: identification of the antigens mediating response. *Ann Surg* 228: 307–319

96 Shi Y, Evans JE, Rock KL (2003) Molecular identification of a danger signal that alerts the immune system to dying cells. *Nature* 425: 516–521

97 Hunt CR, Dix DJ, Sharma GG et al (2004) Genomic instability and enhanced radiosensitivity in Hsp70.1- and Hsp70.3-deficient mice. *Mol Cell Biol* 24: 899–911

98 Millar DG, Garza KM, Odermatt B et al (2003) Hsp70 promotes antigen-presenting cell function and converts T-cell tolerance to autoimmunity *in vivo*. *Nat Med* 9: 1469–1476

99 Noessner E, Gastpar R, Milani V et al (2002) Tumor-derived heat shock protein 70 peptide complexes are cross-presented by human dendritic cells. *J Immunol* 169: 5424–5432

100 Buttiglieri S, Galetto A, Forno S, De Andrea M, Matera L (2003) Influence of drug-induced apoptotic death on processing and presentation of tumor antigens by dendritic cells. *Int J Cancer* 106: 516–520

101 Yaglom JA, Ekhterae D, Gabai VL, Sherman MY (2003) Regulation of necrosis of H9c2 myogenic cells upon transient energy deprivation: rapid deenergization of mitochondria recedes necrosis and is controlled by reactive oxygen species, stress kinas JNK, HSP72, and ARC. *J Biol Chem* 278: 50483–50496

102 Bretscher P, Cohn M (1970) A theory of self-nonself discrimination. *Science* 169: 1042–1049

103 Janeway C (1989) Immunogenicity signals 1,2,3 ... and 0. *Immunol Today* 10: 283–286

104 Shurin MR, Lu L, Kalinski P, Stewart-Akers AM, Lotze MT (1999) Th1/Th2 balance in cancer, transplantation and pregnancy. *Springer Semin Immunopathol* 21: 339–359

105 Fukao T, Matsuda S, Koyasu S (2000) Synergistic effects of IL-4 and IL-18 on IL-12-dependent IFN-gamma production by dendritic cells. *J Immunol* 164: 64–71

106 Matsuda H, Suda T, Hashizume H et al (2002) Alteration of balance between myeloid dendritic cells and plasmacytoid dendritic cells in peripheral blood of patients with asth-

ma. *Am J Respir Crit Care Med* 166: 1050–1054
107 Kaser A, Kaser S, Kaneider NC, Enrich B, Wiedermann CJ, Tilg H (2004) Interleukin-18 attracts plasmacytoid dendritic cells (DC2s) and promotes Th1 induction by DC2s through IL-18 receptor expression. *Blood* 103: 648–655
108 Gran B, Zhang GX, Yu S et al (2002) IL-12p35-deficient mice are susceptible to experimental autoimmune encephalomyelitis: evidence for redundancy in the IL-12 system in the induction of central nervous system autoimmune demyelination. *J Immunol* 169: 7104–7110
109 Becher B, Durell BG, Noelle RJ (2003) IL-23 produced by CNS-resident cells controls T cell encephalitogenicity during the effector phase of experimental autoimmune encephalomyelitis. *J Clin Invest* 112: 1186–1191
110 Kalinski P, Hilkens CM, Snijders A, Snijdewint FG, Kapsenberg ML (1997) IL-12-deficient dendritic cells, generated in the presence of prostaglandin E2, promote type 2 cytokine production in maturing human naive T helper cells. *J Immunol* 159: 28–35
111 Kalinski P, Hilkens CM, Snijders A, Snijdewint FG, Kapsenberg ML (1997) Dendritic cells, obtained from peripheral blood precursors in the presence of PGE2, promote Th2 responses. *Adv Exp Med Biol* 417: 363–367
112 Kapsenberg ML, Hilkens CM, Wierenga EA, Kalinski P (1999) The paradigm of type 1 and type 2 antigen-presenting cells. Implications for atopic allergy. *Clin Exp Allergy* 29: 33–36
113 Johansson-Lindbom B, Svensson M, Wurbel MA, Malissen B, Marquez G, Agace W (2003) Selective generation of gut tropic T cells in gut-associated lymphoid tissue (GALT): requirement for GALT dendritic cells and adjuvant. *J Exp Med* 198: 963–969
114 Thomson AW, Lu L, Subbotin VM et al (1995) *In vitro* propagation and homing of liver-derived dendritic cell progenitors to lymphoid tissues of allogeneic recipients. Implications for the establishment and maintenance of donor cell chimerism following liver transplantation. *Transplantation* 59: 544–551
115 Penna G, Vulcano M, Sozzani S, Adorini L (2002) Differential migration behavior and chemokine production by myeloid and plasmacytoid dendritic cells. *Hum Immunol* 63: 1164–1171
116 Loza MJ, Perussia B (2004) The IL-12 signature: NK cell terminal CD56(+high) stage and effector functions. *J Immunol* 172: 88–96
117 Hart AL, Kamm MA, Knight SC, Stagg AJ (2004) Quantitative and functional characteristics of intestinal-homing memory T cells: analysis of Crohn's disease patients and healthy controls. *Clin Exp Immunol* 135: 137–145
118 Mule JJ, Schwarz SL, Roberts AB, Sporn MB, Rosenberg SA (1998) Transforming growth factor-beta inhibits the *in vitro* generation of lymphokine-activated killer cells and cytotoxic T cells. *Cancer Immunol Immunother* 26: 95–100
119 Su HC, Leite-Morris KA, Braun L, Biron CA (1991) A role for transforming growth factor-beta 1 in regulating natural killer cell and T lymphocyte proliferative responses during acute infection with lymphocytic choriomeningitis virus. *J Immunol* 147: 2717–2727

120 Defrance T, Vanbervliet B, Briere F, Durand I, Rousset F, Banchereau J (1992) Interleukin 10 and transforming growth factor beta cooperate to induce anti-CD40-activated naive human B cells to secrete immunoglobulin A. *J Exp Med* 175: 671–682

121 Lotze MT (1992) T-cell growth factors and the treatment of patients with cancer. *Clin Immunol Immunopathol* 62: S47–S54

122 Chomarat P, Vannier E, Dechanet J et al (1995) Balance of IL-1 receptor antagonist/IL-1 beta in rheumatoid synovium and its regulation by IL-4 and IL-10. *J Immunol* 154: 1432–1439

123 Berman RM, Suzuki T, Tahara H, Robbins PD, Narula SK, Lotze MT (1996) Systemic administration of cellular IL-10 induces an effective, specific, and long-lived immune response against established tumors in mice. *J Immunol* 157: 231–238

124 Kalinski P, Schuitemaker JH, Hilkens CM, Wierenga EA, Kapsenberg ML (1999) Final maturation of dendritic cells is associated with impaired responsiveness to IFN-gamma and to bacterial IL-12 inducers: decreased ability of mature dendritic cells to produce IL-12 during the interaction with Th cells. *J Immunol* 162: 3231–3236

125 Gorelik L, Flavell RA (2001) Immune-mediated eradication of tumors through the blockade of transforming growth factor-beta signaling in T cells. *Nat Med* 7: 1118–1122

126 Lawrance IC, Wu F, Leite AZ et al (2003) A murine model of chronic inflammation-induced intestinal fibrosis down-regulated by antisense NF-kappa B. *Gastroenterology* 125: 1750–1761

127 Wojtowicz-Praga S (2003) Reversal of tumor-induced immunosuppression by TGF-beta inhibitors. *Invest New Drugs* 21: 21–32

128 Lucas M, Stuart LM, Savill J, Lacy-Hulbert A (2003) Apoptotic cells and innate immune stimuli combine to regulate macrophage cytokine secretion *J Immunol* 171: 2610–2615

129 Oppenheim MH, Lotze MT (1994) Interleukin-2: solid-tumor therapy. *Oncology* 51: 154–169

130 Leder GH, Oppenheim M, Rosenstein M et al (1996) Inhibition of nitric oxide synthesis does not improve interleukin-2-mediated antitumor effects *in vivo*. *Eur Surg Res* 28: 167–178

131 Xiong H, Zhu C, Li F, Hegazi R, He K, Babyatsky M, Bauer AJ, Plevy SE (2003) Inhibition of interleukin-12 p40 transcription and NF-kappa B activation by nitric oxide in murine macrophages and dendritic cells. *J Biol Chem* 279: 10776–10783

132 Kim J-E, Tannenbaum SR (2003) S-nitrosation regulates the activation of endogenous procaspase-9 in HT-29 human colon carcinoma cells. *J Biol Chem; in press*

133 Miljkovic D, Markovic M, Bogdanovic N, Mostarica Stojkovic M, Trajkovic V (2002) Necrotic tumor cells oppositely affect nitric oxide production in tumor cell lines and macrophages. *Cell Immunol* 215: 72–77

134 Caux C, Massacrier C, Vanbervliet B, Barthelemy C, Liu YJ, Banchereau J (1994) Interleukin 10 inhibits T cell alloreaction induced by human dendritic cells. *Int Immunol* 6: 1177–1185

135 Fluckiger AC, Durand I, Banchereau J (1994) Interleukin 10 induces apoptotic cell death of B-chronic lymphocytic leukemia cells. *J Exp Med* 179: 91–99
136 Maeurer MJ, Martin DM, Castelli C et al (1995) Host immune response in renal cell cancer: interleukin-4 (IL-4) and IL-10 mRNA are frequently detected in freshly collected tumor-infiltrating lymphocytes. *Cancer Immunol Immunother* 41: 111–121
137 Suzuki T, Tahara H, Narula S, Moore KW, Robbins PD, Lotze MT (1995) Viral interleukin 10 (IL-10), the human herpes virus 4 cellular IL-10 homologue, induces local anergy to allogeneic and syngeneic tumors. *J Exp Med* 182: 477–486
138 Li W, Lu L, Li Y et al (1997) High-dose cellular IL-10 exacerbates rejection and reverses effects of cyclosporine and tacrolimus in Mouse cardiac transplantation. *Transplant Proc* 29: 1081–1082
139 Wu MS, Wu CY, Chen CJ, Lin MT, Shun CT, Lin JT (2003) Interleukin-10 genotypes associate with the risk of gastric carcinoma in Taiwanese Chinese. *Int J Cancer* 104: 617–623
140 Hurme M, Haanpaa M, Nurmikko T et al (2003) IL-10 gene polymorphism and herpesvirus infections. *J Med Virol* 70: S48–S50
141 Klingemann HG, Tsoi MS, Storb R (1986) Inhibition of prostaglandin E2 restores defective lymphocyte proliferation and cell-mediated lympholysis in recipients after allogeneic marrow grafting. *Blood* 68: 102–107
142 Kalinski P, Schuitemaker JH, Hilkens CM, Kapsenberg ML (1998) Prostaglandin E2 induces the final maturation of IL-12-deficient CD1a+CD83+ dendritic cells: the levels of IL-12 are determined during the final dendritic cell maturation and are resistant to further modulation. *J Immunol* 161: 2804–2809
143 Snijdewint FG, Kalinski P, Wierenga EA, Bos JD, Kapsenberg ML (1993) Prostaglandin E2 differentially modulates cytokine secretion profiles of human T helper lymphocytes. *J Immunol* 150: 5321–5329
144 Peron JM, Esche C, Subbotin VM, Maliszewski C, Lotze MT, Shurin MR (1998) FLT3-ligand administration inhibits liver metastases: role of NK cells. *J Immunol* 161: 6164–6170
145 Lotze MT, Rubin JT, Zeh HJ (1992) New biologic agents come to bat for cancer therapy. *Curr Opin Oncol* 4: 1116–1123
146 Bindon C, Czerniecki M, Ruell P et al (1983) Clearance rates and systemic effects of intravenously administered interleukin 2 (IL-2) containing preparations in human subjects. *Br J Cancer* 47: 123–133
147 Lotze MT, Frana LW, Sharrow SO, Robb RJ, Rosenberg SA (1985) *In vivo* administration of purified human interleukin 2. I. Half-life and immunologic effects of the Jurkat cell line-derived interleukin 2. *J Immunol* 134: 157–166
148 Davis ID, Maher DW, Cebon JS et al (2000) A phase I and pharmacokinetic study of subcutaneously-administered recombinant human interleukin-4 (rhuIL-4) in patients with advanced cancer. *Growth Factors* 17: 287–300
149 Gilleece MH, Scarffe JH, Ghosh A et al (1992) Recombinant human interleukin 4 (IL-

4) given as daily subcutaneous injections – a phase I dose toxicity trial. *Br J Cancer* 66: 204–210
150 Custer MC, Lotze MT (1990) A biologic assay for IL-4. Rapid fluorescence assay for IL-4 detection in supernatants and serum. *J Immunol Methods* 128: 109–117
151 Weber J, Yang JC, Topalian SL et al (1993) Phase I trial of subcutaneous interleukin-6 in patients with advanced malignancies. *J Clin Oncol* 11: 499–506
152 D'Hondt V, Humblet Y, Guillaume T et al (1995) Thrombopoietic effects and toxicity of interleukin-6 in patients with ovarian cancer before and after chemotherapy: a multicentric placebo-controlled, randomized phase Ib study. *Blood* 85: 2347–2353
153 Gordon MS, Nemunaitis J, Hoffman R et al (1995) A phase I trial of recombinant human interleukin-6 in patients with myelodysplastic syndromes and thrombocytopenia. *Blood* 85: 3066–3076
154 Bouffet E, Philip T, Negrier C et al (1997) Phase I study of interleukin-6 in children with solid tumours in relapse. *Eur J Cancer* 33: 1620–1626
155 Sosman JA, Aronson FR, Sznol M et al (1997) Concurrent phase I trials of intravenous interleukin 6 in solid tumor patients: reversible dose-limiting neurological toxicity. *Clin Cancer Res* 3: 39–46
156 Schuler M, Bruntsch U, Spath-Schwalbe E et al (1998) Lack of efficacy of recombinant human interleukin-6 in patients with advanced renal cell cancer: results of a phase II study. *Eur J Cancer* 34: 754–756
157 Olencki T, Finke J, Tubbs R et al (2000) Phase 1 trial of subcutaneous IL-6 in patients with refractory cancer: clinical and biologic effects. *J Immunother* 23: 549–56
158 Moller P, Sun Y, Dorbic T et al (1998) Vaccination with IL-7 gene-modified autologous melanoma cells can enhance the anti-melanoma lytic activity in peripheral blood of patients with a good clinical performance status: a clinical phase I study. *Br J Cancer* 77: 1907–1916
159 Ghalib R, Levine C, Hassan M et al (2003) Recombinant human interleukin-11 improves thrombocytopenia in patients with cirrhosis. *Hepatology* 37: 1165–1171
160 Gordon MS, McCaskill-Stevens WJ, Battiato LA et al (1996) A phase I trial of recombinant human interleukin-11 (neumega rhIL-11 growth factor) in women with breast cancer receiving chemotherapy. *Blood* 87: 3615–3624
161 Tepler I, Elias L, Smith JW, 2nd et al (1996) A randomized placebo-controlled trial of recombinant human interleukin-11 in cancer patients with severe thrombocytopenia due to chemotherapy. *Blood* 87: 3607–3614
162 Isaacs C, Robert NJ, Bailey FA et al (1997) Randomized placebo-controlled study of recombinant human interleukin-11 to prevent chemotherapy-induced thrombocytopenia in patients with breast cancer receiving dose-intensive cyclophosphamide and doxorubicin. *J Clin Oncol* 15: 3368–3377
163 Reynolds CH (2000) Clinical efficacy of rhIL-11. *Oncology (Huntingt)* 14: 32–40
164 Bussel JB, Mukherjee R, Stone AJ (2001) A pilot study of rhuIL-11 treatment of refractory ITP. *Am J Hematol* 66: 172–177
165 Atkins MB, Robertson MJ, Gordon M et al (1997) Phase I evaluation of intravenous

recombinant human interleukin 12 in patients with advanced malignancies. *Clin Cancer Res* 3: 409–417
166 Robertson MJ, Cameron C, Atkins MB et al (1999) Immunological effects of interleukin 12 administered by bolus intravenous injection to patients with cancer. *Clin Cancer Res* 5: 9–16
167 Kang WK, Park C, Yoon HL et al (2001) Interleukin 12 gene therapy of cancer by peritumoral injection of transduced autologous fibroblasts: outcome of a phase I study. *Hum Gene Ther* 12: 671–684
168 Gajewski TF, Fallarino F, Ashikari A, Sherman M (2001) Immunization of HLA-A2+ melanoma patients with MAGE-3 or MelanA peptide-pulsed autologous peripheral blood mononuclear cells plus recombinant human interleukin 12. *Clin Cancer Res* 7: 895s–901s
169 Portielje JE, Gratama JW, van Ojik HH, Stoter G, Kruit WH (2003) IL-12: a promising adjuvant for cancer vaccination. *Cancer Immunol Immunother* 52: 133–144
170 Hashimoto W, Osaki T, Okamura H et al (1999) Differential antitumor effects of administration of recombinant IL-18 or recombinant IL-12 are mediated primarily by Fas-Fas ligand- and perforin-induced tumor apoptosis, respectively. *J Immunol* 163: 583–589
171 Osaki T, Hashimoto W, Gambotto A et al (1999) Potent antitumor effects mediated by local expression of the mature form of the interferon-gamma inducing factor, interleukin-18 (IL-18). *Gene Ther* 6: 808–815
172 Hashimoto W, Tanaka F, Robbins PD et al (2003) Natural killer, but not natural killer T, cells play a necessary role in the promotion of an innate antitumor response induced by IL-18. *Int J Cancer* 103: 508–513
173 Tanaka F, Hashimoto W, Robbins PD, Lotze MT, Tahara H (2002) Therapeutic and specific antitumor immunity induced by co-administration of immature dendritic cells and adenoviral vector expressing biologically active IL-18. *Gene Ther* 9: 1480–1486
174 Son YI, Dallal RM, Lotze MT (2003) Combined treatment with interleukin-18 and low-dose interleukin-2 induced regression of a murine sarcoma and memory response. *J Immunother* 26: 234–240
175 Redlinger RE, Jr., Mailliard RB, Lotze MT, Barksdale EM, Jr. (2003) Synergistic interleukin-18 and low-dose interleukin-2 promote regression of established murine neuroblastoma *in vivo*. *J Pediatr Surg* 38: 301–307
176 Kirkwood JM, Ernstoff MS (1984) Interferons in the treatment of human cancer. *J Clin Oncol* 2: 336–352
177 Kirkwood JM, Richards T, Zarour HM et al (2002) Immunomodulatory effects of high-dose and low-dose interferon alpha2b in patients with high-risk resected melanoma: the E2690 laboratory corollary of intergroup adjuvant trial E1690. *Cancer* 95: 1101–1112
178 Agarwala SS, Kirkwood JM (2003) Temozolomide in combination with interferon alpha-2b in patients with metastatic melanoma: a phase I dose-escalation study. *Cancer* 97: 121–127
179 Bock SN, Cameron RB, Kragel P, Mule JJ, Rosenberg SA (1991) Biological and antitu-

mor effects of recombinant human macrophage colony-stimulating factor in mice. *Cancer Res* 51: 2649–2654
180 Schwartzentruber DJ, Topalian SL, Mancini M, Rosenberg SA (1991) Specific release of granulocyte-macrophage colony-stimulating factor, tumor necrosis factor-alpha, and IFN-gamma by human tumor-infiltrating lymphocytes after autologous tumor stimulation. *J Immunol* 146: 3674–3681
181 Sanda MG, Yang JC, Topalian SL et al (1992) Intravenous administration of recombinant human macrophage colony-stimulating factor to patients with metastatic cancer: a phase I study. *J Clin Oncol* 10: 1643–1649
182 Shurin MR, Pandharipande PP, Zorina TD et al (1997) FLT3 ligand induces the generation of functionally active dendritic cells in mice. *Cell Immunol* 179: 174–184
183 Gitlitz BJ, Figlin RA, Kiertscher SM, Moldawer N, Rosen F, Roth MD (2003) Phase I trial of granulocyte macrophage-colony stimulating factor and interleukin-4 as a combined immunotherapy for patients with cancer. *J Immunother* 26: 171–178
184 Epoetin: for better or for worse? (2004) *Lancet Oncol* 5: 1
185 Brower V (2003) Epoetin for cancer patients: a boon or a danger? *J Natl Cancer Inst* 95: 1820–1821
186 Weiss MJ (2003) New insights into erythropoietin and epoetin alfa: mechanisms of action, target tissues, and clinical applications. *Oncologist* 8 (Suppl 3): 18–29
187 Bommer J, Kugel M, Schoeppe W et al (1988) Dose-related effects of recombinant human erythropoietin on erythropoiesis. Results of a multicenter trial in patients with end-stage renal disease. *Contrib Nephrol* 66: 85–93
188 Eschbach JW, Egrie JC, Downing MR, Browne JK, Adamson JW (1987) Correction of the anemia of end-stage renal disease with recombinant human erythropoietin. Results of a combined phase I and II clinical trial. *N Engl J Med* 316: 73–78
189 Jablons DM, Mule JJ, McIntosh JK et al (1989) IL-6/IFN-beta-2 as a circulating hormone. Induction by cytokine administration in humans. *J Immunol* 142: 1542–1547
190 Saarinen UM, Koskelo EK, Teppo AM, Siimes MA (1990) Tumor necrosis factor in children with malignancies. *Cancer Res* 50: 592–595
191 Logan TF, Gooding W, Kirkwood JM, Shadduck RK (1996) Tumor necrosis factor administration is associated with increased endogenous production of M-CSF and G-CSF but not GM-CSF in human cancer patients. *Exp Hematol* 24: 49–53
192 Jackson SH, Yu CR, Mahdi RM, Ebong S, Egwuagu CE (2004) Dendritic cell maturation requires STAT1 and is under feedback regulation by suppressors of cytokine signaling. *J Immunol* 172: 2307–2315
193 Roman-Gomez J, Jimenez-Velasco A, Castillejo JA et al (2004) The suppressor of cytokine signaling-1 is constitutively expressed in chronic myeloid leukemia and correlates with poor cytogenetic response to interferon-alpha. *Haematologica* 89: 42–48
194 Gatto L, Berlato C, Poli V, Tininini S, Kinjyo I, Yoshimura A, Cassatella MA, Bazzoni F (2004) Analysis of suppressor of cytokine signaling (SOCS)-3 promoter responses to interferon. *J Biol Chem; in press*

195 Yoshimura A, Ohishi HMM, Aki D, Hanada T (2004) Regulation of TLR signaling and inflammation by SOCS family proteins. *J Leukoc Biol; in press*

196 Lin SY, Yeh KT, Chen WT et al (2004) Promoter CpG methylation of tumor suppressor genes in colorectal cancer and its relationship to clinical features. *Oncol Rep* 11: 341–348

197 Bayle J, Letard S, Frank R, Dubreuil P, De Sepulveda P (2004) Suppressor of cytokine signaling 6 associates with KIT and regulates KIT receptor signaling. *J Biol Chem* 279: 12249–12259

198 Johnston JA (2003) SOCS suppressors, regulators, and degraders. *J Leukoc Biol* 75: 743–748

199 Kubo M, Hanada T, Yoshimura A (2003) Suppressors of cytokine signaling and immunity. *Nat Immunol* 4: 1169–1176

200 Osaki T, Peron JM, Cai Q et al (1998) IFN-gamma-inducing factor/IL-18 administration mediates IFN-gamma- and IL-12-independent antitumor effects. *J Immunol* 160: 1742–1749

201 Tanaka F, Hashimoto W, Okamura H, Robbins PD, Lotze MT, Tahara H (2002) Rapid generation of potent and tumor-specific cytotoxic T lymphocytes by interleukin 18 using dendritic cells and natural killer cells. *Cancer Res* 60: 4838–4844

202 Son YI, Dallal RM, Mailliard RB, Egawa S, Jonak ZL, Lotze MT (2001) Interleukin-18 (IL-18) synergizes with IL-2 to enhance cytotoxicity, interferon-gamma production, and expansion of natural killer cells. *Cancer Res* 61: 884–888

203 Jonak ZL, Trulli S, Maier C, et al (2002) High-dose recombinant interleukin-18 induces an effective Th1 immune response to murine MOPC-315 plasmacytoma. *J Immunother* 25: S20–S27

204 Towne JE, Garka KE, Renshaw BR, Virca GD, Sims JE (2004) IL-1F6, IL-1F8 and IL-1F9 signal through IL-1Rrp2 and IL-1RAcP to activate the pathway leading to NFkappa B and mitogen-activated protein kinases. *J Biol Chem* 279: 13677–13688

205 Gao W, Kumar S, Lotze MT, Hanning C, Robbins PD, Gambotto A (2003) Innate immunity mediated by the cytokine IL-1 homologue 4 (IL-1H4/IL-1F7) induces IL-12-dependent adaptive and profound antitumor immunity. *J Immunol* 170: 107–113

206 Kumar S, Hanning CR, Brigham-Burke MR et al (2002) Interleukin-1F7B (IL-1H4/IL-1F7) is processed by caspase-1 and mature IL-1F7B binds to the IL-18 receptor but does not induce IFN-gamma production. *Cytokine* 18: 61–71

207 Arend WP (2002) The balance between IL-1 and IL-1Ra in disease. *Cytokine Growth Factor Rev* 13: 323–340

208 Wong HL, Costa GL, Lotze MT, Wahl SM (1993) Interleukin (IL) 4 differentially regulates monocyte IL-1 family gene expression and synthesis *in vitro* and *in vivo*. *J Exp Med* 177: 775–781

209 Rodriguez-Calvillo M, Duarte M, Tirapu I et al (2002) Upregulation of natural killer cells functions underlies the efficacy of intratumorally injected dendritic cells engineered to produce interleukin-12. *Exp Hematol* 30: 195–204

210 Ziske C, Marten A, Schottker B et al (2001) Resistance of pancreatic carcinoma cells is

reversed by coculturing NK-like T cells with dendritic cells pulsed with tumor-derived RNA and CA 19-9. *Mol Ther* 3: 54–60

211 Rosenberg SA, Eberlein TJ, Grimm EA, Lotze MT, Mazumder A, Rosenstein M (1982) Development of long-term cell lines and lymphoid clones reactive against murine and human tumors: a new approach to the adoptive immunotherapy of cancer. *Surgery* 92: 328–336

212 Lotze MT, Rayner AA, Grimm EA (1985) Problems with the isolation of lymphoid clones with reactivity to human tumors. *Behring Inst Mitt* 77: 105–114

213 Fox BA, Spiess PJ, Kasid A et al (1990) *In vitro* and *in vivo* antitumor properties of a T-cell clone generated from murine tumor-infiltrating lymphocytes. *J Biol Response Mod* 9: 499–511

214 Hwu P, Rosenberg SA (1994) The genetic modification of T cells for cancer therapy: an overview of laboratory and clinical trials. *Cancer Detect Prev* 18: 43–50

215 Bartels CJ, Rosenberg SA, Yang JC (1996) Adoptive cellular immunotherapy of cancer in mice using allogeneic T-cells. *Ann Surg Oncol* 3: 67–73

216 Dudley ME, Ngo LT, Westwood J, Wunderlich JR, Rosenberg SA (2000) T-cell clones from melanoma patients immunized against an anchor-modified gp100 peptide display discordant effector phenotypes. *Cancer J* 6: 69–77

217 Mailliard RB, Dallal RM, Son YI, Lotze MT (2000) Dendritic cells promote T-cell survival or death depending upon their maturation state and presentation of antigen. *Immunol Invest* 29: 177–185

218 Dudley ME, Wunderlich JR, Robbins PF et al (2002) Cancer regression and autoimmunity in patients after clonal repopulation with antitumor lymphocytes. *Science* 298: 850–854

219 Dudley ME, Wunderlich JR, Yang JC et al (2002) A phase I study of nonmyeloablative chemotherapy and adoptive transfer of autologous tumor antigen-specific T lymphocytes in patients with metastatic melanoma. *J Immunother* 25: 243–251

220 Phan GQ, Yang JC, Sherry RM et al (2003) Cancer regression and autoimmunity induced by cytotoxic T lymphocyte-associated antigen 4 blockade in patients with metastatic melanoma. *Proc Natl Acad Sci USA* 100: 8372–8377

221 Hodi FS, Mihm MC, Soiffer RJ et al (2003) Biologic activity of cytotoxic T lymphocyte-associated antigen 4 antibody blockade in previously vaccinated metastatic melanoma and ovarian carcinoma patients. *Proc Natl Acad Sci USA* 100: 4712–4717

222 Herberman RB, Bartram S, Haskill JS, Nunn M, Holden HT, West WH (1997) Fc receptors on mouse effector cells mediating natural cytotoxicity against tumor cells. *J Immunol* 119: 322–326

223 Alvarez JM, de Landazuri MO, Bonnard GD, Herberman RB (1978) Cytotoxic activities of normal cultured human T cells. *J Immunol* 121: 1270–1275

224 Riccardi C, Puccetti P, Santoni A, Herberman RB (1979) Rapid *in vivo* assay of mouse natural killer cell activity. *J Natl Cancer Inst* 63: 1041–1045

225 Herberman RB (1982) Natural killer cells. *Hosp Pract (Hosp Ed)* 17: 93–103

226 Basse PH, Goldfarb RH, Herberman RB, Hokland ME (1994) Accumulation of adop-

tively transferred A-NK cells in murine metastases: kinetics and role of interleukin-2. *In vivo* 8: 17–24
227 Yasumura S, Lin WC, Hirabayashi H, Vujanovic NL, Herberman RB, Whiteside TL (1994) Immunotherapy of liver metastases of human gastric carcinoma with interleukin 2-activated natural killer cells. *Cancer Res* 54: 3808–3816
228 Okada K, Nannmark U, Vujanovic NL et al (1996) Elimination of established liver metastases by human interleukin 2-activated natural killer cells after locoregional or systemic adoptive transfer. *Cancer Res* 56: 1599–1608
229 Vujanovic NL, Basse P, Herberman RB, Whiteside TL (1996) Antitumor functions of natural killer cells and control of metastases. *Methods* 9: 394–408
230 Basse PH, Whiteside TL, Chambers W, Herberman RB (2001) Therapeutic activity of NK cells against tumors. *Int Rev Immunol* 20: 439–501
231 Yang Q, Hokland ME, Bryant JL et al (2003) Tumor-localization by adoptively transferred, interleukin-2-activated NK cells leads to destruction of well-established lung metastases. *Int J Cancer* 105: 512–519
232 Stift A, Friedl J, Dubsky P et al (2003) Dendritic cell-based vaccination in solid cancer. *J Clin Oncol* 21: 135–142
233 Smithers M, O'Connell K, MacFadyen S et al (2003) Clinical response after intradermal immature dendritic cell vaccination in metastatic melanoma is associated with immune response to particulate antigen. *Cancer Immunol Immunother* 52: 41–52
234 Nencioni A, Muller MR, Grunebach F et al (2003) Dendritic cells transfected with tumor RNA for the induction of antitumor CTL in colorectal cancer. *Cancer Gene Ther* 10: 209–214
235 Iwashita Y, Tahara K, Goto S et al (2003) A phase I study of autologous dendritic cell-based immunotherapy for patients with unresectable primary liver cancer. *Cancer Immunol Immunother* 52: 155–161
236 Morse MA, Nair SK, Boczkowski D et al (2002) The feasibility and safety of immunotherapy with dendritic cells loaded with CEA mRNA following neoadjuvant chemoradiotherapy and resection of pancreatic cancer. *Int J Gastrointest Cancer* 32: 1–6
237 Krause SW, Neumann C, Soruri A, Mayer S, Peters JH, Andreesen R (2002) The treatment of patients with disseminated malignant melanoma by vaccination with autologous cell hybrids of tumor cells and dendritic cells. *J Immunother* 25: 421–428
238 Chang AE, Redman BG, Whitfield JR et al (2002) A phase I trial of tumor lysate-pulsed dendritic cells in the treatment of advanced cancer. *Clin Cancer Res* 8: 1021–1032
239 Alejandro Lopez J, Crosbie G, Kelly C et al (2002) Monitoring and isolation of blood dendritic cells from apheresis products in healthy individuals: a platform for cancer immunotherapy. *J Immunol* Methods 267: 199–212
240 Lau R, Wang F, Jeffery G et al (2001) Phase I trial of intravenous peptide-pulsed dendritic cells in patients with metastatic melanoma. *J Immunother* 24: 66–78
241 Geiger JD, Hutchinson RJ, Hohenkirk LF et al (2001) Vaccination of pediatric solid tumor patients with tumor lysate-pulsed dendritic cells can expand specific T cells and mediate tumor regression. *Cancer Res* 61: 8513–8519

242 Banchereau J, Palucka AK, Dhodapkar M et al (2001) Immune and clinical responses in patients with metastatic melanoma to CD34(+) progenitor-derived dendritic cell vaccine. *Cancer Res* 61: 6451–6458
243 Panelli MC, Wunderlich J, Jeffries J et al (2000) Phase 1 study in patients with metastatic melanoma of immunization with dendritic cells presenting epitopes derived from the melanoma-associated antigens MART-1 and gp100. *J Immunother* 23: 487–498
244 Nestle FO, Alijagic S, Gilliet M et al (1998) Vaccination of melanoma patients with peptide- or tumor lysate-pulsed dendritic cells. *Nat Med* 4: 328–332
245 Mayordomo JI, Zorina T, Storkus WJ et al (1997) Bone marrow-derived dendritic cells serve as potent adjuvants for peptide-based antitumor vaccines. *Stem Cells* 15: 94–103
246 Mayordomo JI, Loftus DJ, Sakamoto H et al (1996) Therapy of murine tumors with p53 wild-type and mutant sequence peptide-based vaccines. *J Exp Med* 183: 1357–1365
247 Celluzzi CM, Mayordomo JI, Storkus WJ, Lotze MT, Falo LD, Jr. (1996) Peptide-pulsed dendritic cells induce antigen-specific CTL-mediated protective tumor immunity. *J Exp Med* 183: 283–287
248 Dworacki G, Meidenbauer N, Kuss I et al (2001) Decreased zeta chain expression and apoptosis in CD3+ peripheral blood T lymphocytes of patients with melanoma. *Clin Cancer Res* 7: 947s–957s
249 Beckebaum S, Cicinnati VR, Dworacki G et al (2002) Reduction in the circulating pDC1/pDC2 ratio and impaired function of *ex vivo*-generated DC1 in chronic hepatitis B infection. *Clin Immunol* 104: 138–150
250 Hoffmann TK, Muller-Berghaus J, Ferris RL, Johnson JT, Storkus WJ, Whiteside TL (2002) Alterations in the frequency of dendritic cell subsets in the peripheral circulation of patients with squamous cell carcinomas of the head and neck. *Clin Cancer Res* 8: 1787–1793
251 Saito T, Dworacki G, Gooding W, Lotze MT, Whiteside TL (2000) Spontaneous apoptosis of CD8+ T lymphocytes in peripheral blood of patients with advanced melanoma. *Clin Cancer Res* 6: 1351–1364
252 Shaw JP, Basch R, Shamamian P (2004) Hematopoietic stem cells and endothelial cell precursors express Tie-2, CD31 and CD45. *Blood Cells Mol Dis* 32: 168–175
253 Bailey AS, Jiang S, Afentoulis M et al (2004) Transplanted adult hematopoietic stems cells differentiate into functional endothelial cells. *Blood* 103: 13–19
254 Plett PA, Frankovitz SM, Orschell-Traycoff CM (2002) *In vivo* trafficking, cell cycle activity, and engraftment potential of phenotypically defined primitive hematopoietic cells after transplantation into irradiated or nonirradiated recipients. *Blood* 100: 3545–3552
255 Imai K, Kobayashi M, Wang J et al (1999) Selective transendothelial migration of hematopoietic progenitor cells: a role in homing of progenitor cells. *Blood* 93: 149–156
256 Rao M, Yang W, Seifalian AM, Winslet MC (2003) Role of cyclooxygenase-2 in the angiogenesis of colorectal cancer. *Int J Colorectal Dis* 3: 3
257 Howe LR, Dannenberg AJ (2003) COX-2 inhibitors for the prevention of breast cancer. *J Mammary Gland Biol Neoplasia* 8: 31–43

258 Goulet AC, Einsphar JG, Alberts DS et al (2003) Analysis of cyclooxygenase 2 (COX-2) expression during malignant melanoma progression. *Cancer Biol Ther* 2: 713–718
259 Lotze MT, Rees RC (2004) Identifying biomarkers and surrogates of tumors (cancer biometrics): correlation with immunotherapies and immune cells. *Cancer Immunol Immunother* 53: 256–261
260 Yasui Y, Pepe M, Thompson ML et al (2003) A data-analytic strategy for protein biomarker discovery: profiling of high-dimensional proteomic data for cancer detection. *Biostatistics* 4: 449–463
261 Mosca PJ, Lyerly HK, Ching CD, Hobeika AC, Clay TM, Morse MA (2003) Proteomics for monitoring immune responses to cancer vaccines. *Curr Opin Mol Ther* 5: 39–43

Inflammatory chemokines: their role in tumor growth and progression

Frances R. Balkwill

Cancer Research UK, Translational Oncology Laboratory, Barts and The London Queen Mary's Medical School, Charterhouse Square, London EC1M 6BQ, UK

Introduction

Chemokines comprise a group of closely related chemotactic cytokines that are primarily involved in movement of cells [1]. Chemokines are small proteins (mostly 8–14 kDa) and can be classified by structure into four groups (C, CC, CXC, CX_3C) defined by the number and spacing of cysteines in highly conserved positions in the N-terminal region of the protein.

All chemokines bind to chemokine receptors that are seven-transmembrane-domain G-coupled proteins. The majority of chemokine receptors can bind more than one chemokine, but the receptors are generally specific for each subfamily, hence receptor nomenclature follows that of the chemokines; e.g. receptors for CC chemokines are designated CCR and those for CXC chemokines CXCR. Figure 1 summarizes the known human chemokine receptors and their families. Chemokine receptor ligand pairs can be categorized into several classes depending on whether the ligand is constitutively produced or inducible. Most pro-inflammatory chemokines are inducible and their receptors bind several different chemokine ligands. Many different cells express chemokine receptors; however, they are predominantly expressed on leukocytes. Subsets of leukocytes express different chemokine receptors and this allows them to respond to a range of inducible or homoeostatic chemokines during normal and pathologic processes.

Many cancers express an extensive network of chemokines and chemokine receptors [1–3]. These tumors are characterized by disregulated production of chemokines and abnormal chemokine receptor signaling and expression [4, 5]. Tumor-associated chemokines are thought to play at least five roles in the biology of primary and metastatic disease: control of the leukocyte infiltrate into the tumor, manipulation of tumor immune response, regulation of angiogenesis, action as autocrine or paracrine growth and survival factors, and control of the movement of tumor cells themselves. Hence, these biological activities of chemokines in the tumor microenvironment are just as likely to contribute to cancer growth and spread as to any host anti-tumor response.

Cancer and Inflammation, edited by Douglas W. Morgan, Ulf J. Forssmann and Marian T. Nakada

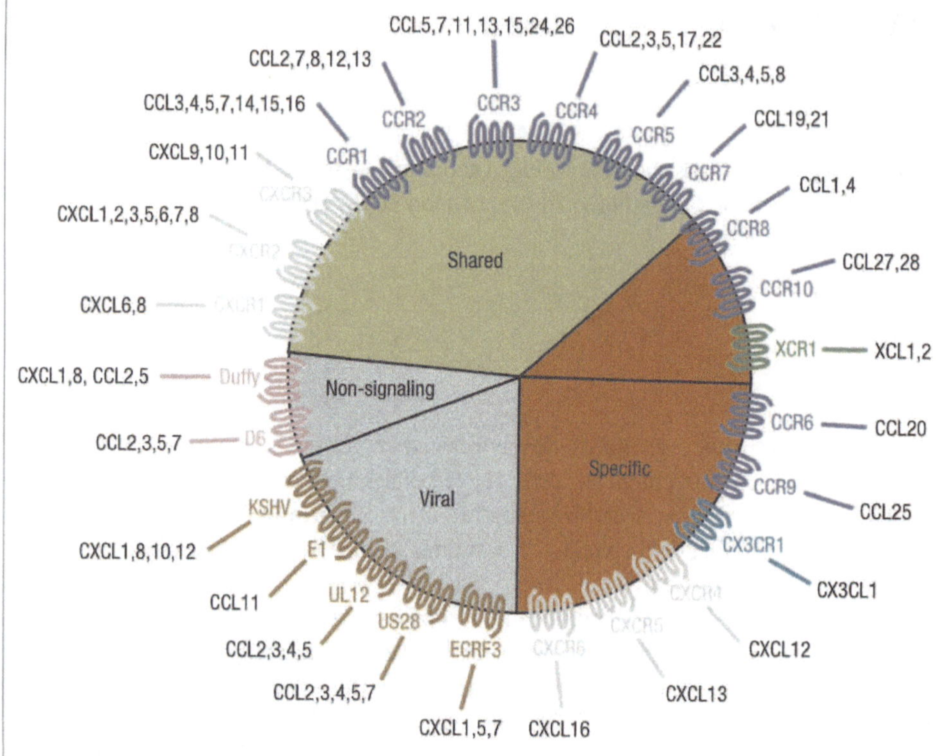

Figure 1
Classification of chemokine receptors and their ligands.
The four chemokine receptor families are grouped as "shared" if they bind more than one ligand, "specific" if they only bind one ligand, and if they bind chemokines but do not signal "non-signalling". Viral chemokine receptors and their chemokine ligands are also shown. A further classification can be made where chemokine receptors are grouped into inducible, inflammatory (in the green area) oder constitutive and basal trafficking/homing (in the red area).

Control of the tumor-associated leukocyte infiltrate by chemokines

Most solid tumors, be they of epithelial, mesothelial or haemopoietic origin, comprise a mixture of malignant cells and host stromal cells. Stromal cells are recruited into the tumor tissue and are integral to growth of primary tumor and spread of metastases [6–8]. Macrophages, lymphocytes, endothelial cells and fibroblasts are found in all solid cancers with eosinophils, granulocytes, natural killer cells and B cells also reported in some tumor types.

Chemokine production in human cancers

The leukocyte infiltrate of malignant lesions may have both positive and negative effects on tumor growth [9–12]. There is increasing evidence that these cells, especially macrophages, are a major source of growth factors, angiogenic factors, inflammatory cytokines and chemokines. Collectively these cytokines have profound effects on endothelial, epithelial and mesenchymal cells within the tumor microenvironment. It is also now clear that the extent and phenotype of the leukocyte infiltrate in solid tumors is related to local production of chemokines by both tumor and stromal cells. CC chemokines in particular are major determinants of macrophage and lymphocyte infiltration, for instance in human carcinomas of the breast and cervix, squamous cell carcinomas, sarcomas and gliomas, and Hodgkin's disease [2, 13].

For instance, the majority of cases of Hodgkin's disease are characterized by a complex chemokine network that includes chemokines CCL17 (TARC), CCL11 (eotaxin), CCL22 (MDC), which attract Th2 lymphocytes, as well as Th1-attracting chemokines CXCL10 (IP-10), CXCL9 (Mig-1), CCL2, CCL3, CCL5 and CXCL1 (*gro*/MGSA) [5]. In chronic lymphocytic leukemia (CLL), there is evidence that CD40 ligand stimulation of leukemic cells leads to production of CCL22 and CCL17. These chemokines caused migration of activated T cells *in vitro* and such T cells are also found in CLL lymph nodes and bone marrow. Thus malignant B cells can chemo-attract $CD4^+$ T cells that in turn induce strong chemokine production by the leukemic clone, leading to progressive accumulation of leukemic cells [14].

The predominant infiltrating cells in ovarian cancer are macrophages and $CD8^+$ T lymphocytes [8]. CCL2 localized to epithelial areas of the tumor [15] and correlated with the extent of lymphocyte and macrophage infiltration [8]. CCL3 (MIP-1α), CCL4 (MIP-1β) and CCL5 (RANTES) were also present in solid ovarian tumors, and localized to tumor-infiltrating leukocytes. CCL5 expression also correlated with the extent of $CD8^+$ T lymphocyte infiltration [8].

Ascites formation is a common occurrence in human epithelial ovarian cancer. mRNA and picomolar to nanomolar levels of protein for CCL2, CCL3, CCL4, CCL5, CCL8 (MCP-2) and CCL22 were found in the ascites cells and ascitic fluid [16]. Ascitic fluid contained variable numbers of tumor cells, macrophages and $CD3^+$ T lymphocytes that were predominantly $CD4^+$. A direct correlation was found between CCL5 concentration in ascitic fluid and $CD3^+$ T cell infiltrate [16]. Most of the data suggest that macrophages and tumor cells produce chemokines but tumor-associated fibroblasts may also be a source of chemokines and be involved in the recruitment of mononuclear cells, e.g. through production of CCL2 [17].

There are conflicting data on the prognostic significance of chemokine production and the tumor-associated leukocyte infiltrate. For instance, in breast cancer there is a positive correlation between macrophages, lymph node metastasis and clinical aggressiveness, and the tumor cells have been reported to produce CCL2 (MCP-1) and CCL5 (RANTES) [18, 19]. CCL5 levels correlated with tumor progression with only minimal chemokine expression found in benign breast disease [20]. Levels of CCL2 expression also correlated with breast cancer progression and macrophage accumulation, but were additionally found to relate to levels of MT1-MMP, the angiogenic factor thymidine phosphorylase and microvessel density in tumor sections [19].

The extent of CCL2 expression by the mononuclear cell infiltrate was significantly associated with tumor cell invasion, and macrophage and vessel counts in squamous cell carcinomas [21]. In contrast, CCL5 expression by tumor cells in non-small-cell lung cancer patients was associated with an "active lymphocyte response" and was a positive predictor of survival in this cancer [22].

Chemokine receptor profiles of infiltrating cells in cancer

Despite abundant chemokine expression in epithelial tumors, available data suggest that there is limited expression of chemokine receptors on tumor-associated leukocytes. CCR1 was the only CC chemokine receptor consistently expressed within the solid ovarian tumors and this localized to infiltrating $CD68^+$ macrophages and $CD8^+$ lymphocytes [23]. Downregulation of chemokine receptors on tumor-associated leukocytes may be due to high levels of chemokine ligands or inflammatory cytokines such as tumor necrosis factor α (TNFα) [24]. Altered physiological conditions such as hypoxia may also alter chemokine receptor profiles and response to chemokines in the tumor microenvironment [25]. The expression of chemokine receptors was markedly different in the ascitic form of ovarian cancer where leukocytes expressed a wide range of chemokine receptors at levels comparable to those found circulating in the periphery [16]. This may reflect the differences in microenvironment between the solid and "liquid" forms of this malignancy.

In Hodgkin's disease CCR3, which binds CCL11, was detected in some but not all cells of the reactive infiltrate [5]. The expression profile of this chemokine receptor was abnormal; not only T cells but also B cells, which do not normally express this receptor, stained positive. The receptor for CXCR3, which binds CXCL10 (IP-10) and CXCL9 (Mig-1), was moderately upregulated on $CD4^+$ T cells in the tumor.

Although the data on chemokine expression by tumor-associated leukocytes are limited, it is possible that in the presence of multiple chemokine gradients restricted expression of chemokine receptors in solid tumors may permit concise control of the extent and movement of the infiltrating leukocytes in the tumor, encouraging their retention within the tumor.

Chemokines and immune suppression in tumors

Infiltrating leukocytes may not only contribute to tumor progression by producing matrix metalloproteinases (MMPs) and growth, angiogenic and immunosuppressive factors, but the profile of the cells attracted by chemokines to the tumor may contribute to an immunosuppressive environment. There is often a prevalence of Th2 cells in tumors and this polarization may be a general strategy to subvert immune responses against tumors [2]. Hodgkin's disease, for instance, is characterized by constitutive activation of nuclear factor κB (NF-κB) and overproduction of Th2 cytokines and chemokines into the tumor, causing an influx of Th2 cells and eosinophils [5]. These reactive cells are thought not only to contribute to proliferation and survival of the malignant cells, but to suppression of cell-mediated immunity. Chronic exposure to high chemokine concentrations in the tumor microenvironment may encourage activated Type II macrophages that release immunosuppressive interleukin-10 and transforming growth factor β (TGFβ) [26]. These macrophages may also release CCL2, which could contribute to a Th2-polarized immunity [27] and stimulate a Type II inflammatory response [2].

Tumors are also known to inhibit dendritic cell 1 (DC1) migration and function, thus suppressing any specific immune response. In ovarian cancer, there is evidence that tumor cell production of CXCL12 weakens immunity by attracting and protecting CXCR4-expressing preDC2 cells, and altering preDC1 distribution, immunity and stimulation of fibrosis [28]. Another example of a strategy to encourage a Th2 environment in tumors comes from Kaposi's sarcoma. The viral genome encodes three chemokines (vMIPI, II and III) that are selective attractants for polarized Th2 cells [29].

Angiogenic and angiostatic chemokines exist in the tumor microenvironment

Chemokines may also regulate angiogenesis in the epithelial tumor microenvironment. CXC chemokines containing the three-amino-acid motif glutamine-leucine-arginine (ELR), such as CXCL8 (interleukin-8), CXCL1, CXCL5 (ENA-78), CXCL6 (GCP-2) and CXCL7 (NAP-2), promote angiogenesis [30]. They are directly chemotactic for endothelial cells and can stimulate angiogenesis in neo-vascularization experiments *in vivo*. Elevated levels of CXCL5 were found, for instance, in primary non-small-cell lung cancer and correlated with the vascularity of the tumors [31]. In contrast CXC chemokines lacking the ELR motif, such as CXCL9 and CXCL10, are often anti-angiogenic [30]. Levels of CXCL10 in human lung cancers were inversely related to tumor progression [30].

Chemokines and tumor cell growth

As well as promoting angiogenesis, deregulated chemokines may contribute directly to transformation of tumor cells by acting as growth and survival factors, generally in an autocrine manner. This action of chemokines has been extensively characterized in malignant melanoma. CXCL1 and CXCL8 are constitutively produced by melanoma cells, but not by untransformed melanocytes [1, 4, 32]. Melanoma cells also show elevated levels of the CXCR2 receptor for these chemokines, and autocrine chemokine stimulation enhances survival, proliferation and tumor cell migration [4, 33]. In addition, CXCL8 and CXCL1, as well as the CC chemokine CCL20 (MIP-3β), all stimulate growth of pancreatic tumor cell lines [34, 35].

In epithelial ovarian cancer, tumor cells express CXCR4 and its ligand CXCL12 enhances tumor cell proliferation in conditions of sub-optimal growth [36]. This autocrine chemokine stimulation may also have paracrine implications because CXCL12 stimulated the production of TNFα by ovarian tumor cells. Production of TNFα in the tumor microenvironment has been implicated in tumor progression [37].

Interactions between CXCL12 and CXCR4 also stimulate growth of prostate cancer cells [38], growth and survival of glioblastoma cells [39, 40], and growth of malignant plasma cells of multiple myeloma [41]. The survival effects of CXCL12/CXCR4 are at least partially regulated by phosphorylation of Akt in many of these cancer cells.

The ability of tumor cells to proliferate in response to chemokines appears to have been exploited by the human Kaposi's sarcoma herpes virus (KSHV). The KSHV genome encodes a G-protein-coupled receptor that signals constitutively and is structurally similar to CXCR2 [42]. Expression of this receptor is associated with cellular transformation. Cells transfected with a constitutively signaling mutated CXCR2 are similarly transformed [43]. Transgenic mice overexpressing the KSHV–GPCR under the control of the CD2 promoter develop lesions with remarkable similarity to Kaposi's sarcoma [44].

Chemokine gradients and the spread of malignant cells

Chemokines are central to trafficking of leukocytes and it seems that mechanisms utilized in homing of leukocytes in both pathological situations and during homeostasis, may also used by tumor cells. Restricted and specific expression of chemokine receptors, especially CXCR4 and CCR7, by tumor cells may be one important step in the development of site-specific metastasis. For example, tumor cells from breast, prostate, pancreatic, gastric and ovarian carcinomas, neuroblastoma, glioblastoma, melanoma, thyroid cancer, multiple myeloma, cutaneous T cell lymphoma and some leukemias express a limited and highly specific range of chemokine receptors (e.g. [45–52]). Generally only one or two of the known chemokine receptors are expressed on each tumor type. In breast, prostate and ovarian cancer, neuroblastoma, melanoma and some forms of leukemia, the respective ligand is strongly expressed at sites of tumor spread. Expression of CCR7 and CCR10 on melanoma cells, for example, was linked to expression of ligands for these receptors at the two major sites of metastasis, skin and lymph nodes [46]. Functional CCR7 and CXCR4 chemokine receptors are found on human breast cancer cells [46]. The ligand for CCR7, CCL21 (SLC), is highly expressed in lymph nodes and in a tissue screen strong expression of the ligand for CXCR4, CXCL12 (SDF-1), was only seen in the target organs for breast cancer metastases. Moreover, breast cancer cells migrated towards tissue extracts from these target organs, and chemotaxis could be partially abrogated by neutralizing antibodies to CXCR4 [46]. Vascular endothelial growth factor (VEGF) expression may be linked to high levels of CXCR4 expression on breast cancer cells [53]. In breast cancer cell lines, a VEGF autocrine pathway induces CXCR4 expression, promoting their migration towards CXCL12. Using high-density tissue microarrays from 600 patients, Sun et al. [38] found that CXCR4 protein expression was significantly elevated in localized and metastatic prostate cancer compared to normal or benign prostate tissue. CXCL12 protein levels were found to be higher in metastatic, compared to normal, prostate tissue.

Gastric cancer cells expressed CCR7 and responded to its chemokine ligands by directed migration *in vitro* [49]. In biopsies from this disease, 66% of cases contained CCR7-positive tumor cells and there was a significant difference in both lymph-node metastasis and lymphatic invasion between CCR7-positive and -negative cases. Stepwise regression analysis showed that the most important factor determining lymph-node metastasis in gastric cancer was CCR7 expression in the primary tumor. Expression of CCR7 in CLL correlated with clinical lymphadenopathy and its ligands CCL21 and CCL19 were located in high endothelial venules [54].

When biopsies from classical Hodgkin's disease where compared to the nodular lymphocyte predominant subtype, differences in chemokine receptor expression by tumor cells and chemokine ligand expression by the reactive cells in the tumor nodules were seen [55]. These differences might contribute to specific localization and confinement of neoplastic cells within the target organs of different types of Hodgkin's disease.

Animal cancer studies provide some experimental proof that cancer cells may co-opt normal mechanisms of chemokine-directed leukocyte homing to lymph nodes. When B16 melanoma cells were transduced with a retroviral vector containing cDNA for the chemokine receptor CCR7, metastasis to lymph nodes was increased [56]. Conversely when the same cells were transfected with the CXCR4 receptor they had a marked increase in the ability to form lung metastases, but spread to lymph node, liver and kidney was rare [57].

However, the process of metastasis is complex multi-step process. There are several stages at which the interaction between tumor cell chemokine receptors and their ligands could be important. For instance, in epithelial ovarian cancer, CXCR4 was the only one of 14 chemokine receptors investigated that was expressed by a panel of ovarian cancer cell lines [45]. The CXCR4 ligand CXCL12 was present in nanogram quantities in ascitic fluid from ovarian cancer patients. Stimulation of CXCR4 induced a calcium flux and directed migration of the tumor cells. Moreover, CXCR4 was expressed on a subset of cells in primary ovarian tumors, and more strongly expressed by tumor cells in ascites. Our initial conclusion was that this chemokine receptor–ligand interaction could be involved in peritoneal spread of this cancer. However, in agreement with Zhou et al. [28], we then found that the CXCR4 ligand CXCL12 was also expressed strongly by tumor cells in the solid ovarian cancer biopsies [36]. As described above, stimulation of CXCR4-expressing ovarian tumor cells with CXCL12 not only promoted invasion of cells through extracellular matrix, but caused production of the pro-inflammatory cytokine TNFα and increased cell proliferation under sub-optimal conditions [36]. Taken together these chemokine actions may allow tumor cells to grow in distant and less favorable sites and, *via* the pro-inflammatory cytokine TNFα, initiate a cytokine network in the surrounding stroma. However, the significance of high levels of tumor-derived CXCL12 at the site of the primary lesion is not understood. Although this may stimulate tumor growth, it could also serve to retain the malignant cells, rather than encourage metastasis. This hypothesis would be supported by observations that CXCR4 antagonists promote the release of stem cells from bone marrow by neutralizing CXCL12–CXCR4 interactions that normally retain cells in this microenvironment [58]. However, migration of primordial germ cells in zebrafish embryos is largely controlled by expression of CXCL12. A remarkable correlation was recorded between spatio-temporal expression of CXCL12 and location of primordial germ cells at different development stages, suggesting that CXCL12 can provide a key directional cue in a very localized manner [59].

To further understand the role of CXCR4 expression in ovarian cancer, we over-expressed CXCR4 in an ovarian cancer cell line, SKOV-3 that had low basal expression of this chemokine receptor (Kulbe et al., unpublished observations). CXCR4-transfected cells responded in a similar fashion to ovarian cancer cells, which naturally express CXCR4; stimulation with the CXCR4 ligand CXCL12 resulted in directed migration and invasion, proliferation under sub-optimal growth conditions, increased adhesion to fibronectin and induction of mRNA for TNFα. However, there were differences between CXCR4-transfected and mock-transfected controls when tumor cells were grown as intraperitoneal xenografts. Although CXCR4 transfectants generated a lower volume of tumor in the abdominal cavity, they formed a greater number of invasive and metastatic foci. CXCR4-expressing tumor deposits were widely disseminated into organs such as the mesenteric tissue, ovaries, lymph nodes, pancreas, thoracic cavity, lungs, and colon. These highly invasive tumors also had poor histological differentiation and higher mitotic index when compared to mock-transfected cells. We believe that acquisition of CXCR4 expression by tumor cells leads to increased adhesion to the extracellular matrix, increased invasiveness and increased survival at distant sites.

Targeting the chemokine network in tumors

There are a number of areas where manipulation of chemokines and their receptors could be therapeutic in cancer. A change in the extent and composition of the leukocyte infiltrate could inhibit angiogenesis, survival and spread of tumor cells. Manipulation of some tumor chemokines could also directly affect angiogenesis. Direct inhibition of the action of tumor cell chemokine receptors may prevent or delay lymph node and haematogenous metastases and may decrease survival of tumor cells at the site of the primary tumor or metastatic deposits. However, in spite of extensive pre-clinical studies of chemokine and chemokine receptor antagonists in inflammatory and infectious disease models [60], there are little published data on such strategies in models of malignant disease.

Manipulation of the leukocyte infiltrate

As described above, the macrophage/lymphocyte balance of the tumor infiltrate appears to be a critical factor in the development of cancer [61]. For instance, overexpression of the cytokine colony-stimulating factor 1 (macrophage-colony-stimulating factor) in a mouse model of mammary cancer increased infiltration of macrophages and accelerated tumor invasion and metastasis [62]. Stromal-cell derived MMP-9, most likely from tumor-associated macrophages, plays a critical role in angiogenesis and growth of ovarian cancer xenografts in nude mice [63]. Direct evidence for the involvement of chemokines in this stromal tumor promotion comes from studies of melanoma cell lines growing in nude mice. The effects of tumor-derived CCL2 depended on the level of secretion [11]. Low-level production of CCL2 was associated with modest macrophage infiltration, tumor formation and neo-vascularization of the tumor mass. High CCL2 secretion led to massive macrophage infiltration and destruction of tumor cells [11]. Attempts to decrease macrophage infiltration in tumors by neutralizing chemokines/receptors or chemokine antagonists seem warranted, but there are little published data.

However, we have recently studied the action of the chemokine receptor antagonist metRANTES in experimental breast cancer [64]. CCL5 (RANTES) was produced by 410.4 transplantable tumor cells and its receptors, CCR1 and CCR5, were expressed by the leukocyte infiltrate. As Met-CCL5 is an antagonist of CCR1 and CCR5 with activity in models of inflammatory disease, we tested its activity against 410.4 tumors. After 5 weeks of daily treatment with Met-CCL5, the volume and weight of 410.4 tumors were significantly decreased compared with control-treated tumors. Met-CCL5 was also active against established tumors. The total cell number obtained after collagenase digestion was decreased in Met-CCL5-treated tumors as was the proportion of infiltrating macrophages. Furthermore, chemokine antagonist treatment increased stromal development and necrosis.

Another approach to chemokine therapy of cancer is to overexpress certain chemokines in the tumor microenvironment. In the past 10 years many experimental animal studies have shown that overexpression of chemokines can increase tumor-associated leukocyte numbers and phenotypes with concomitant stimulation of destructive immune or inflammatory responses. This was first shown by overexpressing CCL2 in experimental tumors and stimulating a destructive macrophage influx [65]. Overexpression of CCL20 (MIP-3β) suppressed tumor growth by attracting dendritic cells to activate tumor-specific cytotoxic T lymphocytes [66]. CCL19 (MIP-3β) overexpression mediated rejection of murine breast tumors in a natural killer (NK) cell- and $CD4^+$ T cell-dependent manner [67] and CCL21 (6Ckine) reduced growth of a colon carcinoma cell line in mice using a similar mechanism [68]. In contrast to the above results, overexpression of CCL3 in B16 melanoma cells did not stimulate an effective anti-tumor response but prevented the initiation of metastases [69]. Direct injection of chemokines may achieve the same effect. When CCL21 was injected into axillary lymph-node-draining experimental lung tumors, extensive lymphocyte and dendritic cell infiltration into the tumors and enhanced mouse survival [70]. Enhanced production of Th1 cytokines and anti-angiogenic chemokines was noted accompanied by decreased lymph node and tumor site production of TGFβ. However, these gene-delivery approaches have not yet been translated into clinical trial.

Chemokines in anti-angiogenic strategies

In experimental models using human non-small-cell lung cancer cell lines grown in SCID mice, neutralization of CXCL5 [31] and CXCL8 [71] reduced tumor growth, vascularity and metastasis but had no direct effect on cell growth *in vitro*. The ELR^+ chemokine CXCL8 was also important in promoting angiogenesis and tumorigenesis in human ovarian cancer xenografts implanted into the peritoneum of nude mice [72]. In this study, mouse survival was inversely associated with CXCL8 expression within the tumor. Overexpression of the ELR^- chemokines CXCL9 and CXCL10 inhibited the growth of Burkitt's lymphoma tumors established in nude mice [73]. Likewise, administration of intra-tumoral CXCL10 inhibited NSCLC tumorigenesis and metastasis in SCID mice [71]. CCL21 (6Ckine) also inhibited growth and angiogenesis of human lung cancer cell lines in SCID mice [74]. Thus chemokines contribute to the network of pro- and anti-angiogenic factors in tumors and could be useful targets.

Chemokine antagonists and metastases

Chemokine receptor antagonists may also have direct actions on tumor cells. In this respect there are three published pre-clinical studies of antibodies that neutralize chemokines or chemokine receptors. As described above, B16 melanoma cells transduced with a retroviral vector containing cDNA for the chemokine receptor CCR7 showed increased lymph-node metastasis [56]. Lymphatic spread of these CCR7-transfected cells was blocked by neutralizing antibodies to the CCR7 ligand, CCL21 [56]. A majority of non-Hodgkin's lymphoma cells express CXCR4 and treatment of cells *in vitro* with neutralizing antibodies to CXCR4 inhibited cell migration and pseudopodium formation, and decreased proliferation [75]. In an animal model of human high-grade NHL, CXCR4 neutralization delayed tumor growth, reduced the weight of any tumors that subsequently developed and significantly increased mouse survival (75]. Finally, neutralizing antibodies to CXCR4 also suppressed lymph-node metastasis in a xenograft model of a CXCR4-expressing breast cancer [46].

Conclusions

The chemokine network in human tumors is complex and its role is only partially understood. There is a great deal of information on potential roles of individual chemokines, but more work is needed to define the overall chemokine and chemokine receptor profile of individual tumor types, and the cells within them. The chemokines that are produced by human tumors are part of an even more complex network of inflammatory, immunomodulating and growth-promoting cytokines, little is known about interactions between all these mediators. A common theme is emerging of the involvement of constitutively activated NF-κB in chemokine disregulation in cancers. Many of the processes that chemokines mediate during wound healing and inflammation are also active in cancer. The only differences are that chemokine production is generally disregulated in cancer and, as in chronic inflammatory disease, chemokine production is sustained and not self-limiting.

Pre-clinical studies of chemokine antagonists in animal cancer models are warranted, as are investigations of tumor development and spread in animals deficient in individual chemokines or receptors. Such experiments could provide a rationale for novel approaches to cancer treatment where manipulation of the chemokine balance could be a useful adjunct to existing biological therapies of cancer.

References

1 Vicari AP, Caux C (2002) Chemokines in cancer. *Cytokine Growth Factor* Rev 13: 143–145

2 Balkwill F, Mantovani A (2001) Inflammation and cancer: back to Virchow. *Lancet* 357: 539–545
3 Murphy PM (2001) Chemokines and molecular basis of cancer metastasis. *N Engl J Med* 354: 833–835
4 Dhawan P, Richmond A (2002) Role of CXCL1 in tumorigenesis of melanoma. *J Leukoc Biol* 72: 9–18
5 Skinnider BF, Mak TW (2002) The role of cytokines in classical Hodgkin lymphoma. *Blood* 99: 4283–4297
6 Brigati C, Noonan DM, Albini A, Benelli R (2002) Tumors and inflammatory infiltrates: Friends or foes? *Clin Exp Metastasis* 19: 247–258
7 Coussens LM, Werb Z (2001) Inflammatory cells and cancer: think different! *J Exp Med* 193: F23–F26
8 Negus RPM, Stamp GWH, Hadley J, Balkwill FR (1997) A quantitative assessment of the leukocyte infiltrate in ovarian cancer and its relationship to the expression of C–C chemokines. *Am J Pathol* 150(5): 1723–1734
9 Zhang L, Conejo-Garcia JR, Katsaros D, Girnotty PA, Massobrio M, Regnani G, Makrigiannakis A, Gray H, Schlienger K, Liebman MN et al (2003) Intratumoral T cells, recurrence, and survival in epithelial ovarian cancer. *N Engl J Med* 348: 203–213
10 Daniel D, Meyer-Morse N, Bergsland EK, Dehne K, Coussens LM, Hanahan D (2003) Immune enhancement of skin carcinogenesis by $CD4^+$ T cells. *J Exp Med* 197: 1017–1028
11 Nesbit M, Schaider H, Miller TH, Herlyn M (2001) Low-level monocyte chemoattractant protein-1 stimulation of monocytes leads to tumour formation in nontumorigenic melanoma cells. *J Immunol* 166: 6483–6490
12 Mantovani A, Sozzani S, Locati M, Allavena P, Sica A (2002) Macrophage polarization: tumor-associated macrophages as a paradigm for polarized M2 mononuclear phagocytes. *Trends Immunol* 23: 549–555
13 Bottazzi B, Polentarutti N, Acero R, Balsari A, Boraschi D, Ghezzi P, Salmona M, Mantovani A (1983) Regulation of the macrophage content of neoplasms by chemoattractants. *Science* 220 (4593): 210–212
14 Ghia P, Strola G, Granziero L, Guena M, Guida G, Sallusto F, Ruffing N, Montagna L, Piccoli P, Chilosi M et al (2002) Chronic lymphocytic leukemia B cells are endowed with the capacity to attract $CD4^+$, $CD40L^+$ T cells by producing CCL22. *Eur J Immunol* 32: 1403–1413
15 Negus RPM, Stamp GWH, Relf MG, Burke F, Malik STA, Bernasconi S, Allavena P, Sozzani S, Mantovani A, Balkwill FR (1995) The detection and localization of monocyte chemoattractant protein-1 (MCP-1) in human ovarian cancer. *J Clin Invest* 95: 2391–2396
16 Milliken D, Scotton C, Raju S, Balkwill F, Wilson J (2002) Analysis of chemokines and chemokine receptor expression in ovarian cancer ascites. *Clin Cancer Res* 8: 1108–1114
17 Silzle T, Kreutz M, Dobler MA, Brockhoff G, Kneuchel R, Kunz-Schughart LA (2003)

tumor-associated fibroblasts recruit blood monocytes into tumor tissue. *Eur J Immunol* 33: 1311–1320
18 Luboshits G, Shina S, Kaplan O, Engelberg S, Nass D, Lifshitz-Mercer B, Chaitchik S, Keydar I, Ben-Baruch A (1999) Elevated expression of the CC chemokine regulated on activation, normal T cell expressed and secreted (RANTES) in advanced breast carcinoma. *Cancer Res* 59: 4681–4687
19 Saji H, Koike M, Yamori T, Saji S, Motoharu S, Matsushima K, Toi M (2001) Significant correlation of monocyte chemoattractant protein-1 expression with neovascularization and progression of breast carcinoma. *Cancer* 92: 1085–1091
20 Azenshtein E, Luboshits G, Shina S, Neumark E, Shahbazian D, Weil M, Wigler N, Keydar I, Ben-Baruch A (2002) The CC chemokine RANTES in breast carcinoma progression: regulation of expression and potential mechanisms of promalignant activity. *Cancer Res* 62: 1093–1102
21 Ohta M, Kitadai Y, Tanaka S, Yoshihara M, Yasui W, Mukaida N, Haruma K, Chayama K (2002) Monocyte chemoattractant protein-1 expression correlates with macrophage infiltration and tumor vascularity in human esophageal squamous cell carcinomas. *Int J Cancer* 102: 220–224
22 Moran CJ, Arenberg DA, Huang CC, Giordano TJ, Thomas DG, Misek DE, Chen G, Iannettoni MD, Orringer MB, Hanash S et al (2002) RANTES expression is a predictor of survival in stage I lung adenocarcinoma. *Clin Cancer Res* 8: 3803–3812
23 Scotton C, Milliken D, Wilson J, Raju S, Balkwill F (2001) Analysis of CC chemokine and chemokine receptor expression in solid ovarian tumours. *Br J Cancer* 85: 891–897
24 Sica A, Saccani A, Bottazzi B, Bernasconi S, Allevena P, Brancatelli G, Fei F, LaRosa G, Scotton C, Balkwill FR et al (2000) Defective expression of the monocyte chemotactic protein-1 receptor CCR2 in macrophages associated with uman ovarian carcinoma. *J Immunol* 164: 733–738
25 Grimshaw MJ, Balkwill FR (2001) Inhibition of monocyte and macrophage chemotaxis by hypoxia and inflammation – a potential mechanism. *Eur J Immunol* 31: 480–489
26 Sica A, Saccani A, Bottazzi B, Polentarutti N, Vecchi A, Van Damme J, Mantovani A (2000b) Autocrine production of IL-10 mediates defective IL-12 production and NF-k activation in tumor-associated macrophages. *J Immunol* 164: 762–767
27 Gu L, Tseng S, Horner RM, Tam C, Loda M, Rollins BJ (2000) Control of TH2 polarization by the chemokine monocyte chemoattractant protein-1. *Nature* 404: 407–411
28 Zhou W, Machelon V, Coulomb-l'Hermin A, Borvak J, Nome F, Isaeva T, Wei S, Krzysiek R, Durand-Gasselin I, Gordon A et al (2001) Stromal-derived factor-1 in human tumors recruits and alters the function of plasmacytoid precursor dendritic cells. *Nature Med* 7: 1339–1346
29 Sozzani S, Luini W, Bianchi G, Allavena P, Wells TN, Napolitano M, Bernardini G, Vecchi A, D'Ambrosio D, Mazzeo D et al (1998) The viral chemokine macrophage inflammatory protein-II is a selective Th2 chemoattractant. *Blood* 92: 4036–4039
30 Belperio JA, Keane MP, Arenberg DA, Addison CL, Ehlert JE, Burdick MD, Strieter RM (2000) CXC chemokines in angiogenesis. *J Leukoc Biol* 68 (1): 1–8

31 Arenberg DA, Keane MP, DiGiovine B, Kunkel SL, Morris SB, Xue YY, Burdick MD, Glass MC, Iannettoni MD, Strieter RM (1998) Epithelial-neutrophil activating peptide (ENA-78) is an important angiogenic factor in non-small cell lung cancer. *J Clin Invest* 102 (3): 465–472
32 Schadendorf D, Moller A, Algermissen B, Worm M, Sticherling M, Czarnetzki BM (1993) IL-8 produced by human malignant melanoma cells *in vitro* is an essential autocrine growth factor. *J Immunol* 151 (5): 2667–2675
33 Luan J, Shattuck-Brandt R, Hyaghnegahdar H, Owen JD, Strieter R, Burdick M, Nirodi C, Beauchamp D, Johnson KN, Richmond A (1997) Mechanism and biological significance on constitutive expression of MGSA/GRO chemokines in malignant melanoma tumor progression. *J Leukoc Biol* 62: 588–597
34 Takamori H, Oades ZG, Hoch OC, Burger M, Schraufstatter IU (2000) Autocrine growth effect of IL-8 and GROalpha on a human pancreatic cancer cell line, Capan-1. *Pancreas* 21 (1): 52–56
35 Kleeff J, Kusama T, Rossi DL, Ishiwata T, Maruyama H, Friess H, Buchler MW, Zlotnik A, Korc M (1999) Detection and localization of MIP-3a/LARC/Exodus, a macrophage proinflammatory chemokine, and its CCR6 receptor in human pancreatic cancer. *Int J Cancer* 81: 650–657
36 Scotton CJ, Wilson JL, Scott K, Stamp G, Wilbanks GD, Fricker S, Bridger G, Balkwill FR (2002) Multiple actions of the chemokine CXCL12 on epithelial tumor cells in human ovarian cancer. *Cancer Res* 62: 5930–5938
37 Balkwill F (2002) Tumor necrosis factor or tumor promoting factor? *Cytokine Growth Factor Rev* 13: 135–141
38 Sun Y-X, Wang J, Shelburne CE, Lopatin DE, Chinnaiyan AM, Rubin MA, Pienta KJ, Taichman RS (2003) Expression of CXCR4 and CXCL12 (SDF-1) in human prostate cancers (PCa) *in vivo*. *J Cell Biochem* 89: 462–473
39 Zhou Y, Larsen PH, Hao C, Yong VW (2002) CXCR4 is a major chemokine receptor on glioma cells and mediates their survival. *J Biol Chem* 277: 49481–49487
40 Barbero S, Bonavia R, Bajetto A, Porcile C, Pirani P, Ravettti JL, Zona GL, Spaziante R, Florio T, Schettini G (2003) Stromal cell-derived factor 1a stimulates human glioblastoma cell growth through the activation of both extracellular signal-regulated kinases 1/2 and Akt. *Cancer Res* 63: 1969–1974
41 Hideshima T, Chauhan D, Hayashi T, Podar K, Akiyama M, Gupta D, Richardson P, Munshi N, Anderson KC (2002) The biological sequelae of stromal cell-derived factor-1alpha in multiple myeloma. *Mol Cancer Ther* 1: 539–544
42 Arvanitakis L, Geras-Raaka E, Varma a, Gershengorn MC, Cesarman E (1997) Human herpesvirus KSHV encodes a constitutively active G-protein-coupled receptor linked to cell proliferation. *Nature* 385: 347–350
43 Burger M, Burger JA, Hoch RC, Oades Z, Takamori H, Schraufstatter IU (1999) Point mutation causing constitutive signaling of CXCR2 leads to transforming activity similar to Kaposi's sarcoma herpesvirus-G protein-coupled receptor. *J Immunol* 163: 2017–2022

44 Yang TY, Chen SC, Leach MW, Manfra D, Homey B, Wiekowski M, Sullivan L, Jenh CH, Narula SK, Chensue SW et al (2000) Transgenic expression of the chemokine receptor encoded by human herpesvirus 8 induces an angioproliferative disease resembling Kaposi's sarcoma. *J Exp Med* 191: 445–453
45 Scotton CJ, Wilson JL, Milliken D, Stamp G, Balkwill FR (2001) Epithelial cancer cell migration: a role for chemokine receptors? *Cancer Res* 61: 4961–4965
46 Muller A, Homey B, Soto H, Ge N, Catron D, Buchanan ME, McClanahan T, Murphy E, Yuan W, Wagner SN et al (2001) Involvement of chemokine receptors in breast cancer metastasis. *Nature* 410: 50–56
47 Rempel SA, Dudas S, Ge S, Gutierrez JA (2000) Identification and localization of the cytokine SDF1 and its receptor, CXC chemokine receptor 4, to regions of necrosis and angiogenesis in human glioblastoma. *Clin Cancer Res* 6: 102–111
48 Taichman RS, Cooper C, Keller Et, Pienta KJ, Taichman NS, McCauley LK (2002) Use of the stromal cell-derived factor-1/CXCR4 pathway in prostate cancer metastasis to bone. *Cancer Res* 62: 1832–1837
49 Mashino K, Sadanaga N, Yamaguchi H, Tanaka F, Ohta M, Shibuta K, Inoue H, Mori M (2002) Expression of chemokine receptor CCR7 is associated with lymph node metastasis of gastric carcinoma. *Cancer Res* 62: 2937–2941
50 Geminder H, Sagi-Assif O, Goldberg L, Meshel t, Rechavi G, Witz IP, Ben-Baruch A (2001) A possible role for CXCR4 and its ligand, the CXC chemokine stromal cell-derived factor-1, in the development of bone marrow metastases and neuroblastoma. *J Immunol* 167: 4747–4757
51 Koshiba T, Hosotani R, Miyamoto Y, Ida J, Tsuji S, Nakajima S, Kawaguchi M, Kobayashi H, Doi R, Hori T et al (2000) Expression of stromal cell-derived factor 1 and CXCR4 ligand receptor system in pancreatic cancer: a possible role for tumor progression. *Clin Cancer Res* 6: 3530–3535
52 Ferenczi K, Fuhlbrigge RC, Pinkus J, Pinkus GS, Kupper TS (2002) Increased CCR4 expression in cutaneous T cell lymphoma. *J Invest Dermatol* 119: 1405–1410
53 Bachelder RE, Wendt MA, Mercurio AM (2002) Vascular endothelial growth factor promotes breast carcinoma invasion in an autocrine manner by regulating the chemokine receptor CXCR4. *Cancer Res* 62: 7203–7206
54 Till KJ, Lin K, Zuzel M, Cawley JC (2002) The chemokine receptor CCR7 and alpha4 integrin are important for migrationn of chronic lymphocytic leukemia cells into lymph nodes. *Blood* 99: 2977–2984
55 Hopken UE, Foss HD, Meyer D, Hinz M, Leder K, Stein H, Lipp M (2002) Up-regulation of the chemokine receptor CCR7 in classical but not in lymphocyte-predominant Hodgkin disease correlates with distinct dissemination of neoplastic cells in lymphoid organs. *Blood* 99: 1109–1116
56 Wiley HE, Gonzalez EB, Maki S, Wu M-t, Hwang ST (2001) Expression of CC chemokine receptor-7 and regional lymph node metastasis of B16 murine melanoma. *J Natl Cancer Inst* 93: 1638–1643
57 Murakami T, Maki W, Cardones AR, Fang H, Kyi AT, Nestle FO, Hwang ST (2002)

Expression of CXC chemokine receptor-4 enhances the pulmonary metastatic potential of murine B16 melanoma cells. *Cancer Res* 62: 7328–7334
58 Broxmeyer HE, Cooper S, Kohli L, Hangoc G, Lee Y, Mantel C, Clapp DW, Kim CH (2003) Transgenic expression of stromal cell-derived factor-1/CXC chemokine ligand 12 enhances myeloid progenitor cell survival/antiapoptosis *in vitro* in response to growth factor withdrawal and enhances myelopoiesis *in vivo*. *J Immunol* 170: 421–429
59 Doitsidou M, Reichman-Fried M, Stebler J, Koprunner M, Dorries J, Meyer D, Esguerra CV, Leung TC, Raz E (2002) Guidance of primordial germ cell migration by the chemokine SDF-1. *Cell* 111: 647–659
60 Proudfoot AEI (2002) Chemokine receptors: multifaceted therapeutic targets. *Nature Rev* 2: 106–115
61 Mantovani A, Bottazzi B, Colotta F, Sozzani S, Ruco L (1992) The origin and function of tumor-associated macrophages. *Immunol Today* 13 (7): 265–270
62 Lin EY, Nguyen AV, Russell RG, Pollard JW (2001) Colony-stimulating factor 1 promotes progression of mammary tumors to malignancy. *J Exp Med* 193: 727–739
63 Huang S, Van Arsdall M, Tedjaranti S, McCarty M, Wu W, Langley R, Fidler IJ (2002) Contributions of stromal metalloproteinase-9 to angiogenesis and growth of human ovarian carcinoma in mice. *J Natl Cancer Inst* 94: 1134–1142
64 Robinson SC, Scott KA, Wilson J, Thompson RG, Proudfoot AEL, Balkwill F (2003) A chemokine receptor antagonist inhibits experimental breast tumor growth. *Cancer Res* 63: 5978–5991
65 Bottazzi B, Walter S, Govoni D, Colotta F, Mantovani A (1992) Monocyte chemotactic cytokine gene transfer modulates macrophage infiltration, growth, and susceptibility to IL-2 therapy of a murine melanoma. *J Immunol* 148 (4): 1280–1285
66 Fushimi T, Kojima A, Moore MAS, Crystal RG (2000) Macrophage inflammatory protein 3a transgene attracts dendritic cells to established murine tumors and suppresses tumor growth. *J Clin Invest* 105: 1383–1393
67 Braun SE, Chen K, Foster RG, Kim CH, Hromas R, Kaplan MH, Broxmeyer HE, Cornetta K (2000) The CC chemokine CKb-11/MIP-3b/ELC/Exodus 3 mediates tumor rejection of murine breast cancer cells through NK cells. *J Immunol* 164: 4025–4031
68 Vicari AP, Ait-Yahia S, Chemin K, Mueller A, Zlotnik A, Caux C (2000) Antitumor effects of the mouse chemokine 6CKine/SLC through angiostatic and immunological mechanisms. *J Immunol* 165: 1992–2000
69 van Deventer HW, Serody JS, McKinnon KP, Clements C, Brickey WJ, Ting JP-Y (2002) Transfection of macrophage inflammatory protein 1a into B16 F10 melanoma cell inhibits growth of pulmonary metastases but not subcutaneous tumors. *J Immunol* 169: 1634–1639
70 Sharma S, Stolina M, Zhu L, Lin Y, Batra R, Huang M, Strieter R, Dubinett SM (2001) Secondary lymphoid organ chemokine reduces pulmonary tumour burden in spontaneous murine bronchoalveolar cell carcinoma. *Cancer Res* 61: 6406–6412
71 Arenberg DA, Kunkel SL, Polverini PJ, Morris SB, Burdick MD, Glass MC, Taub DT, Iannettonni MD, Whyte RI, Strieter RM (1996) Interferon-γ-inducible protein 10 (IP-

10) is an agionstatic factor that inhibits human non-small cell lung cancer (NSCLC) tumorigenesis and spontaneous metastases. *J Exp Med* 184: 981–992
72 Yoneda J, Kuniyasu H, Crispens MA, Price JE, Bucana CD, Fidler IJ (1998) Expression of angiogenesis-related genes and progression of human ovarian carcinomas in nude mice. *J Natl Cancer Inst* 90(6): 447–454
73 Teruya-Feldstein J, Jaffe ES, Burd PR, Kanegane H, Kingma DW, Wilson WH, Longo DL, Tosato G (1997) The role of Mig, the monokine induced by interferon-gamma, and IP-10, the interferon-gamma-inducible protein-10, in tissue necrosis and vascular damage associated with Epstein-Barr virus-positive lymphoproliferative disease. *Blood* 90 (10): 4099–105
74 Arenberg DA, Zlotnick A, Strom SR, Burdick MD, Strieter RM (2001) The murine CC chemokine, 6C-kine, inhibits tumor growth and angiogenesis in a human lung cancer SCID mouse model. *Cancer Immunol Immunother* 49 (11): 587–592
75 Bertolini F, Dell'Agnola C, Mancuso P, Rabascio C, Burlini A, Monestiroli S, Gobbi A, Pruneri G, Martinelli G (2002) CXCR4 neutralization, a novel therapeutic approach for non-Hodgkin's lymphoma. *Cancer Res* 62: 3106–3112

Inflammation and matrix metalloproteinases: implications for cancer development

Karin E. de Visser[1] *and Lisa M. Coussens*[1,2,3]

[1]Cancer Research Institute, [2]Department of Pathology, and [3]Comprehensive Cancer Center, University of California, San Francisco 2340 Sutter St., San Francisco, CA 94143, USA

Matrix metalloproteinases (MMPs): structure, regulation, localization, and function

MMPs are a family of at least 25 highly homologous secreted or plasma membrane-associated zinc-binding proteinases (reviewed in [1, 2]). MMPs can be produced by virtually all cell types, and regulate many developmental processes and a variety of pathological conditions, including, but not limited to, cancer, auto-immune diseases, and periodontitis.

Structure

Based on their domain organization, MMPs can be classified into eight groups, five of which are secreted and three of which contain transmembrane domains and are expressed as cell surface enzymes (membrane-type MMPs (MT-MMPs)) (Fig. 1). All MMPs are expressed as pre-pro proteins where the N-terminal signal sequence (pre-domain) directs transport to the endoplasmic reticulum. Propeptide domains contain a zinc-interacting sulfhydryl group and maintain enzyme latency. In addition, MMPs contain a catalytic domain with a conserved zinc-binding site [1]. With the exception of the minimal-domain MMPs (MMP-7 and MMP-26) and the Type II transmembrane MMP (MMP-23), all MMPs contain a hemopexin domain adjacent to the catalytic domain linked *via* a hinge region. Hemopexin domains are believed to mediate interactions with tissue inhibitors of MMPs (TIMPs), some cell-surface molecules and proteolytic substrates [3, 4]. The MT-MMPs have a transmembrane domain, or a C-terminal glycosylphosphatidylinositol-anchoring domain with which they are covalently linked to plasma membranes, and are thought to play a crucial role in localizing some proteolytic activities to the cell surface [5, 6]. Other MMP structural classes are distinguished by the presence of additional functional domains, such as collagen-binding fibronectin type II inserts within the catalytic domain of the gelatin-binding MMPs (Fig. 1). Although MMP family members

Cancer and Inflammation, edited by Douglas W. Morgan, Ulf J. Forssmann and Marian T. Nakada

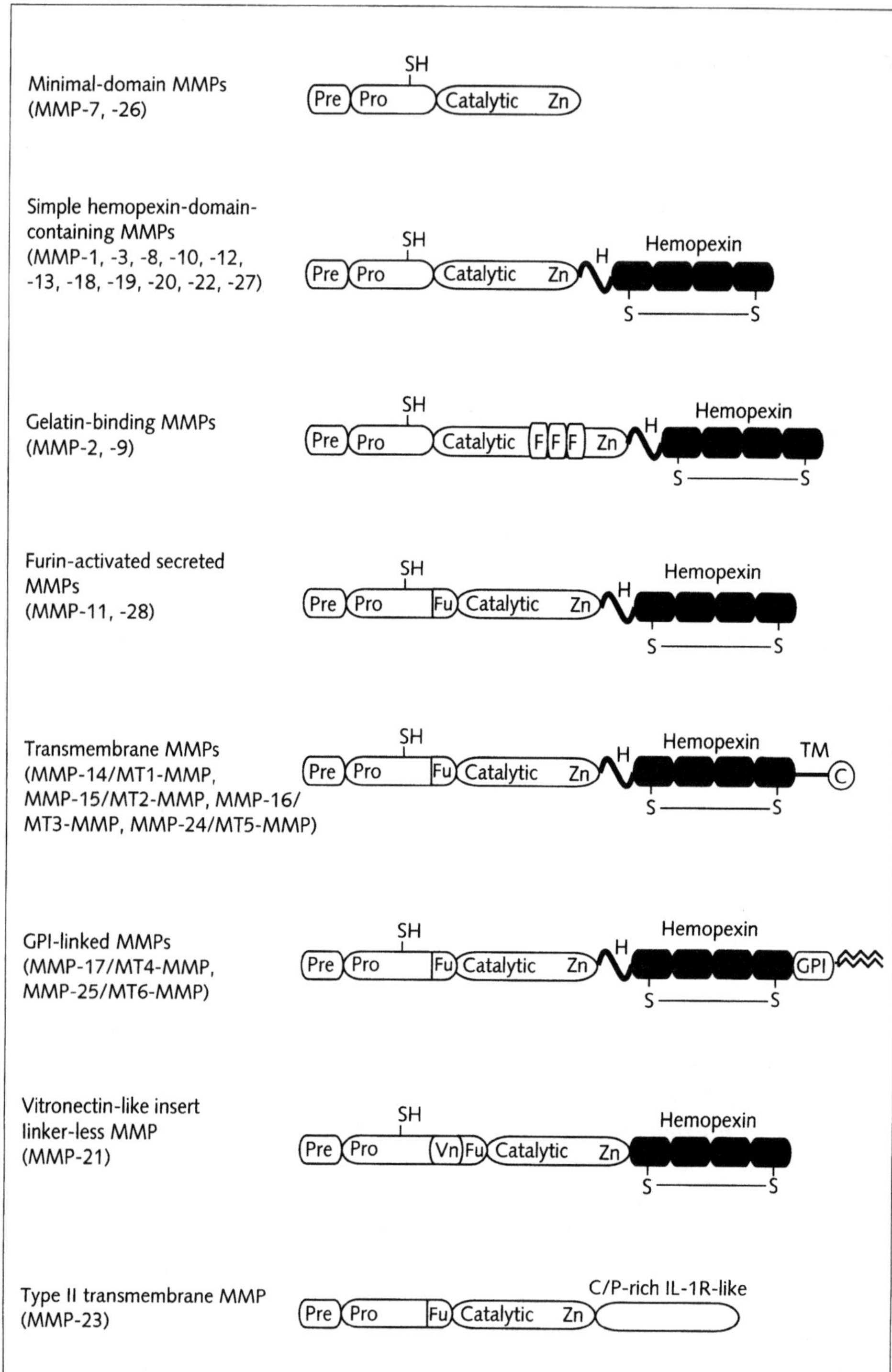
Minimal-domain MMPs
(MMP-7, -26)
SH
Pre
Pro
Catalytic
Zn
Simple hemopexin-domain-containing MMPs
(MMP-1, -3, -8, -10, -12, -13, -18, -19, -20, -22, -27)
H
Hemopexin
S
S
Gelatin-binding MMPs
(MMP-2, -9)
F F F
Furin-activated secreted MMPs
(MMP-11, -28)
Fu
Transmembrane MMPs
(MMP-14/MT1-MMP, MMP-15/MT2-MMP, MMP-16/MT3-MMP, MMP-24/MT5-MMP)
TM
C
GPI-linked MMPs
(MMP-17/MT4-MMP, MMP-25/MT6-MMP)
GPI
Vitronectin-like insert linker-less MMP
(MMP-21)
Vn
Type II transmembrane MMP
(MMP-23)
C/P-rich IL-1R-like

share structural organization, they differ in their patterns of mRNA expression, mechanisms of activation, tissue localization, and substrate specificity.

Regulation of MMP expression and activity

Expression of MMP mRNA is tightly regulated and controlled in a cell-type-dependent process. MMP mRNAs are regulated by numerous stimulatory and inhibitory mediators such as growth factors (e.g. vascular endothelial growth factor (VEGF), transforming growth factor β (TGF-β), and epidemial growth factor (EGF)), hormones (e.g. glucocorticoids), cytokines (e.g. interleukin-1 (IL-1), tumor necrosis factor α (TNF-α)), chemical agents (e.g. phorbol esters), and physical stress [7–9]. These factors modulate MMP mRNA expression by regulating expression and/or activity of transcription factors that interact with activator protein-1 (AP-1) sites and/or the polyoma enhancer activator (PEA3) sites within MMP promotor regions [8, 10, 11], although other mechanisms also exist.

MMP mRNA expression is also influenced by genetic variation [12]. Naturally occurring single-nucleotide polymorphisms (SNPs) have been identified in the promoters of a number of MMP genes [12]. These sequence variations have been shown to contribute to inter-individual differences in MMP transcription levels that have been linked to susceptibility of various diseases including cancer and coronary heart disease [13–15]. As an example, the presence of an additional guanine residue in the MMP-1 promoter results in higher MMP-1 transcription levels [16]. This polymorphism has been found more frequently in patients with ovarian and colorectal cancer [13, 14], suggesting a role for MMP-1 expression in disease susceptibility.

The biological activity of MMPs is tightly regulated posttranslationally. Activation of latent MMPs requires interaction between the cysteine sulfhydryl group in the propeptide domain with a zinc ion bound to the catalytic domain, otherwise known as the "cysteine switch" (reviewed in [1, 17, 18]). Following sulfhydryl-zinc interaction, propeptide domains are proteolyticaly removed by proteases, including

Figure 1
The MMP family.
Based on their domain organization, MMPs can be classified into eight groups. Pre, signal sequence; Pro, propeptide containing a zinc-interacting sulfhydryl (SH) group; Fu, furin-susceptible site; Vn, vitronectin-like insert; catalytic domain containing a zinc-binding site (Zn); F, collagen-binding fibronectin type II insert; H, hinge region; Hemopexin-like domain with the first and last repeat linked by a disulfide bond; TM, transmembrane domain; C, cytoplasmic tail; GPI, glycosylphosphatidylinositol-anchoring domain; C/P-rich IL-1R-like, cysteine/proline-rich interleukin-1 receptor-like domain.

other active MMPs, serine and cysteine proteases, and the MMP itself (reviewed in [1]). Activation of latent MMP-11, -21, and -28, and the MT-MMPs is distinctive in that they contain a furin-susceptible insert and are therefore activated intracellularly by Golgi-associated furin proteases [19]. Pro-MMP-2 is activated in multiple steps through a unique pathway involving interaction with active MT-MMP-1/MMP-14 and TIMP-2 [20].

Both latent and active MMPs are further regulated by endogenous MMP inhibitors. A major endogenous inhibitor of MMPs is the abundant plasma protein α2-macroglobulin [21]. After forming a complex with α2-macroglobulin, MMPs are irreversibly cleared from tissue fluid [21]. Reversible inhibition of MMPs is achieved *via* binding to tissue-localized TIMPs (reviewed in [22, 23]). Four members of the TIMP family have been identified, designated as TIMP-1–4. TIMPs exert their MMP-inhibitory function by binding to MMPs in a 1:1 molar stoichiometric fashion, resulting in a complex that then renders the MMP unable to bind substrate molecules. Individual TIMPs differ in their ability to inhibit various MMPs. As will be discussed in more detail below, TIMPs can inhibit as well as stimulate cell invasion, proliferation, metastasis, and angiogenesis through MMP-dependent and -independent mechanisms [20, 23–28]. Recent work has identified a new cell-surface inhibitor of MMPs, termed reversion-inducing-cysteine-rich protein with Kazal motifs (RECK; reviewed in [29]). RECK encodes a secreted glycoprotein containing a serine protease-inhibitor-like domain, two domains containing EGF-like repeats and a C-terminal domain encoding a glycosylphosphatidylinositol modification anchoring RECK to the plasma membrane [30]. To date, at least three members of the MMP family have been found to be inhibited by RECK [30, 31]. Membrane-anchored RECK inhibits secretion of pro-MMP-9 and both membrane-anchored and soluble RECK inhibit the catalytic activity of MMP-2, -9, and -14. In addition, RECK inhibits the final processing step of pro-MMP-2 activation; however, the exact mechanisms involved in inhibiting MMP secretion and/or activity by RECK are still unclear. Interestingly, RECK mRNA is abundantly expressed in many normal adult tissues, whereas its expression is suppressed in several tumor cell lines [30]. Importantly, restored expression of RECK in tumor cells results in decreased secretion of MMP-9 and a suppression of tumor cell invasive activity [30].

MMP localization and function

MMP activity is often found localized at or near cell surfaces. Mechanisms for localizing MMPs to this locale include covalent interaction of MT-MMPs to the cell surface, binding of MMPs to cell-surface receptors, such as the hyaluronan receptor CD44, integrins and extracellular matrix metalloproteinase inducer (EMMPRIN) [32, 33], and concentration of MMPs on pericellular ECM molecules [34]. MMPs can also be stored in the granules of inflammatory cells – e.g. granulocytes, macrophages, neutrophils, and mast cells – and are released following inflammatory cell degranulation [35–40].

One important function ascribed to MMP family members is induction of extracellular matrix (ECM) and basement membrane remodeling. MMPs cleave virtually all structural ECM proteins (reviewed in [2, 41]). Besides inducing and/or regulating structural and barrier changes, MMP-mediated matrix degradation also results in release of a variety of factors with distinct biological activities that are sequestered in the ECM.

It has recently become clear that MMP function is more complex than mere ECM remodeling. A number of non-matrix substrates have been identified, including other proteinases, proteinase inhibitors, clotting factors, chemotactic molecules, latent growth factors, growth factor-binding proteins, cell-surface receptors, and cell–cell and cell–matrix adhesion molecules (reviewed in [42]). For instance, MMP-14 contributes to the activation pathway of MMP-2 by cleaving the N-terminal prodomain of pro-MMP-2 [43]. MMP-9 and MMP-2 can proteolytically cleave latent TGFβ [44], and several osteoclast-derived MMPs can release TGFβ from bone ECM *via* cleavage of latent TGFβ-binding protein-1 [45]. MMP-8, -12, -13, and -14 have the capacity to proteolytically process fibrinogen and factor XII of the plasma-clotting system [46]. In a coculture of intervertebral discs and macrophages, it was shown that MMP-7 is required for release of TNFα from peritoneal macrophages [47]. In addition, multiple MMPs can modulate immune responses by processing of chemoattractant proteins [48, 49]; thus, beyond connective-tissue remodeling functions, MMPs regulate the function of bioactive mediators by proteolytic processing. As a consequence of these very diverse activities, MMPs participate in many biological (e.g. embryogenesis, angiogenesis, endometrial cycling, and wound healing) and pathological (e.g. cancer, arthritis, and cardiovascular disease) processes. The net effect of active MMPs is mainly determined by the concentration of enzyme and substrate, the tissue distribution and the interplay of regulatory proteins.

MMPs and inflammation

Based on the specificity of target recognition and on the timing of activation, the immune system can be divided into two subsets, innate and acquired. The first line of defense against pathogens is referred to as the innate immune system, and several immune cells, including neutrophils, macrophages, mast cells, and natural killer (NK) cells, are involved. The innate immune system is relatively non-specific and is not intrinsically affected by prior contact with infectious agents. The second line of defense is the acquired immune system and is characterized by antigen-specificity and immunological memory. T lymphocytes are involved in the cellular acquired immune response and with B lymphocytes in the humoral (antibody-mediated) acquired immune response. In order to provide optimal protection against infectious threats, the innate immune system is intimately linked to the acquired immune system [50, 51].

Inflammation is a multi-step process that begins with the recruitment and activation of inflammatory cells by chemotactic mediators released at the site of tissue injury or infection [52]. In response to chemoattractants, leukocytes, dendritic cells (DCs), and lymphocytes migrate from the bloodstream and lymphatics and enter affected tissues by extravasating through vessel walls into the ECM [53, 54]. At the site of tissue damage, inflammatory cells exert their effector function by releasing pre-formed and newly synthesized inflammatory mediators including cytokines, proteases, and membrane-perforating agents, or by direct and specific killing of aberrant cells. Subsequently, clearance of recruited immune cells is necessary to re-establish normal tissue integrity. As will be discussed below, each of these steps in inflammation can be regulated directly or indirectly by MMPs.

Regulation of MMP levels by inflammatory cells

MMPs are important effectors and regulators of inflammation. It is therefore not surprising that inflammatory cells such as macrophages, neutrophils, mast cells, eosinophils, and lymphocytes are important sources of MMPs and MMP activators [37, 55–57]. MMP levels, at sites of inflammation, are modulated by inflammatory cells *via* direct and indirect pathways. Activation of immune cells can result in direct release of activated MMPs or latent MMP precursors, whereas production of MMPs by inflammatory cells is controlled by various types of stimuli. As an example, MMP-1 and MMP-9 production by macrophages is enhanced by contact with matrix proteins such as laminin and collagens I and III [56, 58]. Mast cells on the other hand secrete pro-MMP-9 upon cell–cell contact with activated T cells [37]. Lipopolysaccharide (LPS) and IL-8 can trigger rapid degranulation of considerable amounts of intracellularly stored pro-MMP-9 and MT6-MMP from neutrophils [36, 38, 57]. Ovarian cancer cells induce pro-MMP-9 secretion by monocytes [59]. Moreover, several cytokines including IL-4, IL-10, and TGF-β suppress MMP production by macrophages, monocytes, and mast cells [40, 60–63]. Inflammatory cell-derived MMPs have been shown to be crucial factors in several pathological situations [39, 64–68]. As an example, macrophages are a primary source of MMP-1 and MMP-9 in a lung injury model where injury is inhibited by treatment with recombinant TIMP-2 [39, 66]. Likewise, neutrophil-derived MMP-9 is required for the induction of experimental autoimmune subepidermal blistering disease [67]. The induction and progression of experimental autoimmune encephalomyelitis (EAE) is reversed by treatment with an MMP inhibitor [65].

An indirect pathway *via* which immune cells influence MMP levels is by secreting inflammatory mediators that have a capacity to activate pro-MMPs. Likewise, immune cells influence MMP levels by expressing surface molecules with proteolytic capacity. Several studies have highlighted the potential role of mast cell-derived endopeptidases (chymase and tryptase) in mediating ECM degradation through the activation of several pro-MMPs [69–72]. In a transgenic mouse model of squamous carcinogenesis, appearance of the active form of MMP-9 in dysplastic skin lesions correlates with dramatic mast cell infiltration and elevated levels of chymase activity [70]. Additional *in vitro* experiments showed that treatment of hyperplastic skin lysates (containing pro-MMP-9) with chymase resulted in an increase in the amount of activated MMP-9 [70]. Neutrophil-derived elastase, cathepsin G, and proteinase-3 activate pro-MMP-2 through mechanisms requiring MT1-MMP [73]. The biological effect of this mechanism of MMP-2 activation is increased invasion of tumor cells through ECM *in vitro* [73]. Taken together, this body of work supports the conclusion that inflammatory cells and their products are crucial modulators of MMP production and activity.

Regulation of inflammation by MMPs

Inflammatory cells not only produce MMPs, but also require MMPs for many of their normal functions. Increasingly it has been recognized that MMPs provide specialized functions in all of the multi-step processes of immunity and inflammation. One of the initial steps in inflammation is recruitment of inflammatory cells by chemokines and cytokines secreted at the site of injury. MMPs modulate chemotaxis of leukocytes to sites of inflammation *via* different mechanisms. First, MMPs can regulate recruitment of immune cells *via* modulation of chemoattractant gradients, as is the case for chondrocyte-derived MMP-3 which is required for the generation of macrophage chemoattractant and macrophage infiltration in a model of herniated disc resorption [74]. Whether MMP-3 directly releases chemokines from the ECM or inactivates chemokine inhibitors remains to be established. A recent study expanded the concept that MMPs are critical in chemotaxis by showing that MMP-7-deficient mice were protected against the lethal pulmonary fibrotic effects of bleomycin-induced injury due to impaired transepithelial migration of neutrophils [75]. The underlying mechanism responsible for the impairment is that without MMP-7, generation of a transepithelial gradient of the CXC chemokine KC by shedding of the cell-bound proteoclycan syndecan-1 does not occur [75]. Conversely, MMPs also provide a suppressive role for recruitment of inflammatory cells. It has recently been shown that several MMPs inactivate monocyte chemoattractant protein (MCP)-1, -2, -3, and -4 *via* cleavage, resulting in a significant reduction in leukocyte infiltration [49, 76]. Likewise, multiple MMPs can cleave the CXC chemokine stromal cell-derived factor-1 (SDF-1), resulting in loss of binding to its cognate receptor CXCR4 [48]. MMP-cleaved SDF-1 is unable to mediate chemotaxis of $CD34^+$ hematopoietic progenitor stem cells and pre-B cells [48].

MMPs also regulate recruitment of immune cells *via* modulation of their migratory capacity. In order to enter sites of injury, or to detect antigen on dendritic cells, inflammatory cells must exit the bloodstream and migrate into tissues and the lymphatic system [53, 54]. During this multi-step migration process, leukocytes undergo adherence to endothelial cells, rolling, and finally extravasation through the endothelial cell layer and basement membrane of high endothelial venules into the ECM. During this process, chemokines and cytokines stimulate secretion of pro-MMPs or *de novo* synthesis of MMPs in a variety of inflammatory cells [77, 78]. In addition, T cell expression of MMP-2 is induced by vascular cell-adhesion molecule-1 (VCAM-1)-dependent adhesion to endothelial cells [79]. It has also become clear that MMPs also play an important role in modulating migration of various inflammatory cells across basement membranes and endothelium. Macrophages from MMP-12-deficient mice have diminished capacity to degrade components of the ECM, resulting in an inability to penetrate basement membranes [80]. Likewise, *in vitro* migration of T lymphocytes across a basal lamina equivalent is inhibited by a hydroxamic acid MMP inhibitor [81]. *In vivo* treatment with MMP inhibitors resulted in a reduced number of lymphocytes that completed transendothelial migration across high endothelial venules into lymph nodes [82]. Dendritic cells transport antigen from the tissues to the lymph nodes where antigens are presented to T lymphocytes. Recently, it was shown that expression of MMP-2 and MMP-9 on the surface of Langerhans cells and skin dendritic cells is necessary for their migration [83]. MMP-3 deficiency resulted in an impaired T cell-mediated contact-hypersensitivity response caused by defective activation of T lymphocytes [84]. Whether MMP-3 is required for the migration of antigen-loaded dendritic cells to the draining lymph nodes, or for the activation or migration of T cells, is not known.

At sites of injury or infection, inflammatory cells perform their effector functions in order to heal afflicted tissues. A recent study underscores the importance of MMP activity in regulating inflammatory cell function. In many human tumors, expression of IL-2 receptor-α (IL-2Rα) on tumor-infiltrating lymphocytes is downregulated [85–87]. Since IL-2Rα expression is required for development and propagation of functional T cells, downregulation results in poor T cell function [88]. It has been found that tumor-derived MMP-9 mediates cleavage of IL-2Rα and thus contributes to tumor-mediated immunosuppression [89]. One of the most important effector functions of T lymphocytes is the capacity to kill target cells in an antigen-specific manner. One mechanism by which T lymphocytes can perform this cytolytic capacity is *via* the Fas/Fas ligand pathway [90]. Since MMP-3 and MMP-7 can cleave and functionally inactivate Fas ligand [91–93], this pathway of target cell killing by T lymphocytes may be inhibited in the presence of MMPs.

Another crucial step in inflammation is the resolving phase, characterized by inflammatory cell death or egression of inflammatory cells from sites of inflammation. Several studies report a critical role for MMPs in resolution of inflammation.

In an experimental model of asthma, MMP-2 deficiency resulted in impaired leukocyte egression from the airway stromal compartment, followed by an increase in mortality [94]. This impaired migration of leukocytes across the epithelium into the airway lumen correlated with a decreased chemoattractant activity for inflammatory cells in the lung interstitium [94]. Likewise, MMP-9-deficient mice exhibited a persistent T cell-mediated contact hypersensitivity upon antigen challenge due to their failure to resolve acute inflammation [84]. These studies suggest that the various steps of the inflammatory process are tightly regulated by local MMP activity.

MMPs and neoplastic progression

Malignant tumors are characterized by their ability to cross tissue boundaries and spread to and thrive in ectopic tissue sites. To do so, neoplastic cells must penetrate multiple ECM barriers as they traverse the epithelial basement membrane and interstitial stroma, enter blood vessels or lymphatics, and extravasate to form metastases at distal sites. There is clinical and experimental evidence that in addition to degradation and/or remodeling of ECM molecules, MMPs participate in additional aspects of tumor evolution, including neoplastic cell initiation and proliferation, angiogenesis, inflammation, ECM remodeling, and metastatic growth. Numerous reports have documented the expression of MMPs in virtually all human cancers [5, 95–100], and a significant correlation has been found between MMP expression levels and clinical outcome [96, 98, 101–104]. For instance, high plasma levels of MMP-9 in patients with colorectal cancer is associated with shortened survival [101].

MMP expression patterns vary depending on the enzyme in question and type of tumor involved. Neoplastic cells often upregulate surface expression of EMMPRIN, a molecule that induces MMP synthesis by adjacent stromal cells and also binds MMP-1 to the tumor cell surface [33]. Interestingly, in epithelial tumors most upregulated MMPs are not expressed by carcinoma cells themselves but instead are primarily expressed by stromal fibroblasts, inflammatory cells, and vascular cells present in the tumor microenvironment [70, 95, 99, 100, 105, 106].

Experimental mouse models have been used to study the nature of MMP involvement in the transformation of cells, as well as in premalignant events leading to primary tumor growth, invasion, and metastasis. In general, overexpression of MMPs in tissues results in the development of a hyperproliferative and/or malignant phenotype, as well as rendering animals more susceptible to oncogene-induced or chemically induced carcinogenesis [107–113], whereas overexpression of TIMPs or MMP deficiency, in some cases, can result in diminished susceptibility to neoplastic progression [114–119]. Transgenic expression of either MMP-3, MT1-MMP, or MMP-7 in mammary epithelial cells triggers a cascade of molecular and functional alterations, and ultimately results in the development of mammary gland tumors

[107–111]. Likewise, overexpression of MMP-1 in mouse skin results in increased susceptibility to chemically induced tumorigenesis [112, 113]. Some studies have shown that by suppressing MMP activity through forced TIMP expression, highly malignant cells can be made less aggressive, and thus provide indirect evidence that MMPs contribute to tumor progression. For instance, transgenic overexpression of TIMP-1 in the liver blocked the development of hepatocellular carcinomas [114]. Additionally, overexpression of TIMP-2 reduced the growth of melanoma cells in murine skin; however, increased TIMP-2 levels did not prevent metastasis formation [115].

Compelling evidence for a functional role of MMPs in cancer development has come from mouse models of *de novo* cancer development harboring homozygous null mutations in various MMPs, where eliminating a single MMP delays tumor progression in a number of mouse tumor models [116–119]. Evidence for involvement of MMP-9 in neoplastic progression has been provided in a transgenic mouse model of squamous carcinogenesis of the skin [116]. The role of MMP-9 during tumorigenesis was addressed by studying the phenotypic consequences of attenuated MMP-9 function in MMP-9-deficient tumor-prone transgenic mice [116]. Transgenic mice lacking MMP-9 had reduced epithelial proliferative indices and altered differentiation characteristics, delayed activation of angiogenesis and, importantly, a dramatic 50% reduction in the incidence of carcinomas as compared to MMP-9-proficient controls [116]. The few tumors that did arise in the absence of MMP-9 displayed a less differentiated phenotype [116]. The development of intestinal tumors is clearly reduced in MMP-7-deficient mice carrying the APC^{min} mutation [117]. In a transgenic model of pancreatic islet cell carcinogenesis, treatment with MMP inhibitors (MPIs) delayed the onset of angiogenesis and tumor growth [119]. Genetic ablation of MMP-2 was found to inhibit tumor formation whereas lack of MMP-9 resulted in suppression of angiogenesis and tumor growth [119]. MMP-11 deficiency resulted in a diminished sensitivity to chemically induced tumorigenesis [118]. In addition, fibroblasts from MMP-11-deficient mice lose the capacity to promote malignant cell implantation in nude mice, suggesting that MMP-11 contributes in a paracrine manner to epithelial cell malignancy [118].

Based on their proven *in vitro* capacity to degrade ECM components, MMPs have been implicated as important mediators of metastasis; however, data supporting a positive role for MMPs in metastasis are limited [120–123]. MMP-2-deficient mice display diminished lung colonization after intravenous inoculation of tumor cells [120]. Likewise, inhibition of MMP activity *via* overexpression of TIMP-1 in melanoma cells results in a reduction in the size and number of micro-metastases in a chick embryo model [121]. Since metastases arise from cancer cells that have escaped from primary tumors *in vivo*, these models may not reflect the physiological process of true metastasis formation. In combination, however, these studies suggest that MMPs contribute to multiple stages of tumor progression, including tumor initiation, angiogenesis, tumor growth, and metastasis formation.

MMPs, inflammation, and the development of cancer

It is well established that cancer is a progressive, multi-stage disease arising as a consequence of accumulating genetic alterations. These genetic mutations are required, but not sufficient, for the outgrowth of tumors. Extensive interaction with the surrounding microenvironment is of prime importance during neoplastic progression [124]. Clinical and experimental data indicate a strong promoting role for inflammatory leukocytes in neoplastic progression [125]. Multiple studies have shown that accumulation of inflammatory cells in solid human cancers correlates strongly with higher tumor grade, metastasis, and poor prognosis [126–131]. Strikingly, inflammatory cells are often localized in the stroma around the invading fronts and around newly formed blood vessels of both experimentally induced tumors and various human tumors and not in the center of the tumors, suggesting that inflammatory cells assist in invasion and angiogenesis [70, 126, 132]. Furthermore, it has become clear that chronic inflammation predisposes humans to the development of carcinomas in several organs [133, 134]. The best established of malignancies associated with chronic inflammation is colon carcinogenesis arising in patients with inflammatory bowel disease [135]. Similarly, chronic *Helicobacter pylori* infection predisposes to gastric cancer [136]. In line with these clinical observations, TGFβ1-deficient mice develop granulocyte inflammatory lesions that progress to colon cancer [137]. Development of colon cancer can be eliminated by maintaining mice free of inflammation in a germ-free environment, indicating that inflammation is required for tumor progression [137]. Perhaps the best clinical evidence for the importance of inflammation during neoplastic progression comes from studies showing reduced risk of cancer among long-term users of anti-inflammatory drugs [138–143]. As an example, a reduced risk of colorectal cancer has been observed among long-term users of non-steroidal anti-inflammatory drugs or aspirin [139]. These clinical data suggest a clear relationship between inflammation and development of cancer; however, many of the molecular and cellular mechanisms mediating this relationship are not provided by such correlative data.

Elucidating the mechanisms by which immune cells participate in neoplastic development will eventually facilitate the rational design of novel therapies against human cancer. What do infiltrating inflammatory cells provide to evolving neoplasms? The inflammatory component of a developing neoplasm includes a diverse leukocyte population, e.g. macrophages, mast cells, neutrophils, and eosinophils. These cells are variably loaded with an assorted array of cytokines, growth factors including VEGF and basic fibroblastic growth factor (bFGF), cytotoxic mediators including reactive oxygen species, various proteases including MMPs, membrane-perforating agents, and soluble mediators of cell killing, such as TNFα, interleukins, and interferons.

As described above, expression of MMPs in cancer correlates with poor prognosis. A closer look at several human and experimental tumors reveals that tumor-associated MMPs are often not synthesized by the tumor cells themselves, but primarily found in inflammatory cells that are present within the tumor microenvironment [99, 100, 105, 106]. Combined expression of MMP-9 and urokinase-type plasminogen activator (uPA) in colorectal cancer and MMP-3 localized at the tumor invasive front with inflammatory cells correlated strongly with metastasis rate and survival [99]. In human basal cell carcinoma, MMP-9 expression was identified in eosinophils within inflammatory infiltrates surrounding the tumor [105]. In human colorectal cancer, a persistent localization of MMP-9-producing macrophages was observed in the interphase between tumor and surrounding stroma [106]. These data suggest that delivery of MMPs by inflammatory cells to the tumor microenvironment may facilitate tumor progression.

Direct evidence that inflammatory cells contribute to tumorigenesis *via* secretion of MMPs has been provided by several recent experimental models. In a transgenic mouse model of pancreatic islet cell cancer in which MMP-9 contributed to the angiogenic switch, MMP-9 could only be detected in infiltrating inflammatory cells and not in neoplastic cells of tumors [119]. MMP-9 deficiency resulted in reduced skin carcinogenesis in tumor-prone transgenic mice where the characteristics of neoplastic development were restored by reconstitution with wild-type bone marrow-derived cells [116]. In this same cancer model, inflammatory cells, specifically mast cells, were found to facilitate the angiogenic switch and the conversion of a normal dermis into an aberrant stromal support in the MMP-9-proficient transgenic mice [70]. These data support the hypothesis that inflammatory cells are important contributors to neoplastic progression, in part, by their deposition of MMP-9 into reactive stroma. Also the group of Huang et al. [144] provided direct evidence that expression of MMP-9 by inflammatory cells promotes tumorigenesis. The growth, vascularization, and macrophage infiltration of xenografted MMP-9-expressing human ovarian cancer cells were clearly reduced in MMP-9-deficient nude mice. Reconstitution with MMP-9-expressing spleen cells resulted in increased angiogenesis and tumorigenicity of the tumor cells, and the tumors in reconstituted mice contained infiltrated MMP-9-expressing macrophages [144]. A recent study by Hiratsuka et al. [122] described a novel mechanism by which inflammatory cell-derived MMPs contribute to metastasis formation. In this study, MMP-9 was specifically induced in macrophages and endothelial cells in prematastatic lung by a distant primary tumor. In line with these findings, patients with distant tumors displayed significantly elevated levels of MMP-9 in lung tissue as compared to those from tumor-free patients [122]. Thus, these studies indicate that inflammatory cells contribute to carcinogenesis by creating an environment that is permissive for primary tumor growth and secondary metastasis formation (Fig. 2).

Implications for prevention and treatment of cancer

With such compelling data supporting a role for MMPs as potentiators of neoplastic progression, synthetic MPIs were developed and tested for anti-cancer properties *in vitro* and *in vivo* (reviewed in [145]). Broad-spectrum (blocking multiple MMPs) and narrow-spectrum (blocking the activity of selected MMPs) MPIs have been developed and tested in experimental pre-clinical and clinical studies with several demonstrating efficacy in experimental mouse transplant models of cancer development [119, 146–149]. For example, treatment of mice with a broad-spectrum MPI was shown to inhibit experimental metastasis formation [146]. Treatment of nude mice with batimastat (a broad-spectrum hydroxamate inhibitor) inhibited local regrowth after resection of human breast cancer xenografts and reduced metastasis [147]. Likewise, in a transgenic mouse model of pancreatic islet cell carcinogenesis, treatment with batimastat or a relatively specific MMP-9 MPI reduced the number and growth of pancreatic islet tumors [119]. In an oral squamous cell carcinoma implantation study, treatment with the broad MPI marimastat resulted in suppression of lymph node metastasis [148]. Treatment with a sulfhydryl-based MPI inhibited the number of experimental lung metastases in a dose-dependent manner [149].

In contrast, several pre-clinical studies have also suggested that inhibition of MMP activity does not result in inhibition of tumor growth, but instead supports tumor progression. Treatment of mice with batimastat promoted metastasis formation of human breast carcinoma cells and murine T lymphoma cells [150]. Whereas treatment of transgenic mice harboring hyperplastic pancreatic islets with batimastat significantly prevented the development of angiogenic islets, treatment of mice bearing established tumors was unsuccessful [151], suggesting that timing and duration of MPI treatment is an important factor. Furthermore, the therapeutic efficacy of MPIs also depends on the type of tumor and its microenvironment. This has recently been underscored by a study of Shiraga et al. [152] showing that MMP expression varies with host microenvironment. In two different metastasis models using human lung cancer cell lines, it was found that tumor-derived MMPs are important for the formation of lung metastasis, whereas MMPs produced by host stroma cells are important for metastasis to the liver [152]. Inhibition of MMPs reduced metastasis formation in the lung and liver, but not in the kidney or lymph nodes [152], in this same report. These experimental studies suggest that the therapeutic efficacy of MPIs largely depends on the time of onset and the duration of treatment, and the type of the targeted tumor and its microenvironment.

These restrictions may explain, in part, why in spite of the encouraging results with MPIs in pre-clinical studies, clinical trials with MPIs have not been successful (reviewed in [145]). As mentioned above, in several mouse models MMPs contributed to early stages of neoplastic development, and MPI treatment in pre-clinical animal models was in general more efficient when initiated during early disease development [151]. In contrast, in most clinical trials, the MPI treatment was applied to patients with advanced cancer. For the future design of MPI clinical trials it will be important to understand if initiating MPI treatment at an earlier stage, or to apply MPIs in a prophylactic setting, will benefit or aid in disease regression

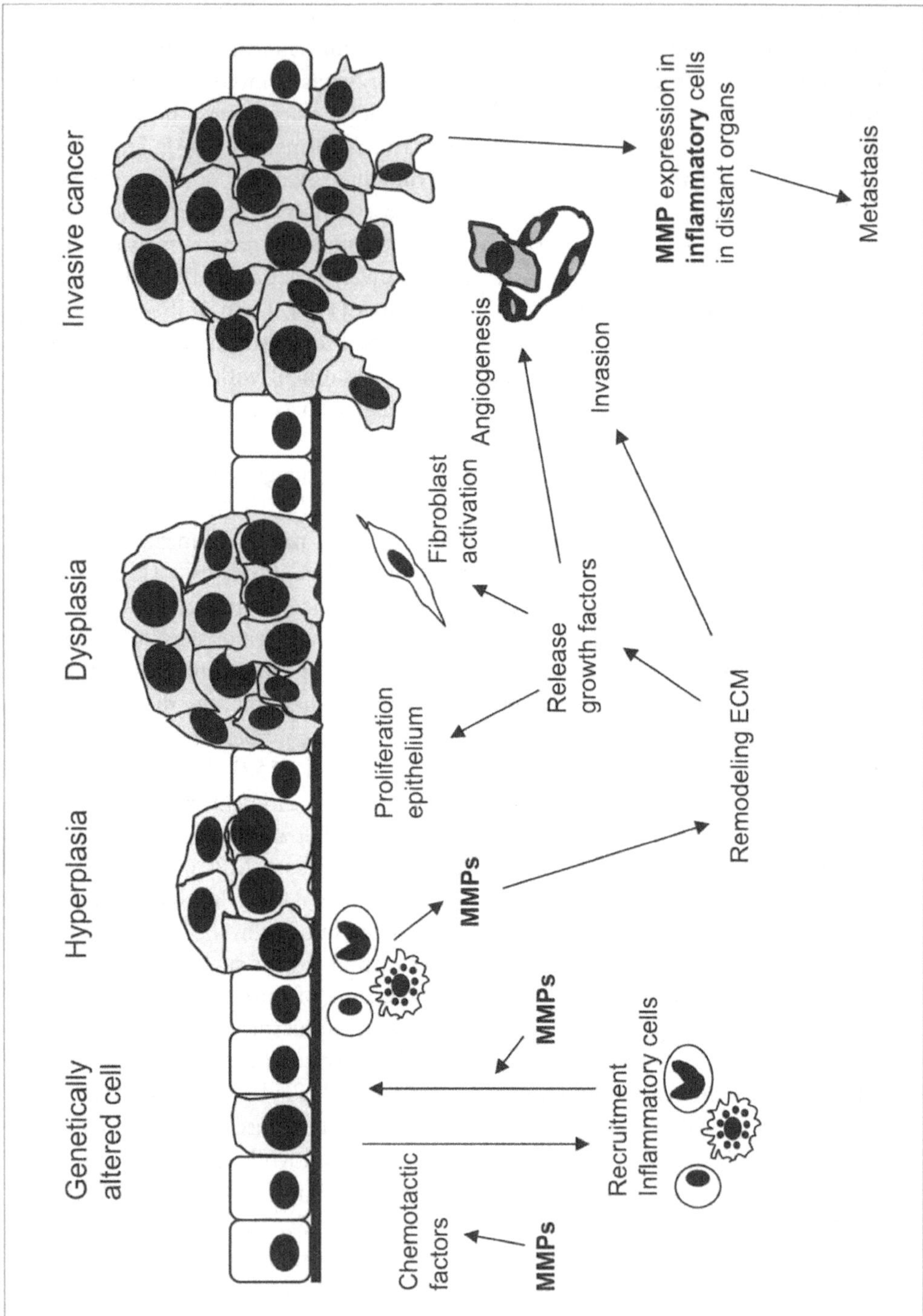
Genetically altered cell
Hyperplasia
Dysplasia
Invasive cancer
Chemotactic factors
MMPs
Recruitment Inflammatory cells
MMPs
MMPs
Proliferation epithelium
Release growth factors
Remodeling ECM
Fibroblast activation
Angiogenesis
Invasion
MMP expression in inflammatory cells in distant organs
Metastasis

or survival. Patients with genetic mutations that predispose for cancer, patients with pre-malignant lesions (e.g. colon polyps), or patients with minimal residual disease are more likely to benefit from MMP inhibition than patients with advanced disease. In addition, a more thorough understanding of organ heterogeneity of host-derived MMP expression and more insight into the biological activities of individual MMPs in different types of cancer will be crucial to develop a more rational clinical trial design.

As discussed in this chapter, the increased presence of MMPs in tumors is largely the result of a host response induced by the growing neoplastic mass. Based on the important contribution of inflammatory cells, another anti-cancer therapeutic opportunity would be to inhibit inflammation. Currently, it is not clear which molecules and mechanisms are involved in elaborating recruitment of inflammatory cells towards the (pre)-malignant lesions. Since these recruitment pathways may represent the best control points in which to target such anti-cancer therapeutics, future studies should be aimed at elucidating the mechanisms responsible for recruitment of inflammatory cells to neoplastic lesions. Alternatively, another approach would be to inhibit the contribution of inflammatory cells to neoplastic progression by blocking their production of MMPs by treatment with stabilizing agents protecting against degranulation.

Concluding remarks

There is a growing body of clinical and experimental evidence showing a strong promoting role of inflammatory cells in neoplastic progression. In this chapter, we have provided an overview of recent literature showing that one of the pathways *via*

Figure 2
Connection between inflammation, MMPs, and cancer development.
Early neoplastic lesions activate the recruitment of several types of inflammatory cells most likely by generating a chemotactic gradient. MMPs can influence recruitment of inflammatory cells by modifying the chemotactic gradient and by regulating the migratory capacity of inflammatory cells. Inflammatory cells recruited towards the tumor microenvironment secrete and/or activate various types of MMPs. MMPs can degrade virtually all components of the ECM and, in doing so, MMPs may change the tumor environment in such a way that invasion of tumor cells is supported. In addition, remodeling of the ECM by MMPs results in the release and activation of various growth factors that are normally sequestered in the ECM. These growth factors can support neoplastic progression by stimulating proliferation of neoplastic cells, by activating fibroblasts, and by activating angiogenesis. In addition, inflammatory cell-derived MMPs contribute to carcinogenesis by creating an environment in premetastatic organs that is permissive for metastasis.

which inflammatory cells can drive tumorigenesis is by regulating MMP levels in the tumor microenvironment. Despite the clear promoting role of MMPs in all stages of cancer development, results from clinical trials targeting MMPs have been disappointing. Deeper understanding of the temporal and spatial expression patterns of MMPs in tumors and an increased insight into their complex functional capacities will be necessary in order to fully optimize the efficacy and minimize the toxicity of therapeutic agents targeting MMPs. As inflammatory cells will not only deliver MMPs, but also other inflammatory cell-derived factors that may play additional promoting roles in tumor development, inhibition of the inflammatory response may be a more effective anti-cancer strategy than targeting MMPs alone. The challenge now is to dissect the mechanisms by which inflammatory cells are recruited to the different stages of neoplastic progression, as these early signalling pathways may be the best control points in which to target the next generation of anti-cancer therapeutics.

Acknowledgments

We gratefully acknowledge Robert Diaz, Jin-Sae Rhee and Daniel Maslyar for their valuable suggestions. KEdV is a fellow of the Dutch Cancer Society. LMC is supported by generous grants from the NIH, AACR and the Edward Malinckrodt, Jr. Foundation.

References

1 Sternlicht MD, Werb Z (2001) How matrix metalloproteinases regulate cell behavior. *Annu Rev Cell Dev Biol* 17: 463–516

2 Egeblad M, Werb Z (2002) New functions for the matrix metalloproteinases in cancer progression. *Nat Rev Cancer* 2: 161–174

3 Kai HS, Butler GS, Morrison CJ, King AE, Pelman GR, Overall CM (2002) Utilization of a novel recombinant myoglobin fusion protein expression system to characterize the tissue inhibitor of metalloproteinase (TIMP)-4 and TIMP-2 C-terminal domain and tails by mutagenesis. The importance of acidic residues in binding the MMP-2 hemopexin C-domain. *J Biol Chem* 277: 48696–48707

4 Roeb E, Schleinkofer K, Kernebeck T, Potsch S, Jansen B, Behrmann I, Matern S, Grotzinger J (2002) The matrix metalloproteinase 9 (mmp-9) hemopexin domain is a novel gelatin binding domain and acts as an antagonist. *J Biol Chem* 277: 50326–50332

5 Sato H, Takino T, Okada Y, Cao J, Shinagawa A, Yamamoto E, Seiki M (1994) A matrix metalloproteinase expressed on the surface of invasive tumour cells. *Nature* 370: 61–65

6 Cao J, Sato H, Takino T, Seiki M (1995) The C-terminal region of membrane type matrix metalloproteinase is a functional transmembrane domain required for pro-gelatinase A activation. *J Biol Chem* 270: 801–805

7 Esteve PO, Chicoine E, Robledo O, Aoudjit F, Descoteaux A, Potworowski EF, St Pierre Y (2002) Protein kinase C-zeta regulates transcription of the matrix metalloproteinase-9 gene induced by IL-1 and TNF-alpha in glioma cells *via* NF-kappa B. *J Biol Chem* 277: 35150–35155
8 Troussard AA, Costello P, Yoganathan TN, Kumagai S, Roskelley CD, Dedhar S (2000) The integrin linked kinase (ILK) induces an invasive phenotype *via* AP-1 transcription factor-dependent upregulation of matrix metalloproteinase 9 (MMP-9). *Oncogene* 19: 5444–5452
9 Fini ME, Cook JR, Mohan R, Brinckerhoff CE (1998). Regulation of matrix metalloproteinase gene expression. In: WC Parks, RP Mecham (eds): *Matrix metalloproteinases*. Academic Press, New York, 299–356
10 Benbow U, Brinckerhoff CE (1997) The AP-1 site and MMP gene regulation: what is all the fuss about? *Matrix Biol* 15: 519–526
11 Crawford HC, Fingleton B, Gustavson MD, Kurpios N, Wagenaar RA, Hassell JA, Matrisian LM (2001) The PEA3 subfamily of Ets transcription factors synergizes with beta-catenin-LEF-1 to activate matrilysin transcription in intestinal tumors. *Mol Cell Biol* 21: 1370–1383
12 Ye S (2000) Polymorphism in matrix metalloproteinase gene promoters: implication in regulation of gene expression and susceptibility of various diseases. *Matrix Biol* 19: 623–629
13 Ghilardi G, Biondi ML, Mangoni J, Leviti S, DeMonti M, Guagnellini E, Scorza R (2001) Matrix metalloproteinase-1 promoter polymorphism 1G/2G is correlated with colorectal cancer invasiveness. *Clin Cancer Res* 7: 2344–2346
14 Kanamori Y, Matsushima M, Minaguchi T, Kobayashi K, Sagae S, Kudo R, Terakawa N, Nakamura Y (1999) Correlation between expression of the matrix metalloproteinase-1 gene in ovarian cancers and an insertion/deletion polymorphism in its promoter region. *Cancer Res* 59: 4225–4227
15 Lamblin N, Bauters C, Hermant X, Lablanche JM, Helbecque N, Amouyel P (2002) Polymorphisms in the promoter regions of MMP-2, MMP-3, MMP-9 and MMP-12 genes as determinants of aneurysmal coronary artery disease. *J Am Coll Cardiol* 40: 43–48
16 Rutter JL, Mitchell TI, Buttice G, Meyers J, Gusella JF, Ozelius LJ, Brinckerhoff CE (1998) A single nucleotide polymorphism in the matrix metalloproteinase-1 promoter creates an Ets binding site and augments transcription. *Cancer Res* 58: 5321–5325
17 Nagase H, Woessner JF (1999) Matrix metalloproteinases. *J Biol Chem* 274: 21491–21494
18 Van Wart HE, Birkedal-Hansen H (1990) The cysteine switch: a principle of regulation of metalloproteinase activity with potential applicability to the entire matrix metalloproteinase gene family. *Proc Natl Acad Sci USA* 87: 5578–5582
19 Pei D, Weiss SJ (1995) Furin-dependent intracellular activation of the human stromelysin-3 zymogen. *Nature* 375: 244–247
20 Butler GS, Butler MJ, Atkinson SJ, Will H, Tamura T, van Westrum SS, Crabbe T,

Clements J, d'Ortho MP, Murphy G (1998) The TIMP2 membrane type 1 metalloproteinase "receptor" regulates the concentration and efficient activation of progelatinase A. A kinetic study. *J Biol Chem* 273: 871–880

21 Woessner JF Jr (1999) Matrix metalloproteinase inhibition. From the Jurassic to the third millennium. *Ann NY Acad Sci* 878: 388–403

22 Brew K, Dinakarpandian D, Nagase H (2000) Tissue inhibitors of metalloproteinases: evolution, structure and function. *Biochim Biophys Acta* 1477: 267–283

23 Gomez DE, Alonso DF, Yoshiji H, Thorgeirsson UP (1997) Tissue inhibitors of metalloproteinases: structure, regulation and biological functions. *Eur J Cell Biol* 74: 111–122

24 Ahonen M, Baker AH, Kahari VM (1998) Adenovirus-mediated gene delivery of tissue inhibitor of metalloproteinases-3 inhibits invasion and induces apoptosis in melanoma cells. *Cancer Res* 58: 2310–2315

25 Baker AH, Zaltsman AB, George SJ, Newby AC (1998) Divergent effects of tissue inhibitor of metalloproteinase-1, -2, or -3 overexpression on rat vascular smooth muscle cell invasion, proliferation, and death *in vitro*. TIMP-3 promotes apoptosis. *J Clin Invest* 101: 1478–1487

26 Blavier L, Henriet P, Imren S, Declerck YA (1999) Tissue inhibitors of matrix metalloproteinases in cancer. *Ann NY Acad Sci* 878: 108–119

27 Murphy AN, Unsworth EJ, Stetler-Stevenson WG (1993) Tissue inhibitor of metalloproteinases-2 inhibits bFGF-induced human microvascular endothelial cell proliferation. *J Cell Physiol* 157: 351–358

28 Oelmann E, Herbst H, Zuhlsdorf M, Albrecht O, Nolte A, Schmitmann C, Manzke O, Diehl V, Stein H, Berdel WE (2002) Tissue inhibitor of metalloproteinases 1 is an autocrine and paracrine survival factor, with additional immune-regulatory functions, expressed by Hodgkin/Reed-Sternberg cells. *Blood* 99: 258–267

29 Rhee JS, Coussens LM (2002) RECKing MMP function: implications for cancer development. *Trends Cell Biol* 12: 209–211

30 Takahashi C, Sheng Z, Horan TP, Kitayama H, Maki M, Hitomi K, Kitaura Y, Sasahara RM, Horimoto A et al (1998) Regulation of matrix metalloproteinase-9 and inhibition of tumor invasion by the membrane-anchored glycoprotein RECK. *Proc Natl Acad Sci USA* 95: 13221–13226

31 Oh J, Takahashi R, Kondo S, Mizoguchi A, Adachi E, Sasahara RM, Nishimura S, Imamura Y, Kitayama H, Alexander DB et al (2001) The membrane-anchored MMP inhibitor RECK is a key regulator of extracellular matrix integrity and angiogenesis. *Cell* 107: 789–800

32 Yu Q, Stamenkovic I (1999) Localization of matrix metalloproteinase 9 to the cell surface provides a mechanism for CD44-mediated tumor invasion. *Genes Dev* 13: 35–48

33 Guo H, Li R, Zucker S, Toole BP (2000) EMMPRIN (CD147), an inducer of matrix metalloproteinase synthesis, also binds interstitial collagenase to the tumor cell surface. *Cancer Res* 60: 888–891

34 Olson MW, Toth M, Gervasi DC, Sado Y, Ninomiya Y, Fridman R (1998) High affini-

ty binding of latent matrix metalloproteinase-9 to the alpha2(IV) chain of collagen IV. *J Biol Chem* 273: 10672–10681

35 Kanbe N, Tanaka A, Kanbe M, Itakura A, Kurosawa M, Matsuda H (1999) Human mast cells produce matrix metalloproteinase 9. *Eur J Immunol* 29: 2645–2649

36 Pugin J, Widmer MC, Kossodo S, Liang CM, Preas HL, Suffredini AF (1999) Human neutrophils secrete gelatinase B *in vitro* and *in vivo* in response to endotoxin and proinflammatory mediators. *Am J Respir Cell Mol Biol* 20: 458–464

37 Baram D, Vaday GG, Salamon P, Drucker I, Hershkoviz R, Mekori YA (2001) Human mast cells release metalloproteinase-9 on contact with activated T cells: juxtacrine regulation by tnf-alpha. *J Immunol* 167: 4008–4016

38 Kang T, Yi J, Guo A, Wang X, Overall CM, Jiang W, Elde R, Borregaard N, Pei D (2001) Subcellular distribution and cytokine- and chemokine-regulated secretion of leukolysin/MT6-MMP/MMP-25 in neutrophils. *J Biol Chem* 276: 21960–21968

39 Gibbs DF, Shanley TP, Warner RL, Murphy HS, Varani J, Johnson KJ (1999) Role of matrix metalloproteinases in models of macrophage-dependent acute lung injury. Evidence for alveolar macrophage as source of proteinases. *Am J Respir Cell Mol Biol* 20: 1145–1154

40 Fang KC, Wolters PJ, Steinhoff M, Bidgol A, Blount JL, Caughey GH (1999) Mast cell expression of gelatinases A and B is regulated by kit ligand and TGF-beta. *J Immunol* 162: 5528–5535

41 Vihinen P, Kahari VM (2002) Matrix metalloproteinases in cancer: prognostic markers and therapeutic targets. *Int J Cancer* 99: 157–166

42 McCawley LJ, Matrisian LM (2001) Matrix metalloproteinases: they're not just for matrix anymore! *Curr Opin Cell Biol* 13: 534–540

43 Deryugina EI, Ratnikov B, Monosov E, Postnova TI, DiScipio R, Smith JW, Strongin AY (2001) MT1-MMP initiates activation of pro-MMP-2 and integrin $\alpha v\beta 3$ promotes maturation of MMP-2 in breast carcinoma cells. *Exp Cell Res* 263: 209–223

44 Yu Q, Stamenkovic I (2000) Cell surface-localized matrix metalloproteinase-9 proteolytically activates TGF-beta and promotes tumor invasion and angiogenesis. *Genes Dev* 14: 163–176

45 Dallas SL, Rosser JL, Mundy GR, Bonewald LF (2002) Proteolysis of latent transforming growth factor-beta (TGF-beta)-binding protein-1 by osteoclasts. A cellular mechanism for release of TGF-beta from bone matrix. *J Biol Chem* 277: 21352–21360

46 Hiller O, Lichte A, Oberpichler A, Kocourek A, Tschesche H (2000) Matrix metalloproteinases collagenase-2, macrophage elastase, collagenase-3, and membrane type 1-matrix metalloproteinase impair clotting by degradation of fibrinogen and factor XII. *J Biol Chem* 275: 33008–33013

47 Haro H, Crawford HC, Fingleton B, Shinomiya K, Spengler DM, Matrisian LM (2000) Matrix metalloproteinase-7-dependent release of tumor necrosis factor-alpha in a model of herniated disc resorption. *J Clin Invest* 105: 143–150

48 McQuibban GA, Butler GS, Gong JH, Bendall L, Power C, Clark-Lewis I, Overall CM

(2001) Matrix metalloproteinase activity inactivates the CXC chemokine stromal cell-derived factor-1. *J Biol Chem* 276: 43503–43508

49 McQuibban GA, Gong JH, Wong JP, Wallace JL, Clark-Lewis I, Overall CM (2002) Matrix metalloproteinase processing of monocyte chemoattractant proteins generates CC chemokine receptor antagonists with anti-inflammatory properties *in vivo*. *Blood* 100: 1160–1167

50 Murphy JE, Robert C, Kupper TS (2000) Interleukin-1 and cutaneous inflammation: a crucial link between innate and acquired immunity. *J Invest Dermatol* 114: 602–608

51 Luster AD (2002) The role of chemokines in linking innate and adaptive immunity. *Curr Opin Immunol* 14: 129–135

52 Zlotnik A, Yoshie O (2000) Chemokines: a new classification system and their role in immunity. *Immunity* 12: 121–127

53 Madri JA, Graesser D (2000) Cell migration in the immune system: the evolving inter-related roles of adhesion molecules and proteinases. *Dev Immunol* 7: 103–116

54 Middleton J, Patterson AM, Gardner L, Schmutz C, Ashton BA (2002) Leukocyte extravasation: chemokine transport and presentation by the endothelium. *Blood* 100: 3853–3860

55 Goetzl EJ, Banda MJ, Leppert D (1996) Matrix metalloproteinases in immunity. *J Immunol* 156: 1–4

56 Shapiro SD, Kobayashi DK, Pentland AP, Welgus HG (1993) Induction of macrophage metalloproteinases by extracellular matrix. Evidence for enzyme- and substrate-specific responses involving prostaglandin-dependent mechanisms. *J Biol Chem* 268: 8170–8175

57 Opdenakker G, Van den Steen PE, Dubois B, Nelissen I, Van Coillie E, Masure S, Proost P, Van Damme J (2001) Gelatinase B functions as regulator and effector in leukocyte biology. *J Leukoc Biol* 69: 851–859

58 Corcoran ML, Kibbey MC, Kleinman HK, Wahl LM (1995) Laminin SIKVAV peptide induction of monocyte/macrophage prostaglandin E2 and matrix metalloproteinases. *J Biol Chem* 270: 10365–10368

59 Leber TM, Balkwill FR (1998) Regulation of monocyte MMP-9 production by TNF-alpha and a tumour- derived soluble factor (MMPSF). *Br J Cancer* 78: 724–732

60 Busiek DF, Baragi V, Nehring LC, Parks WC, Welgus HG (1995) Matrilysin expression by human mononuclear phagocytes and its regulation by cytokines and hormones. *J Immunol* 154: 6484–6491

61 Mertz PM, DeWitt DL, Stetler-Stevenson WG, Wahl LM (1994) Interleukin 10 suppression of monocyte prostaglandin H synthase-2. Mechanism of inhibition of prostaglandin-dependent matrix metalloproteinase production. *J Biol Chem* 269: 21322–21329

62 Vaday GG, Schor H, Rahat MA, Lahat N, Lider O (2001) Transforming growth factor-beta suppresses tumor necrosis factor alpha- induced matrix metalloproteinase-9 expression in monocytes. *J Leukoc Biol* 69: 613–621

63 Feinberg MW, Jain MK, Werner F, Sibinga NE, Wiesel P, Wang H, Topper JN, Perrella

MA, Lee ME (2000) Transforming growth factor-beta 1 inhibits cytokine-mediated induction of human metalloelastase in macrophages. *J Biol Chem* 275: 25766–25773
64 Conway JG, Wakefield JA, Brown RH, Marron BE, Sekut L, Stimpson SA, McElroy A, Menius JA, Jeffreys JJ, Clark RL et al (1995) Inhibition of cartilage and bone destruction in adjuvant arthritis in the rat by a matrix metalloproteinase inhibitor. *J Exp Med* 182: 449–457
65 Gijbels K, Galardy RE, Steinman L (1994) Reversal of experimental autoimmune encephalomyelitis with a hydroxamate inhibitor of matrix metalloproteases. *J Clin Invest* 94: 2177–2182
66 Ferrari-Lacraz S, Nicod LP, Chicheportiche R, Welgus HG, Dayer JM (2001) Human lung tissue macrophages, but not alveolar macrophages, express matrix metalloproteinases after direct contact with activated T lymphocytes. *Am J Respir Cell Mol Biol* 24: 442–451
67 Liu Z, Shipley JM, Vu TH, Zhou X, Diaz LA, Werb Z, Senior RM (1998) Gelatinase B-deficient mice are resistant to experimental bullous pemphigoid. *J Exp Med* 188: 475–482
68 Dubois B, Masure S, Hurtenbach U, Paemen L, Heremans H, van den Oord J, Sciot R, Meinhardt T, Hammerling G, Opdenakker G et al (1999) Resistance of young gelatinase B-deficient mice to experimental autoimmune encephalomyelitis and necrotizing tail lesions. *J Clin Invest* 104: 1507–1515
69 Lees M, Taylor DJ, Woolley DE (1994) Mast cell proteinases activate precursor forms of collagenase and stromelysin, but not of gelatinases A and B. *Eur J Biochem* 223: 171–177
70 Coussens LM, Raymond WW, Bergers G, Laig-Webster M, Behrendtsen O, Werb Z, Caughey GH, Hanahan D (1999) Inflammatory mast cells up-regulate angiogenesis during squamous epithelial carcinogenesis. *Genes Dev* 13: 1382–1397
71 Saarinen J, Kalkkinen N, Welgus HG, Kovanen PT (1994) Activation of human interstitial procollagenase through direct cleavage of the Leu83-Thr84 bond by mast cell chymase. *J Biol Chem* 269: 18134–18140
72 Fang KC, Raymond WW, Blount JL, Caughey GH (1997) Dog mast cell alpha-chymase activates progelatinase B by cleaving the Phe88-Gln89 and Phe91-Glu92 bonds of the catalytic domain. *J Biol Chem* 272: 25628–25635
73 Shamamian P, Schwartz JD, Pocock BJ, Monea S, Whiting D, Marcus SG, Mignatti P (2001) Activation of progelatinase A (MMP-2) by neutrophil elastase, cathepsin G, and proteinase-3: a role for inflammatory cells in tumor invasion and angiogenesis. *J Cell Physiol* 189: 197–206
74 Haro H, Crawford HC, Fingleton B, MacDougall JR, Shinomiya K, Spengler DM, Matrisian LM (2000) Matrix metalloproteinase-3-dependent generation of a macrophage chemoattractant in a model of herniated disc resorption. *J Clin Invest* 105: 133–141
75 Li Q, Park PW, Wilson CL, Parks WC (2002) Matrilysin shedding of syndecan-1 regu-

lates chemokine mobilization and transepithelial efflux of neutrophils in acute lung injury. *Cell* 111: 635–646
76 McQuibban GA, Gong JH, Tam EM, McCulloch CA, Clark-Lewis I, Overall CM (2000) Inflammation dampened by gelatinase A cleavage of monocyte chemoattractant protein-3. *Science* 289: 1202–1206
77 Robinson SC, Scott KA, Balkwill FR (2002) Chemokine stimulation of monocyte matrix metalloproteinase-9 requires endogenous TNF-alpha. *Eur J Immunol* 32: 404–412
78 Johnatty RN, Taub DD, Reeder SP, Turcovski-Corrales SM, Cottam DW, Stephenson TJ, Rees RC (1997) Cytokine and chemokine regulation of proMMP-9 and TIMP-1 production by human peripheral blood lymphocytes. *J Immunol* 158: 2327–2333
79 Romanic AM, Madri JA (1994) The induction of 72-kD gelatinase in T cells upon adhesion to endothelial cells is VCAM-1 dependent. *J Cell Biol* 125: 1165–1178
80 Shipley JM, Wesselschmidt RL, Kobayashi DK, Ley TJ, Shapiro SD (1996) Metalloelastase is required for macrophage-mediated proteolysis and matrix invasion in mice. *Proc Natl Acad Sci USA* 93: 3942–3964
81 Leppert D, Waubant E, Galardy R, Bunnett NW, Hauser SL (1995) T cell gelatinases mediate basement membrane transmigration *in vitro*. *J Immunol* 154: 4379–4389
82 Faveeuw C, Preece G, Ager A (2001) Transendothelial migration of lymphocytes across high endothelial venules into lymph nodes is affected by metalloproteinases. *Blood* 98: 688–695
83 Ratzinger G, Stoitzner P, Ebner S, Lutz MB, Layton GT, Rainer C, Senior RM, Shipley JM, Fritsch P, Schuler G et al (2002) Matrix metalloproteinases 9 and 2 are necessary for the migration of Langerhans cells and dermal dendritic cells from human and murine skin. *J Immunol* 168: 4361–4371
84 Wang M, Qin X, Mudgett JS, Ferguson TA, Senior RM, Welgus HG (1999) Matrix metalloproteinase deficiencies affect contact hypersensitivity: stromelysin-1 deficiency prevents the response and gelatinase B deficiency prolongs the response. *Proc Natl Acad Sci USA* 96: 6885–6889
85 Kolenko V, Wang Q, Riedy MC, O'Shea J, Ritz J, Cathcart MK, Rayman P, Tubbs R, Edinger M, Novick A et al (1997) Tumor-induced suppression of T lymphocyte proliferation coincides with inhibition of Jak3 expression and IL-2 receptor signaling: role of soluble products from human renal cell carcinomas. *J Immunol* 159: 3057–3067
86 Coventry BJ, Weeks SC, Heckford SE, Sykes PJ, Bradley J, Skinner JM (1996) Lack of IL-2 cytokine expression despite Il-2 messenger RNA transcription in tumor-infiltrating lymphocytes in primary human breast carcinoma: selective expression of early activation markers. *J Immunol* 156: 3486–3492
87 Sheu BC, Lin RH, Ho HN, Huang SC (1997) Down-regulation of CD25 expression on the surface of activated tumor-infiltrating lymphocytes in human cervical carcinoma. *Hum Immunol* 56: 39–48
88 Waldmann TA (1993) The IL-2/IL-2 receptor system: a target for rational immune intervention. *Trends Pharmacol Sci* 14: 159–164

89 Sheu BC, Hsu SM, Ho HN, Lien HC, Huang SC, Lin RH (2001) A novel role of metalloproteinase in cancer-mediated immunosuppression. *Cancer Res* 61: 237–242

90 Shresta S, Pham CT, Thomas DA, Graubert TA, Ley TJ (1998) How do cytotoxic lymphocytes kill their targets? *Curr Opin Immunol* 10: 581–587

91 Fingleton B, Vargo-Gogola T, Crawford HC, Matrisian LM (2001) Matrilysin [MMP–7] expression selects for cells with reduced sensitivity to apoptosis. *Neoplasia* 3: 459–468

92 Mitsiades N, Yu WH, Poulaki V, Tsokos M, Stamenkovic I (2001) Matrix metalloproteinase-7-mediated cleavage of Fas ligand protects tumor cells from chemotherapeutic drug cytotoxicity. *Cancer Res* 61: 577–581

93 Matsuno H, Yudoh K, Watanabe Y, Nakazawa F, Aono H, Kimura T (2001) Stromelysin-1 (MMP-3) in synovial fluid of patients with rheumatoid arthritis has potential to cleave membrane bound Fas ligand. *J Rheumatol* 28: 22–28

94 Corry DB, Rishi K, Kanellis J, Kiss A, Song Lz LZ, Xu J, Feng L, Werb Z, Kheradmand F (2002) Decreased allergic lung inflammatory cell egression and increased susceptibility to asphyxiation in MMP2-deficiency. *Nat Immunol* 3: 347–353

95 Okada A, Bellocq JP, Rouyer N, Chenard MP, Rio MC, Chambon P, Basset P (1995) Membrane-type matrix metalloproteinase (MT-MMP) gene is expressed in stromal cells of human colon, breast, and head and neck carcinomas. *Proc Natl Acad Sci USA* 92: 2730–2734

96 Cai M, Onoda K, Takao M, Kyoko IY, Shimpo H, Yoshida T, Yada I (2002) Degradation of tenascin-C and activity of matrix metalloproteinase-2 are associated with tumor recurrence in early stage non-small cell lung cancer. *Clin Cancer Res* 8: 1152–1156

97 Zeng ZS, Shu WP, Cohen AM, Guillem JG (2002) Matrix metalloproteinase-7 expression in colorectal cancer liver metastases: evidence for involvement of MMP-7 activation in human cancer metastases. *Clin Cancer Res* 8: 144–148

98 Brinckerhoff CE, Rutter JL, Benbow U (2000) Interstitial collagenases as markers of tumor progression. *Clin Cancer Res* 6: 4823–4830

99 Inuzuka K, Ogata Y, Nagase H, Shirouzu K (2000) Significance of coexpression of urokinase-type plasminogen activator, and matrix metalloproteinase 3 (stromelysin) and 9 (gelatinase B) in colorectal carcinoma. *J Surg Res* 93: 211–218

100 Basset P, Bellocq JP, Wolf C, Stoll I, Hutin P, Limacher JM, Podhajcer OL, Chenard MP, Rio MC, Chambon P (1990) A novel metalloproteinase gene specifically expressed in stromal cells of breast carcinomas. *Nature* 348: 699–704

101 Zucker S, Hymowitz M, Conner C, Zarrabi HM, Hurewitz AN, Matrisian L, Boyd D, Nicolson G, Montana S (1999) Measurement of matrix metalloproteinases and tissue inhibitors of metalloproteinases in blood and tissues. Clinical and experimental applications. *Ann NY Acad Sci* 878: 212–227

102 Nikkola J, Vihinen P, Vlaykova T, Hahka-Kemppinen M, Kahari VM, Pyrhonen S (2002) High expression levels of collagenase-1 and stromelysin-1 correlate with shorter disease-free survival in human metastatic melanoma. *Int J Cancer* 97: 432–438

103 Kallakury BV, Karikehalli S, Haholu A, Sheehan CE, Azumi N, Ross JS (2001) Increased expression of matrix metalloproteinases 2 and 9 and tissue inhibitors of metallopro-

teinases 1 and 2 correlate with poor prognostic variables in renal cell carcinoma. *Clin Cancer Res* 7: 3113–3119

104 Inoue K, Kamada M, Slaton JW, Fukata S, Yoshikawa C, Tamboli P, Dinney CP, Shuin T (2002) The prognostic value of angiogenesis and metastasis-related genes for progression of transitional cell carcinoma of the renal pelvis and ureter. *Clin Cancer Res* 8: 1863–1870

105 Stahle-Backdahl M, Sudbeck BD, Eisen AZ, Welgus HG, Parks WC (1992) Expression of 92-kDa type IV collagenase mRNA by eosinophils associated with basal cell carcinoma. *J Invest Dermatol* 99: 497–503

106 Zeng ZS, Guillem JG (1996) Colocalisation of matrix metalloproteinase-9-mRNA and protein in human colorectal cancer stromal cells. *Br J Cancer* 74: 1161–1167

107 Lochter A, Galosy S, Muschler J, Freedman N, Werb Z, Bissell MJ (1997) Matrix metalloproteinase stromelysin-1 triggers a cascade of molecular alterations that leads to stable epithelial-to-mesenchymal conversion and a premalignant phenotype in mammary epithelial cells. *J Cell Biol* 139: 1861–1872

108 Ha HY, Moon HB, Nam MS, Lee JW, Ryoo ZY, Lee TH, Lee KK, So BJ, Sato H, Seiki M et al (2001) Overexpression of membrane-type matrix metalloproteinase-1 gene induces mammary gland abnormalities and adenocarcinoma in transgenic mice. *Cancer Res* 61: 984–990

109 Sympson CJ, Bissell MJ, Werb Z (1995) Mammary gland tumor formation in transgenic mice overexpressing stromelysin-1. *Semin Cancer Biol* 6: 159–163

110 Rudolph-Owen LA, Chan R, Muller WJ, Matrisian LM (1998) The matrix metalloproteinase matrilysin influences early-stage mammary tumorigenesis. *Cancer Res.* 58: 5500–5506

111 Sternlicht MD, Lochter A, Sympson CJ, Huey B, Rougier JP, Gray JW, Pinkel D, Bissell MJ, Werb Z (1999) The stromal proteinase MMP3/stromelysin-1 promotes mammary carcinogenesis. *Cell* 98: 137–146

112 D'Armiento J, DiColandrea T, Dalal SS, Okada Y, Huang MT, Conney AH, Chada K (1995) Collagenase expression in transgenic mouse skin causes hyperkeratosis and acanthosis and increases susceptibility to tumorigenesis. *Mol Cell Biol* 15: 5732–5739

113 Colandrea TD, D'Armiento J, Kesari KV, Chada KK (2000) Collagenase induction promotes mouse tumorigenesis by two independent pathways. *Mol Carcinog* 29: 8–16

114 Martin DC, Ruther U, Sanchez-Sweatman OH, Orr FW, Khokha R (1996) Inhibition of SV40 T antigen-induced hepatocellular carcinoma in TIMP-1 transgenic mice. *Oncogene* 13: 569–576

115 Montgomery AM, Mueller BM, Reisfeld RA, Taylor SM, DeClerck YA (1994) Effect of tissue inhibitor of the matrix metalloproteinases-2 expression on the growth and spontaneous metastasis of a human melanoma cell line. *Cancer Res* 54: 5467–5473

116 Coussens LM, Tinkle CL, Hanahan D, Werb Z (2000) MMP-9 supplied by bone marrow-derived cells contributes to skin carcinogenesis. *Cell* 103: 481–490

117 Wilson CL, Heppner KJ, Labosky PA, Hogan BL, Matrisian LM (1997) Intestinal

tumorigenesis is suppressed in mice lacking the metalloproteinase matrilysin. *Proc Natl Acad Sci USA* 94: 1402–1407
118 Masson R, Lefebvre O, Noel A, Fahime ME, Chenard MP, Wendling C, Kebers F, LeMeur M, Dierich A, Foidart JM et al (1998) *In vivo* evidence that the stromelysin-3 metalloproteinase contributes in a paracrine manner to epithelial cell malignancy. *J Cell Biol* 140: 1535–1541
119 Bergers G, Brekken R, McMahon G, Vu TH, Itoh T, Tamaki K, Tanzawa K, Thorpe P, Itohara S, Werb Z et al (2000) Matrix metalloproteinase-9 triggers the angiogenic switch during carcinogenesis. *Nat Cell Biol* 2: 737–744
120 Itoh T, Tanioka M, Yoshida H, Yoshioka T, Nishimoto H, Itohara S (1998) Reduced angiogenesis and tumor progression in gelatinase A-deficient mice. *Cancer Res* 58: 1048–1051
121 Koop S, Khokha R, Schmidt EE, MacDonald IC, Morris VL, Chambers AF, Groom AC (1994) Overexpression of metalloproteinase inhibitor in B16F10 cells does not affect extravasation but reduces tumor growth. *Cancer Res* 54: 4791–4797
122 Hiratsuka S, Nakamura K, Iwai S, Murakami M, Itoh T, Kijima H, Shipley JM, Senior RM, Shibuya M (2002) MMP9 induction by vascular endothelial growth factor receptor-1 is involved in lung-specific metastasis. *Cancer Cell* 2: 289–300
123 van Kempen LC, Coussens LM (2002) MMP9 potentiates pulmonary metastasis formation. Cancer Cell 2: 251–252
124 Bissell MJ, Radisky D (2001) Putting tumours in context. *Nat Rev Cancer* 1: 46–54
125 Coussens LM, Werb Z (2002) Inflammation and cancer. *Nature* 420: 860–867
126 Duncan LM, Richards LA, Mihm MC, Jr. (1998) Increased mast cell density in invasive melanoma. *J Cutan Pathol* 25: 11–15
127 Takanami I, Takeuchi K, Naruke M (2000) Mast cell density is associated with angiogenesis and poor prognosis in pulmonary adenocarcinoma. *Cancer* 88: 2686–2692
128 Tomita M, Matsuzaki Y, Onitsuka T (2000) Effect of mast cells on tumor angiogenesis in lung cancer. *Ann Thorac Surg* 69: 1686–1690
129 Toth-Jakatics R, Jimi S, Takebayashi S, Kawamoto N (2000) Cutaneous malignant melanoma: correlation between neovascularization and peritumor accumulation of mast cells overexpressing vascular endothelial growth factor. *Hum Pathol* 31: 955–960
130 Imada A, Shijubo N, Kojima H, Abe S (2000) Mast cells correlate with angiogenesis and poor outcome in stage I lung adenocarcinoma. *Eur Respir J* 15: 1087–1093
131 Benitez-Bribiesca L, Wong A, Utrera D, Castellanos E (2001) The role of mast cell tryptase in neoangiogenesis of premalignant and malignant lesions of the uterine cervix. *J Histochem Cytochem* 49: 1061–1062
132 Shea CR, Prieto VG (1994) Mast cells in angiolipomas and hemangiomas of human skin: are they important for angiogenesis? *J Cutan Pathol* 21: 247–251
133 Weitzman SA, Gordon LI (1990) Inflammation and cancer: role of phagocyte-generated oxidants in carcinogenesis. *Blood* 76: 655–663
134 Ness RB, Cottreau C (1999) Possible role of ovarian epithelial inflammation in ovarian cancer. *J Natl Cancer Inst* 91: 1459–1467

135 Shacter E, Weitzman SA (2002) Chronic inflammation and cancer. *Oncology* 16: 217–226

136 Ernst PB, Gold BD (2000) The disease spectrum of *Helicobacter pylori*: the immunopathogenesis of gastroduodenal ulcer and gastric cancer. *Annu Rev Microbiol* 54: 615–640

137 Engle SJ, Ormsby I, Pawlowski S, Boivin GP, Croft J, Balish E, Doetschman T (2002) Elimination of colon cancer in germ-free transforming growth factor beta 1-deficient mice. *Cancer Res.* 62: 6362–6366

138 Williams CS, Mann M, DuBois RN (1999) The role of cyclooxygenases in inflammation, cancer, and development. *Oncogene* 18: 7908–7916

139 Garcia-Rodriguez LA, Huerta-Alvarez C (2001) Reduced risk of colorectal cancer among long-term users of aspirin and nonaspirin nonsteroidal antiinflammatory drugs. *Epidemiology* 12: 88–93

140 Meier CR, Schmitz S, Jick H (2002) Association between acetaminophen or nonsteroidal antiinflammatory drugs and risk of developing ovarian, breast, or colon cancer. *Pharmacotherapy* 22: 303–309

141 Sharpe CR, Collet JP, McNutt M, Belzile E, Boivin JF, Hanley JA (2000) Nested case-control study of the effects of non-steroidal anti- inflammatory drugs on breast cancer risk and stage. *Br J Cancer* 83: 112–120

142 Cotterchio M, Kreiger N, Sloan M, Steingart A (2001) Nonsteroidal anti-inflammatory drug use and breast cancer risk. *Cancer Epidemiol Biomarkers Prev* 10: 1213–1217

143 Akre K, Ekstrom AM, Signorello LB, Hansson LE, Nyren O (2001) Aspirin and risk for gastric cancer: a population-based case-control study in Sweden. *Br J Cancer* 84: 965–968

144 Huang S, Van Arsdall M, Tedjarati S, McCarty M, Wu W, Langley R, Fidler IJ (2002) Contributions of stromal metalloproteinase-9 to angiogenesis and growth of human ovarian carcinoma in mice. *J Natl Cancer Inst* 94: 1134–1142

145 Coussens LM, Fingleton B, Matrisian LM (2002) Matrix metalloproteinase inhibitors and cancer: trials and tribulations. *Science* 295: 2387–2392

146 Reich R, Thompson EW, Iwamoto Y, Martin GR, Deason JR, Fuller GC, Miskin R (1988) Effects of inhibitors of plasminogen activator, serine proteinases, and collagenase IV on the invasion of basement membranes by metastatic cells. *Cancer Res* 48: 3307–3312

147 Sledge GW, Jr., Qulali M, Goulet R, Bone EA, Fife R (1995) Effect of matrix metalloproteinase inhibitor batimastat on breast cancer regrowth and metastasis in athymic mice. *J Natl Cancer Inst* 87: 1546–1550

148 Maekawa K, Sato H, Furukawa M, Yoshizaki T (2002) Inhibition of cervical lymph node metastasis by marimastat (BB-2516) in an orthotopic oral squamous cell carcinoma implantation model. *Clin Exp Metastasis* 19: 513–518

149 Naglich JG, Jure-Kunkel M, Gupta E, Fargnoli J, Henderson AJ, Lewin AC, Talbott R, Baxter A, Bird J, Savopoulos R et al (2001) Inhibition of angiogenesis and metastasis in

two murine models by the matrix metalloproteinase inhibitor, BMS-275291. *Cancer Res* 61: 8480–8485

150 Kruger A, Soeltl R, Sopov I, Kopitz C, Arlt M, Magdolen V, Harbeck N, Gansbacher B, Schmitt M (2001) Hydroxamate-type matrix metalloproteinase inhibitor batimastat promotes liver metastasis. *Cancer Res* 61: 1272–1275

151 Bergers G, Javaherian K, Lo KM, Folkman J, Hanahan D (1999) Effects of angiogenesis inhibitors on multistage carcinogenesis in mice. *Science* 284: 808–812

152 Shiraga M, Yano S, Yamamoto A, Ogawa H, Goto H, Miki T, Miki K, Zhang H, Sone S (2002) Organ heterogeneity of host-derived matrix metalloproteinase expression and its involvement in multiple-organ metastasis by lung cancer cell lines. *Cancer Res* 62: 5967–5973

Interplay between inflammation and tumor angiogenesis

Li Yan, Xiao-yu R. Song and Marian T. Nakada

Centocor, Inc., 200 Great Valley Parkway, Malvern, PA 19355, USA

Inflammation and angiogenesis in cancer

The association of inflammation and neoplasia was first observed when Westphal reported dense areas of mast cells at the periphery of tumors in 1891 [1]. These inflammatory cells infiltrating tumor tissues were believed to mediate phagocytic functions to aid in host defense against the tumor. Now a new paradigm is being widely accepted that inflammation at the site of a tumor may actually facilitate tumor progression instead of promoting anti-tumor immunity. The diverse contributions of tumor-infiltrating inflammatory cells to neoplastic progression include promoting epithelial cell proliferation, rendering tumor angiogenic potential, and enabling tumor invasiveness [2]. The most direct evidence supporting the role of inflammatory cells in promoting disease progression comes from epidemiological studies of cancer risk among long-term users of aspirin and non-steroidal anti-inflammatory drugs (NSAIDs). Significant reduction in the risk of developing colon, lung, esophagus, and stomach cancers was observed in these users [3, 4].

This chapter will describe the inflammatory components and processes involved in tumor angiogenesis. The general model that will be elaborated is shown in Figure 1. Tumors secrete pro-inflammatory chemokines and cytokines, and they also activate local stromal cell elements to do the same. These chemokines and cytokines act either directly or indirectly through stimulation of the vascular endothelium to recruit leukocytes to the tumor. Indeed, for some tumor types, >70% of the tumor mass consists of infiltrating leukocytes. After activation, these tumor-associated leukocytes, primarily macrophages, release angiogenic factors, mitogens, proteolytic enzymes, and chemotactic factors, recruiting more inflammatory cells and sustaining tumor growth, invasion, and angiogenesis. The new vessels that form in turn provide greater access for more inflammatory cells to enter the tumor.

Angiogenesis is a complex process involving an extensive interplay between cells, soluble factors, and extracellular matrix (ECM) components. In this chapter, we will highlight the cross-talk between malignant, inflammatory, and stromal compartments with an emphasis on the stimulation of tumor angiogenesis by tumor-infil-

Cancer and Inflammation, edited by Douglas W. Morgan, Ulf J. Forssmann and Marian T. Nakada

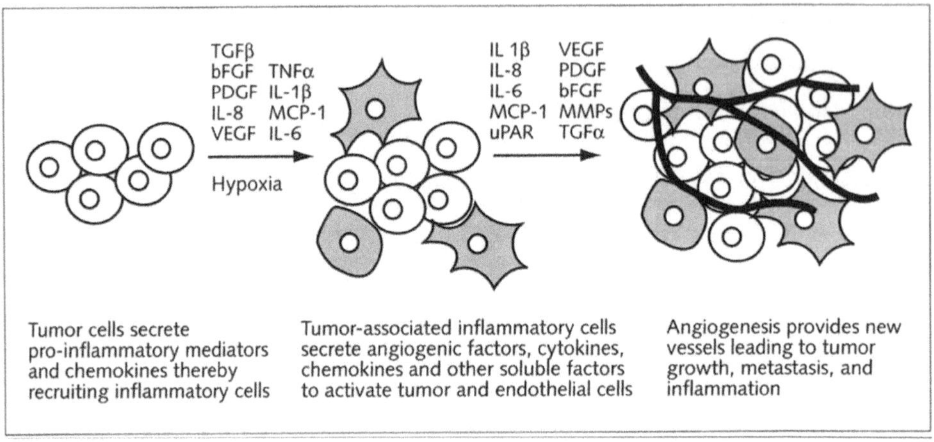

Figure 1
Inflammation and tumor-induced angiogenesis.
TGFβ, transforming growth factor β; bFGF, basic fibroblast growth factor; PDGF, platelet-derived growth factor; IL, interleukin; VEGF, vascular endothelial growth factor; TNFα, tumor necrosis factor α; MCP-1, monocyte chemotactic protein-1; uPAR, urokinase plasminogen activator receptor.

trating inflammatory cells. The regulation of key inflammatory components and mediators involved in tumor angiogenesis and their effects on tumor growth and metastasis will be reviewed. In addition, recent advances in the development of specific anti-inflammatory agents with anti-angiogenesis activity for oncologic indications will be discussed.

An overview of angiogenesis

Angiogenesis, the formation of new blood vessels from an existing vasculature, is essential for tumor growth beyond 1–2 mm in diameter. This process occurs in all types of tumor and the intensity of the angiogenic process, as assessed by microvessel counting methods, correlates with primary tumor growth, invasiveness, and metastatic spread of disease [5, 6]. Tumor angiogenesis provides a means to supply oxygen and nutrients and to remove waste products from tissues that are hypoxic or hypovascularized [7]. Angiogenesis is essential for certain physiologic functions such as embryonic development, wound healing, and the female menstrual cycle. These physiologic processes are tightly regulated by a balance of anti-angiogenic and pro-angiogenic factors. In contrast, unregulated angiogenesis occurs in pathologic conditions [8], such as tumor growth and metastasis [9], atherosclerosis, rheumatoid arthritis (RA), Crohn's disease, psoriasis, endometriosis [10, 11], diabetic nephropathy [12], and adiposity.

An overview of inflammation

To understand the role of inflammation in cancer angiogenesis, it is important to first understand what inflammation is and how it contributes to angiogenesis under both physiological and pathological conditions. In response to tissue injury, a multifactorial network of chemical signals initiates and maintains a host response designed to "heal" the afflicted tissue. This involves activation and directed migration of leukocytes from the blood to sites of damage. The four-step mechanism for leukocyte recruitment involves activation of members of the selectin family of adhesion molecules that facilitate rolling along the vascular endothelium, triggering of signals that activate and upregulate leukocyte integrins mediated by cytokines and leukocyte-activating molecules, immobilization of leukocytes on the surface of the vascular endothelium by means of tight adhesion through $\alpha_4\beta_1$ and $\alpha_4\beta_7$ integrins binding to endothelial vascular cell-adhesion molecule-1 (VCAM-1) and mucosal addressin cell adhesion molecule-1 (MadCAM-1), respectively, and transmigration through the endothelium to sites of injury, presumably facilitated by extracellular proteases such as matrix metalloproteinases (MMPs) [13].

A family of chemotactic cytokines called chemokines possess a relatively high degree of specificity for chemoattraction of specific leukocyte populations [14–16], recruit downstream effector cells, and dictate the natural evolution of the inflammatory response. The profile of cytokine/chemokines persisting at an inflammatory site is important in the development of chronic diseases. The pro-inflammatory cytokine tumor necrosis factor α (TNFα) controls the composition of the inflammatory cell population and mediates many other aspects of the inflammatory process. TNFα stimulates the expression of adhesion molecules by the endothelium and also primes leukocytes for degranulation. Transforming growth factor β1 (TGFβ1) is another important soluble factor in inflammation, both positively and negatively influencing the processes of inflammation and repair. The key concept is that normal inflammation, such as that associated with wound healing, is usually self-limiting; however, deregulation of any of the converging factors can lead to abnormalities and ultimately pathogenesis, which seems to be the case during neoplastic progression.

Leukocyte recruitment to the tumor

The inflammatory microenvironment of tumors is characterized by the presence of host leukocytes both in the supporting stroma and within tumor tissues. The inflammatory component of a developing neoplasm may include a diverse leukocyte population including macrophages, neutrophils, dendritic cells, lymphocytes, eosinophils, and mast cells, all of which are capable of producing an assorted array of cytokines. These inflammatory cells traffic to the tumor site following the cues released by tumor cells, mainly secreted factors such as cytokines and chemokines.

Chemokines were initially defined as soluble factors regulating directional migration of leukocytes during inflammation. Chemokines produced by most tumors belong to the two major groups, the CXC and the CC chemokines. Typically, CXC chemokines attract neutrophils and lymphocytes whereas CC chemokines act on several leukocyte subsets including monocytes, eosinophils, dendritic cells, lymphocytes, and natural killer cells, but not neutrophils. Evidence from animal studies and human tumor studies suggest that CC chemokines are major determinants of macrophage and lymphocyte infiltration in melanoma, carcinoma of the ovary, breast, and cervix, and in sarcomas and gliomas [17, 18].

The immune system plays an important role in the regulation of angiogenesis. Multiple studies indicate that leukocytes can induce vascular proliferation [19–21], and specific leukocyte-derived cytokines such as interleukin-6 (IL-6) have been identified to induce angiogenesis [22–24]. In addition, angiogenic processes can in turn impact the immune system. Normal endothelial cells contribute to the recruitment of immune cells to the inflammatory site through the expression of adhesion molecules, which then sets the inflammatory process in motion.

Inflammatory cell compartment in tumors

Monocytes/macrophages

Macrophages infiltrated into tumor tissues, known as tumor-associated macrophages (TAMs), are a major component of inflammatory infiltrates in neoplastic tissues. These TAMs differentiate from monocytes that are recruited to tumor sites by tumor cell-derived chemokines, most significantly by monocyte chemotactic protein-1 (MCP-1), macrophage colony-stimulating factor (M-CSF or CSF-1), and vascular endothelial growth factor (VEGF). The presence of multiple areas of hypoxia and the accumulation of TAM in these poorly vascularized, hypoxic and necrotic areas suggests that tumor hypoxia functions as a potent stimulation of TAM infiltration [25, 26].

In addition to being a key regulatory molecule of monocyte trafficking to sites of inflammation, MCP-1 is also a potent pro-angiogenic factor. In a corneal angiogenesis assay, MCP-1 was able to elicit angiogenic responses with similar potency to the well-known angiogenic mediator VEGF-A [27]. Angiogenesis induced by MCP-1 is associated with prominent recruitment of macrophages, whereas that induced by VEGF is devoid of inflammatory cell recruitment. Tumor expression of MCP-1 is correlated with the degree of TAM infiltration in human gastric carcinomas [28], esophageal squamous cell carcinomas [29], gliomas [30, 31] and meningioma [32], and breast carcinoma [27, 33, 34]. After activation these TAMs produce a variety of cytokines, complement components, reactive oxygen species, proteases, and growth factors, including VEGF, platelet-derived growth factor (PDGF), thymidine phosphorylase (TP; also known as platelet-derived endothelial cell growth factor (PD-ECGF)), basic fibroblast growth factor (bFGF), TNFα, IL-1β, IL-6, IL-8, MMPs, and urokinase plasminogen activator and its receptor (uPA/uPAR) that modulate tumor angiogenesis [35]. In primary human breast cancer, MCP-1 concentration correlated significantly with the levels of VEGF, TP, TNFα, and IL-8, all of which are potent angiogenic factors. However, in the Matrigel angiogenesis assay, tumor angiogenic potential was found to be primarily associated with tumor cell MCP-1 expression level [36]. Furthermore, neutralizing MCP-1 biologic activity with function-blocking monoclonal antibodies was able to effectively inhibit *in vivo* tumor angiogenesis despite the complexity and redundancy of angiogenic growth factors expressed by tumor cells [36]. In addition, prognostic analysis revealed that a high expression of MCP-1, as well as of VEGF, was a significant indicator of early relapse, further supporting the hypothesis that MCP-1 plays an important role in regulating tumor angiogenesis and disease progression [34].

Expression levels of M-CSF and its receptor, a tyrosine kinase receptor encoded by the *cfms* proto-oncogene, have been associated with high TAM infiltration in breast cancer, and further correlated with tumor metastasis and poor prognosis [37, 38]. High levels of circulating M-CSF have also been detected in patients with breast, endometrial, or ovarian carcinomas, and are associated with disease progression and correlated with poor prognosis [39, 40]. In addition to stimulating macrophage infiltration into the tumor, M-CSF may also induce the differentiation of monocytes into macrophages, and like MCP-1 it can also activate these TAM cells, resulting in production and release of such angiogenic factors as IL-8 [41] and MMPs [42]. Finally, genetic studies demonstrated that M-CSF is essential for the development of late-stage invasive carcinoma and pulmonary metastases [43]. Tumor growth is impaired in M-CSF-deficient mice, accompanied by increased tumor necrosis and decreased mitosis, apparently resulting from diminished angiogenesis and diminished stromal formation [44].

Besides being a potent angiogenic factor for endothelial cells, tumor cell-derived VEGF [45] is also a chemotactic factor for tumor cells, macrophages, and T cells [46]. In fact, VEGF expression in human breast cancer [25], and lung, ovarian, and breast ascites [47] often correlates with macrophage content and vascular density.

Dendritic cells

Monocytes, in the presence of granulocyte-macrophage colony-stimulating factor (GM-CSF) and IL-4, differentiate into immature dendritic cells [48]. Dendritic cells play a crucial role in both the activation of antigen-specific immunity and the maintenance of tolerance. They migrate into inflamed peripheral tissue where they capture antigens, and after maturation migrate to lymph nodes to stimulate T-lymphocyte activation. Soluble factors such as IL-6 and CSF-1, derived from neoplastic cells, push myeloid precursors toward a macrophage-like phenotype [49]. Interestingly, dendritic cells found in neoplastic infiltrates are frequently immature and defective in T-cell stimulatory capacity. Therefore, these infiltrating dendritic cells are likely poor inducers of effective immune response to tumor antigens.

Mast cells

Mast cells were the first inflammatory cell population to be associated with human tumors. Back in 1891, Westphal reported that mast cells are always found at the periphery of malignant human tumors [1]. Recent studies confirmed and extended this finding by demonstrating the accumulation of increased numbers of mast cells within and around colorectal tumors, breast tumors, pulmonary adenocarcinomas, basal cell carcinomas, soft tissue tumors, and melanomas [50]. Mast cells are capable of producing and releasing a variety of pro-angiogenic factors, including VEGF, bFGF, TGFβ, TNFα, IL-8, heparin, and histamine [51]. At the same time, mast cells also secrete enzymes, such as MMPs, chymase, and tryptase, that facilitate neovascularization by stimulating endothelial migration and by releasing extracellular matrix-bound growth factors [50, 51]. In fact, the number of tryptase-positive mast cells correlates with neovascularization in cervical cancer, pulmonary adenocarcinoma, and malignant lymphoma [50]. The most compelling evidence supporting the role of mast cells in tumor angiogenesis arises from mast cell-deficient mice, in which a decreased rate and intensity of tumor angiogenesis results in a reduction in experimental tumor metastasis [52].

Polymorphonuclear neutrophils (PMNs)

Neutrophils are the most abundant circulating blood leukocytes. They provide first-line defense against infection and are potent effectors of inflammation. In addition, their release of soluble chemotactic factors guides the recruitment of both non-specific and specific immune effector cells [53]. Finally, since these cells both respond to and produce cytokines [54], they also modulate the balance between humoral and cell-mediated immunity. In doing so, neutrophils are engaged in a complex cross-talk with immune and endothelial cells in an inflammatory response.

Neutrophils are usually the first type of inflammatory cell found at the site of injury/inflammation. In addition to their well-accepted function of phagocytosis, several lines of evidence suggest that neutrophils may also be involved in the early induction of angiogenesis. Gaudry et al. [55] found that various compounds, including phorbol-12-myristate-13-acetate, fMet-Leu-Phe, and TNFα, could induce the time-dependent release of intracellular VEGF by human neutrophils. Upon stimulation by lipopolysaccharide or TNFα, PMN release significantly increased levels of biologically active VEGF that stimulates endothelial cell proliferation and tubule formation [56]. In addition, Kibbey et al. [57] found that neutrophils can be induced to migrate toward laminin peptides containing the amino acid sequence SKIVAV, and that these neutrophils then secreted angiogenic factors and matrix-degrading enzymes. PMN-derived elastase, cathepsin G, and proteinase-3 collectively activate pro-MMP-2, a critical enzyme for tumor invasion and angiogenesis [58]. Finally, neutrophils are known to produce a number of other angiogenic factors including TNFα and IL-1 [59]. Therefore, it is reasonable to hypothesize that neutrophils may also contribute to early angiogenesis.

The essential role of neutrophils in angiogenesis was demonstrated in neutropenic mice in which IL-8, macrophage-inflammatory protein-2 (MIP-2) (CXCL2), and growth-related oncogene α (GROα) were not able to induce angiogenic reactions [60]. In fact, angiostatin, an anti-angiogenesis factor, may inhibit angiogenesis by blocking chemotaxis of neutrophils to CXCR2 chemokine receptor agonists, including IL-8, MIP-2, and GROα [60].

Lymphocytes

T lymphocytes can activate endothelial expression of various metalloproteinases *via* CD40–CD40-ligand interactions. As a result, increased tube formation in a three-dimensional gel was observed [61]. IL-17 produced by CD4 T cells promotes tumor angiogenesis and growth by stimulating endothelial cell migration, differentiation, as well as by inducing tumor stromal fibroblasts and tumor cells to produce such pro-angiogenic factors as VEGF, keratinocyte-deived chemokine, MIP-2, prostaglandin E_1 and E_2, and nitric oxide [62].

Stimulation of tumor angiogenesis by angiogenic growth factors, cytokines, chemokines, and other soluble mediators produced by infiltrating leukocytes in tumors

After leukocytes infiltrate into tumor tissues, they are prone to activation and in some instances degranulation, thereby producing an array of growth factors, cytokines, chemokines and other soluble mediators that stimulate angiogenesis.

VEGF

VEGF is a potent angiogenic growth factor that plays a key regulatory role during the tumor angiogenic process, and its expression has been correlated with tumor disease staging and prognosis [63]. In a variety of human tumors, VEGF is expressed by both tumor cells and infiltrating TAMs [25, 64]. VEGF expression is readily stimulated by the hypoxic conditions often observed in the center of neoplasia, *via* a transcription factor hypoxia-inducible factor 1 (HIF1) [65]. In invasive breast carcinomas, a large number of TAMs accumulate in poorly vascularized and hypoxic regions. VEGF expressed by tumor cells or TAMs directly stimulates endothelial cell proliferation and migration. VEGF expression by TAMs was only detected in regions where tumor cells also express VEGF induced by hypoxia [25, 64]. Taken together with the finding that VEGF is chemotactic for monocytes across collagen membranes and endothelial cell monolayers [66], it is speculated that hypoxia-induced VEGF expression by tumor cells may also exert a chemotactic effect on TAMs *in vivo*.

In addition, VEGF is also an extremely potent vasopermeability stimulant [67]. In fact, VEGF was initially identified as vascular permeability factor (VPF). Increased vessel permeability could lead to extravasation of macromolecules which may further augment inflammatory responses.

bFGF

bFGF is another potent pro-angiogenic growth factor produced by activated TAMs infiltrated into the tumor tissue [68], and by mast cells commonly found in the peripheral regions of solid tumors [51]. The biological role of bFGF during neoplasm angiogenesis has been well demonstrated [69], and its expression in human tumors, especially by TAMs, has been correlated with tumor vascularization [70].

PD-ECGF

PD-ECGF is a 45 kDa polypeptide also known as TP because of its sequence identity to TP and its enzymatic activity converting thymidine to thymine [71]. PD-ECGF has been shown to stimulate mitosis [72] and migration [73] of endothelial cells in the presence of thymidine. In human tumors, PD-ECGF is expressed by tumor cells as well as by infiltrating lymphocytes [74] and macrophages [34]. The expression of PD-ECGF is correlated with microvessel density and disease progression [75–78].

IL-1

IL-1α and IL-1β are two multifunctional and pro-inflammatory cytokines produced mainly by activated monocytes and macrophages. They affect nearly all types of cells, often in concert with other cytokines or small mediator molecules [79]. Soluble IL-1β in the tumor milieu induces several angiogenic factors, including VEGF, MIP-2, and hepatocyte growth factor (HGF), from tumor and stromal cells and thus promotes tumor growth through stimulating angiogenesis [80]. IL-1 expression at the site of tumor development enhances the expression of adhesion molecules on endothelial and malignant cells and facilitates the invasion of malignant cells into the circulation and their dissemination to remote tissues [81]. In IL-1 gene-knockout mice tumor angiogenesis, growth and lung metastasis are significantly reduced compared to wild-type mice, demonstrating the importance of host-derived IL-1 in these processes [82].

IL-4

IL-4 has been shown to directly stimulate capillary endothelial cell proliferation [83], and induce endothelial cell tube formation [84]. The pro-angiogenic activity of IL-4 is postulated to be mediated by its ability to stimulate the expression of the adhesion molecules VCAM-1 and P-selectin in endothelial cells [85], and uPA [86]. However, a recent report suggested that IL-4 could indeed inhibit *in vitro* angiogenesis induced by VEGF or bFGF, suggesting that the role of IL-4 in angiogenesis might be dependent on the endothelial cell types [87].

IL-6

IL-6 is a secreted, multifunctional glycoprotein that performs various biological functions. The pro-angiogenic effects of IL-6 expressed by TAMs have been attributed to the stimulation of VEGF expression [88, 89].

IL-8

IL-8 is an 8 kDa chemokine of the Glu-Leu-Arg (ELR^+)CXC family with endothelial cell chemotactic and proliferative activity [22]. Recombinant IL-8 potently stimulated angiogenesis when implanted in the rat cornea and induced proliferation and chemotaxis of human umbilical vein endothelial cells. Angiogenic activity present in the conditioned media of inflamed human rheumatoid synovial tissue macrophages or lipopolysaccharide-stimulated blood monocytes was equally blocked by antibodies to either IL-8 or TNFα. An IL-8 antisense oligonucleotide specifically blocked the production of monocyte-induced angiogenic activity. High IL-8 expression levels render tumor cells highly tumorigenic, angiogenic, and invasive [90, 91]. IL-8 expression in human tumors significantly correlates with angiogenesis, as determined by intratumor microvessel density [92]. Finally, expression of IL-8 correlates with angiogenesis in non-small-cell lung carcinoma [93], metastatic growth pattern in melanoma [94], and disease staging and prognosis in head and neck squamous cell carcinoma [95].

It is well established that CXC chemokines with the three amino acids Glu-Leu-Arg (ELR) immediately amino-terminal to the CXC motif (ELR^+) are pro-angiogenic and stimulate endothelial cell chemotaxis, whereas ELR^- CXC chemokines possess angiostatic activities [96, 97]. ELR^+ CXC ligands bind to CXCR2 and to a lesser degree to CXCR1, whereas ELR^- CXC ligands bind to CXCR3, CXCR4, and CXCR5 [16]. Compared to VEGF-A, murine MCP-5/CCL12 exhibits only modest mitogenic properties towards endothelial cells; however, it is a potent chemoattractant. In contrast, stromal-cell-derived factor (SDF-1/CXCL12) induces endothelial expression of VEGF-A which in turn upregulates CXCR4 on endothelial cells [15]. Although it is not always clear if the angiostatic and angiogenic effects of chemokines are direct or indirect, it is accepted that the balance between the two regulates neoplastic cell physiology.

MCP-1

MCP-1 is a potent chemoattractant of monocytes that has recently been suggested to play a pivotal role in tumor angiogenesis. Tumor cell-secreted MCP-1 levels have been correlated with blood vessel density in a number of tumors, including breast cancer [33, 34], squamous cell carcinoma of head, neck [98] and esophagus [29], gastric carcinoma [28], and hemangioma [99]. Furthermore, high levels of tumor MCP-1 were also found to serve as a prognostic biomarker indicating poor prognosis and early relapse [34, 98]. It has been postulated that MCP-1 in tumor tissues may stimulate angiogenesis by recruiting tumor-infiltrating macrophages and subsequently the production of angiogenic growth factors such as VEGF, TNFα, IL-6, and IL-8 [34, 98]. It also appears that MCP-1 may also act on endothelial cells directly *via* cell-surface CCR2 receptor [100].

Other chemokines that have been implicated in stimulating angiogenesis include epithelial neutrophil-activating protein-78, growth-related gene alpha, growth-related gene beta, growth-related gene gamma, granulocyte chemotactic protein-2, and platelet basic protein [101].

Besides the above-mentioned angiogenic growth factors, cytokines and chemokines, leukocytes infiltrated into tumor tissues also make other factors that stimulate angiogenesis.

Angiogenin

Angiogenin is a 14-kDa single-chain polypeptide composed of 123 amino acids

[102]. The pro-angiogenic activity of angiogenin appears to be mediated through its direct interactions with endothelial cells [103, 104]]. Expression of angiogenin by both tumor cells and TAMs is regulated by pro-inflammatory cytokines, including IL-1β and TNFα. High levels of angiogenin in tumor tissues have been correlated with vascular involvement, lymph node metastases, liver metastases, and advanced stages of colon cancer [105]. Serum levels of angiogenin were significantly elevated in patients with endometrial cancer in all stages of tumor progression [106], and in patients with ovarian cancer of stages II and III [107].

Remodeling of ECM by leukocyte-derived proteinases

In addition to secreting soluble growth factors, cytokines, and chemokines to directly stimulate endothelial cells and promote angiogenesis, tumor-associated leukocytes also contribute to the angiogenic process by generating proteinases that remodel the ECM and therefore facilitate neovascularization. These proteinases include MMP-1, MMP-2, MMP-3, MMP-9, and MMP-12, as well as cathepsins, uPA, uPAR, plasmin [58, 108–110], and heparanase [111]. Cleavage of ECM macromolecules by various proteinases also releases various ECM-bound pro-angiogenic factors [112] and fragments of fibrin and collagen [113]. These precisely coordinated events subsequently result in the degradation of the basement membrane and other ECM components, destabilizing the local vasculature and permitting the migration and proliferation of endothelial cells, and eventually leading to tumor angiogenesis, growth, and metastasis.

Endothelial cells

Endothelial cells form a monolayer lining every blood vessel in the circulation and are actively involved in several regulatory processes in the body. Endothelial cells not only are important for transporting peptides/proteins and small solutes to the tissues, they also regulate blood coagulation and vascular remodeling. In addition, they contribute to the recruitment of the immune cells to the inflammatory site through a concerted process involving adhesion molecules, chemokines, and cytokines as detailed below.

Adhesion molecules

Cell adhesion molecules can be classified into four families depending on their biochemical and structural characteristics. These families are the selectins, the immunoglobulin supergene family, the cadherins, and the integrins. Members of each family are implicated in neovascularization.

Integrins are a group of cell-adhesion receptors consisting of non-covalently associated α and β subunits that can heterodimerize in more than 20 combinations. Endothelial cells express several distinct integrins, allowing attachment to a wide variety of ECM proteins [114]. To initiate the angiogenic process, endothelial cells must dissociate from neighboring cells before they can invade the underlying tissue. During invasion and migration, the interaction of the endothelial cells with the ECM is mediated by integrins. Cell–cell contact and cell–ECM interactions are also essential during the final phases of angiogenesis, when endothelial cell polarity is defined and capillary loops are formed [115].

Integrin $\alpha_v\beta_3$ was found to be particularly important during angiogenesis. $\alpha_v\beta$ is a receptor for a number of proteins with an exposed RGD sequence, including fibronectin, vitronectin, laminin, von Willebrand factor (vWF), fibrinogen, and denatured collagen. In addition, $\alpha_v\beta_3$ has been shown to bind MMP-2 in an RGD-independent manner, thereby localizing MMP-2-mediated matrix degradation to the endothelial cell surface [114, 116]. $\alpha_v\beta_3$ is nearly undetectable on quiescent endothelium, but is highly upregulated during cytokine- or tumor-induced angiogenesis. In activated endothelium, $\alpha_v\beta_3$ suppresses the activity of both p53 and the p53-inducible cell-cycle inhibitor $p21^{WAF1/CIP1}$, while increasing the ratio of the anti-apoptotic Bcl-2 to pro-apoptotic Bax proteins, resulting in an anti-apoptotic effect [117]. Consequently, $\alpha_v\beta_3$ was found to promote melanoma growth by regulating tumor cell survival [118].

Another receptor that has been implicated in angiogenesis is integrin $\alpha_v\beta_5$. Antibodies directed against $\alpha_v\beta_3$ were found to specifically block FGF-1- or TNFα-induced angiogenesis, whereas antagonists of $\alpha_v\beta_5$ blocked VEGF-induced angiogenesis [119]. Finally, a human antibody in clinical development against both $\alpha_v\beta_3$ and $\alpha_v\beta_5$ has also been shown to inhibit angiogenesis and tumor growth in pre-clinical models [120].

Besides integrins, a number of other cell-adhesion molecules are involved in angiogenesis. Vascular endothelial cadherin mediates calcium-dependent homophilic interactions between endothelial cells. Recently, knockout studies in mice demonstrated that a deficiency or truncation of vascular endothelial cadherin induces endothelial cell apoptosis and inhibits transmission of the endothelial survival signal by VEGF, leading to embryonic lethality [121]. Members of the immunoglobulin superfamily mediate heterophilic cell–cell adhesion. Intercellular adhesion molecule-1 (ICAM-1) and VCAM-1 are expressed on quiescent endothelium, but are upregulated after stimulation with TNFα, IL-1, or interferon γ (IFNγ) [122]. Moreover, VCAM-1 can induce chemotaxis in endothelial cells *in vitro* and angiogenesis *in vivo* [123]. Also, members of the selectin family, in particular P-selectin and E-selectin, which promote adhesion of leukocytes to cytokine-activated vascular endothelium, have been shown to play a role in angiogenesis [123]. E-selectin was found to induce endothelial migration and tube formation *in vitro* and angiogenesis *in vivo* [124]. However, little is known about the mechanism of action of these molecules, and mice deficient in both E-selectin and P-selectin are viable and fertile [125].

Anti-inflammation as an anti-cancer therapeutic opportunity

Because of the essential tumor-promoting functions played by the large variety of pro-angiogenic growth factors, cytokines, chemokines, and proteinases secreted by tumor-infiltrating leukocytes, it is tempting to explore the utility of anti-inflammatory drugs as anti-cancer therapeutics to inhibit tumor angiogenesis and metastasis. This rationale is strongly supported by the significant correlation between long-term use of aspirin and NSAIDs and the reduction of cancer risks [3, 4]. It is now becoming clear that NSAIDs inhibit tumor angiogenesis by their ability to attenuate cyclooxygenase-2 (COX-2) activity, a key enzyme in converting arachidonic acid to prostaglandins, which in turn induce inflammatory reactions [126]. In a recent study, a specific COX-2 inhibitor, celecoxib, was tested on familial adenomatous polyposis patients in a double-blind placebo-controlled study [127]. Six months of twice-daily treatment with 400 mg led to a significant reduction in the colorectal polyp burden.

TNFα is one of the most important mediators of inflammation and has been linked to the stimulation of angiogenesis by inducing the production of angiogenic factors, chemokines, and MMPs and by stimulating fibroblast growth and function [128]. Therefore, blocking TNFα bioactivity or inhibiting TNFα production may represent an attractive anti-cancer therapy. In rheumatoid arthritis patients, anti-TNFα antibody inhibited cytokine production, reduced angiogenesis, prevented leukocyte infiltrate into the joints, reduced plasma levels of MMPs, and improved bone marrow function. All these actions would be useful in a biological therapy for cancer [128].

In addition to TNFα antagonists, less-specific anti-inflammatory agents may also have some place in cancer therapy. Thalidomide inhibits the processing of mRNA for cytokines such as TNFα and VEGF. Continuous low-dose thalidomide has shown activity in a study of 84 previously treated patients with advanced myeloma [129]. Thalidomide also induced modest anti-tumor responses in malignant glioma [130].

As our understanding and appreciation of the role of inflammation in cancer progression evolves, it is clear that new therapeutic opportunities for treating cancer are emerging. Tumor angiogenesis is a complex process that is intimately linked to inflammation. Inflammation induces angiogenesis and angiogenesis further stimulates inflammation, both processes leading to tumor growth, metastasis and disease progression. Breaking this cycle by inhibiting targets such as cytokines, chemokines, and other inflammatory mediators, either alone or more realistically in combination with other therapies such as anti-angiogenics or classic cytotoxics, may provide highly efficacious therapies for the treatment of malignancies. With recent encouraging progress in the development of anti-angiogenic therapeutics, exampled by the clinical success of Avastin (an anti-VEGF monoclonal antibody) [131], it becomes more attractive to explore the use of anti-inflammatory drugs for oncology by testing their anti-angiogenic properties. However, when considering using anti-inflammatory strategies for anti-cancer therapies, one should carefully consider the potential consequences of inhibiting immune and inflammatory cells which also participate in anti-tumor immune surveillance. With their capacity to elicit cytotoxic responses and phagocytic activity, these cells undoubtedly are integral components of the first-line defense system of the body's response to fight cancer, and are the basis for anti-cancer immunotherapy. In addition, various proteinases expressed by tumor-infiltrating leukocytes are also capable of cleaving endogenous proteins to generate protein fragments with anti-angiogenic properties [132, 133]. Therefore, the challenge for clinical oncologists and experimental cancer researchers will be to identify the appropriate molecular targets, cancer types and disease stages for this type of therapy, and to optimize the therapeutic windows and regimens of anti-inflammatory cancer therapies. It is likely that a combination of these agents with another mode of therapy such as a cytotoxic, cytostatic, or anti-angiogenic drug may prove to be most effective. Selecting the appropriate patient population will likely involve the identification of a set of biomarkers to accurately reflect the nature of inflammatory responses in tumor tissues, and to reliably predict the benefits of such therapies.

References

1 Westphal E, Mastzellen U (eds) (1891) *Farbenanalytische Untersuchuugen zur Histologie und Klinik des Blutes: Gesammelte Mitt(h)eilungen.* Hirschwald Press, Berlin

2 Coussens LM, Werb Z (2002) Inflammation and cancer. *Nature* 420: 860–867

3 Baron JA, Sandler RS (2000) Nonsteroidal anti-inflammatory drugs and cancer prevention. *Annu Rev Med* 51: 511–523

4 Bosetti C, Gallus S, La Vecchia C (2002) Aspirin and cancer risk: an update to 2001. *Eur J Cancer Prev* 11: 535–542

5 Folkman J (1995) Seminars in Medicine of the Beth Israel Hospital, Boston. Clinical applications of research on angiogenesis. *N Engl J Med* 333: 1757–1763

6 O'Byrne KJ, Dalgleish AG, Browning MJ, Steward WP, Harris AL (2000) The relationship between angiogenesis and the immune response in carcinogenesis and the progression of malignant disease. *Eur J Cancer* 36: 151–169

7 Hyder SM, Stancel GM (1999) Regulation of angiogenic growth factors in the female reproductive tract by estrogens and progestins. *Mol Endocrinol* 13: 806–811

8 Folkman J (1995) Angiogenesis in cancer, vascular, rheumatoid and other disease. *Nat Med* 1: 27–31

9 Hanahan D (1998) A flanking attack on cancer. *Nat Med* 4: 13–14

10 Koch AE (1998) Review: angiogenesis: implications for rheumatoid arthritis. *Arthritis Rheum* 41: 951–962
11 Creamer D, Sullivan D, Bicknell R, Barker J (2002) Angiogenesis in psoriasis. *Angiogenesis* 5: 231–236
12 Ferrara N, Alitalo K (1999) Clinical applications of angiogenic growth factors and their inhibitors. *Nat Med* 5: 1359–1364
13 Madri JA, Graesser D (2000) Cell migration in the immune system: the evolving interrelated roles of adhesion molecules and proteinases. *Dev Immunol* 7: 103–116
14 Balkwill F, Mantovani A (2001) Inflammation and cancer: back to Virchow? *Lancet* 357: 539–545
15 Homey B, Muller A, Zlotnik A (2002) Chemokines: agents for the immunotherapy of cancer? *Nat Rev Immunol* 2: 175–184
16 Rossi D, Zlotnik A (2000) The biology of chemokines and their receptors. *Annu Rev Immunol* 18: 217–242
17 Negus RP, Stamp GW, Relf MG, Burke F, Malik ST, Bernasconi S, Allavena P, Sozzani S, Mantovani A, Balkwill FR (1995) The detection and localization of monocyte chemoattractant protein-1 (MCP-1) in human ovarian cancer. *J Clin Invest* 95: 2391–2396
18 Luboshits G, Shina S, Kaplan O, Engelberg S, Nass D, Lifshitz-Mercer B, Chaitchik S, Keydar I, Ben-Baruch A (1999) Elevated expression of the CC chemokine regulated on activation, normal T cell expressed and secreted (RANTES) in advanced breast carcinoma. *Cancer Res* 59: 4681–4687
19 Sidky YA, Auerbach R (1975) Lymphocyte-induced angiogenesis: a quantitative and sensitive assay of the graft-vs.-host reaction. *J Exp Med* 141: 1084–1100
20 Polverini PJ, Cotran PS, Gimbrone MA Jr, Unanue ER (1977) Activated macrophages induce vascular proliferation. *Nature* 269: 804–806
21 Camussi G, Montrucchio G, Lupia E, Soldi R, Comoglio PM, Bussolino F (1997) Angiogenesis induced *in vivo* by hepatocyte growth factor is mediated by platelet-activating factor synthesis from macrophages. *J Immunol* 158: 1302–1309
22 Koch AE, Polverini PJ, Kunkel SL, Harlow LA, DiPietro LA, Elner VM, Elner SG, Strieter RM (1992) Interleukin-8 as a macrophage-derived mediator of angiogenesis. *Science* 258: 1798–1801
23 Hashimoto M, Shingu M, Ezaki I, Nobunaga M, Minamihara M, Kato K, Sumioki H (1994) Production of soluble ICAM-1 from human endothelial cells induced by IL-1 beta and TNF-alpha. *Inflammation* 18: 163–173
24 Freeman MR, Schneck FX, Gagnon ML, Corless C, Soker S, Niknejad K, Peoples GE, Klagsbrun M (1995) Peripheral blood T lymphocytes and lymphocytes infiltrating human cancers express vascular endothelial growth factor: a potential role for T cells in angiogenesis. *Cancer Res* 55: 4140–4145
25 Lewis JS, Landers RJ, Underwood JC, Harris AL, Lewis CE (2000) Expression of vascular endothelial growth factor by macrophages is up-regulated in poorly vascularized areas of breast carcinomas. *J Pathol* 192: 150–158

26 Lewis JS, Lee JA, Underwood JC, Harris AL, Lewis CE (1999) Macrophage responses to hypoxia: relevance to disease mechanisms. *J Leukoc Biol* 66: 889–900
27 Goede V, Brogelli L, Ziche M, Augustin HG (1999) Induction of inflammatory angiogenesis by monocyte chemoattractant protein-1. *Int J Cancer* 82: 765–770
28 Ohta M, Kitadai Y, Tanaka S, Yoshihara M, Yasui W, Mukaida N, Haruma K, Chayama K (2003) Monocyte chemoattractant protein-1 expression correlates with macrophage infiltration and tumor vascularity in human gastric carcinomas. *Int J Oncol* 22: 773–778
29 Ohta M, Kitadai Y, Tanaka S, Yoshihara M, Yasui W, Mukaida N, Haruma K, Chayama K (2002) Monocyte chemoattractant protein-1 expression correlates with macrophage infiltration and tumor vascularity in human esophageal squamous cell carcinomas. *Int J Cancer* 102: 220–224
30 Leung SY, Wong MP, Chung LP, Chan AS, Yuen ST (1997) Monocyte chemoattractant protein-1 expression and macrophage infiltration in gliomas. *Acta Neuropathol (Berl)* 93: 518–527
31 Takeshima H, Kuratsu J, Takeya M, Yoshimura T, Ushio Y (1994) Expression and localization of messenger RNA and protein for monocyte chemoattractant protein-1 in human malignant glioma. *J Neurosurg* 80: 1056–1062
32 Sato K, Kuratsu J, Takeshima H, Yoshimura T, Ushio Y (1995) Expression of monocyte chemoattractant protein-1 in meningioma. *J Neurosurg* 82: 874–878
33 Saji H, Koike M, Yamori T, Saji S, Seiki M, Matsushima K, Toi M (2001) Significant correlation of monocyte chemoattractant protein-1 expression with neovascularization and progression of breast carcinoma. *Cancer* 92: 1085–1091
34 Ueno T, Toi M, Saji H, Muta M, Bando H, Kuroi K, Koike M, Inadera H, Matsushima K (2000) Significance of macrophage chemoattractant protein-1 in macrophage recruitment, angiogenesis, and survival in human breast cancer. *Clin Cancer Res* 6: 3282–3289
35 Crowther M, Brown NJ, Bishop ET, Lewis CE (2001) Microenvironmental influence on macrophage regulation of angiogenesis in wounds and malignant tumors. *J Leukoc Biol* 70: 478–490
36 Yan L, Kesavan P, Stowell N, McCabe F, Griswold D, Das A, Nakada M (2003) Contribution of inflammatory cells in tumor angiogenesis: MCP-1 and tumor angiogenesis. *Proceedings of AACR-NCI-EORTC International Conference, Molecular Targets and Cancer Therapeutics* 132
37 Tang R, Beuvon F, Ojeda M, Mosseri V, Pouillart P, Scholl S (1992) M-CSF (monocyte colony stimulating factor) and M-CSF receptor expression by breast tumour cells: M-CSF mediated recruitment of tumour infiltrating monocytes? *J Cell Biochem* 50: 350–356
38 Scholl SM, Pallud C, Beuvon F, Hacene K, Stanley ER, Rohrschneider L, Tang R, Pouillart P, Lidereau R (1994) Anti-colony-stimulating factor-1 antibody staining in primary breast adenocarcinomas correlates with marked inflammatory cell infiltrates and prognosis. *J Natl Cancer Inst* 86: 120–126

39 Kacinski BM (1995) CSF-1 and its receptor in ovarian, endometrial and breast cancer. *Ann Med* 27: 79–85
40 Chambers SK, Wang Y, Gertz RE, Kacinski BM (1995) Macrophage colony-stimulating factor mediates invasion of ovarian cancer cells through urokinase. *Cancer Res* 55: 1578–1585
41 Varney ML, Olsen KJ, Mosley RL, Bucana CD, Talmadge JE, Singh RK (2002) Monocyte/macrophage recruitment, activation and differentiation modulate interleukin-8 production: a paracrine role of tumor-associated macrophages in tumor angiogenesis. *In Vivo* 16: 471–477
42 Aharinejad S, Abraham D, Paulus P, Abri H, Hofmann M, Grossschmidt K, Schafer R, Stanley ER, Hofbauer R (2002) Colony-stimulating factor-1 antisense treatment suppresses growth of human tumor xenografts in mice. *Cancer Res* 62: 5317–5324
43 Lin EY, Nguyen AV, Russell RG, Pollard JW (2001) Colony-stimulating factor 1 promotes progression of mammary tumors to malignancy. *J Exp Med* 193: 727–740
44 Nowicki A, Szenajch J, Ostrowska G, Wojtowicz A, Wojtowicz K, Kruszewski AA, Maruszynski M, Aukerman SL, Wiktor-Jedrzejczak W (1996) Impaired tumor growth in colony-stimulating factor 1 (CSF-1)-deficient, macrophage-deficient op/op mouse: evidence for a role of CSF-1-dependent macrophages in formation of tumor stroma. *Int J Cancer* 65: 112–119
45 Leek RD, Harris AL, Lewis CE (1994) Cytokine networks in solid human tumors: regulation of angiogenesis. *J Leukoc Biol* 56: 423–435
46 Leek RD, Hunt NC, Landers RJ, Lewis CE, Royds JA, Harris AL (2000) Macrophage infiltration is associated with VEGF and EGFR expression in breast cancer. *J Pathol* 190: 430–436
47 Yeo KT, Wang HH, Nagy JA, Sioussat TM, Ledbetter SR, Hoogewerf AJ, Zhou Y, Masse EM, Senger DR, Dvorak HF et al (1993) Vascular permeability factor (vascular endothelial growth factor) in guinea pig and human tumor and inflammatory effusions. *Cancer Res* 53: 2912–2918
48 Talmor M, Mirza A, Turley S, Mellman I, Hoffman LA, Steinman RM (1998) Generation or large numbers of immature and mature dendritic cells from rat bone marrow cultures. *Eur J Immunol* 28: 811–817
49 Allavena P, Sica A, Vecchi A, Locati M, Sozzani S, Mantovani A (2000) The chemokine receptor switch paradigm and dendritic cell migration: its significance in tumor tissues. *Immunol Rev* 177: 141–149
50 Hiromatsu Y, Toda S (2003) Mast cells and angiogenesis. Microsc Res Tech 60: 64–69
51 Norrby K (2002) Mast cells and angiogenesis. *APMIS* 110: 355–371
52 Starkey JR, Crowle PK, Taubenberger S (1988) Mast-cell-deficient W/Wv mice exhibit a decreased rate of tumor angiogenesis. *Int J Cancer* 42: 48–52
53 Lillard JW Jr, Boyaka PN, Chertov O, Oppenheim JJ, McGhee JR (1999) Mechanisms for induction of acquired host immunity by neutrophil peptide defensins. *Proc Natl Acad Sci USA* 96: 651–656
54 Lloyd AR, Oppenheim JJ (1992) Poly's lament: the neglected role of the polymor-

phonuclear neutrophil in the afferent limb of the immune response. *Immunol Today* 13: 169–172
55 Gaudry M, Bregerie O, Andrieu V, El Benna J, Pocidalo MA, Hakim J (1997) Intracellular pool of vascular endothelial growth factor in human neutrophils. *Blood* 90: 4153–4161
56 McCourt M, Wang JH, Sookhai S, Redmond HP (1999) Proinflammatory mediators stimulate neutrophil-directed angiogenesis. *Arch Surg* 134: 1325–1331; discussion 1331–1332
57 Kibbey MC, Corcoran ML, Wahl LM, Kleinman HK (1994) Laminin SIKVAV peptide-induced angiogenesis *in vivo* is potentiated by neutrophils. *J Cell Physiol* 160: 185–193
58 Shamamian P, Schwartz JD, Pocock BJ, Monea S, Whiting D, Marcus SG, Mignatti P (2001) Activation of progelatinase A (MMP-2) by neutrophil elastase, cathepsin G, and proteinase-3: a role for inflammatory cells in tumor invasion and angiogenesis. *J Cell Physiol* 189: 197–206
59 Hubner G, Brauchle M, Smola H, Madlener M, Fassler R, Werner S (1996) Differential regulation of pro-inflammatory cytokines during wound healing in normal and glucocorticoid-treated mice. *Cytokine* 8: 548–556
60 Benelli R, Morini M, Carrozzino F, Ferrari N, Minghelli S, Santi L, Cassatella M, Noonan DM, Albini A (2002) Neutrophils as a key cellular target for angiostatin: implications for regulation of angiogenesis and inflammation. *FASEB J* 16: 267–269
61 Mach F, Schonbeck U, Fabunmi RP, Murphy C, Atkinson E, Bonnefoy JY, Graber P, Libby P (1999) T lymphocytes induce endothelial cell matrix metalloproteinase expression by a CD40L-dependent mechanism: implications for tubule formation. *Am J Pathol* 154: 229–238
62 Numasaki M, Fukushi J, Ono M, Narula SK, Zavodny PJ, Kudo T, Robbins PD, Tahara H, Lotze MT (2003) Interleukin-17 promotes angiogenesis and tumor growth. *Blood* 101: 2620–2627
63 Ferrara N (1997) The role of vascular endothelial growth factor in the regulation of blood vessel growth. In: Bicknell R, Lewis CE, Ferrara N (eds): *Tumor angiogenesis*. Oxford University Press, Oxford, 185–199
64 Dvorak HF (2002) Vascular permeability factor/vascular endothelial growth factor: a critical cytokine in tumor angiogenesis and a potential target for diagnosis and therapy. *J Clin Oncol* 20: 4368–4380
65 Harris AL (2002) Hypoxia – a key regulatory factor in tumour growth. *Nat Rev Cancer* 2: 38–47
66 Clauss M, Gerlach M, Gerlach H, Brett J, Wang F, Familletti PC, Pan YC, Olander JV, Connolly DT, Stern D (1990) Vascular permeability factor: a tumor-derived polypeptide that induces endothelial cell and monocyte procoagulant activity, and promotes monocyte migration. *J Exp Med* 172: 1535–1545
67 Dvorak HF, Sioussat TM, Brown LF, Berse B, Nagy JA, Sotrel A, Manseau EJ, Van de Water L, Senger DR (1991) Distribution of vascular permeability factor (vascular

endothelial growth factor) in tumors: concentration in tumor blood vessels. *J Exp Med* 174: 1275–1278

68 Sunderkotter C, Steinbrink K, Goebeler M, Bhardwaj R, Sorg C (1994) Macrophages and angiogenesis. *J Leukoc Biol* 55: 410–422

69 Kandel J, Bossy-Wetzel E, Radvanyi F, Klagsbrun M, Folkman J, Hanahan D (1991) Neovascularization is associated with a switch to the export of bFGF in the multistep development of fibrosarcoma. *Cell* 66: 1095–1104

70 Alvarez JA, Baird A, Tatum A, Daucher J, Chorsky R, Gonzalez AM, Stopa EG (1992) Localization of basic fibroblast growth factor and vascular endothelial growth factor in human glial neoplasms. *Mod Pathol* 5: 303–307

71 Sumizawa T, Furukawa T, Haraguchi M, Yoshimura A, Takeyasu A, Ishizawa M, Yamada Y, Akiyama S (1993) Thymidine phosphorylase activity associated with platelet-derived endothelial cell growth factor. *J Biochem (Tokyo)* 114: 9–14

72 Miyadera K, Sumizawa T, Haraguchi M, Yoshida H, Konstanty W, Yamada Y, Akiyama S (1995) Role of thymidine phosphorylase activity in the angiogenic effect of platelet derived endothelial cell growth factor/thymidine phosphorylase. *Cancer Res* 55: 1687–1690

73 Haraguchi M, Miyadera K, Uemura K, Sumizawa T, Furukawa T, Yamada K, Akiyama S, Yamada Y (1994) Angiogenic activity of enzymes. *Nature* 368: 198

74 Giatromanolaki A, Koukourakis MI, Kakolyris S, Kaklamanis L, Barbatis K, O'Byrne KJ, Theodosssiou D, Harris AL, Gatter KC (1998) Focal expression of thymidine phosphorylase associates with CD31 positive lymphocytic aggregation and local neo-angiogenesis in non-small cell lung cancer. *AntiCancer Res* 18: 71–76

75 Matsumura M, Chiba Y, Lu C, Amaya H, Shimomatsuya T, Horiuchi T, Muraoka R, Tanigawa N (1998) Platelet-derived endothelial cell growth factor/thymidine phosphorylase expression correlated with tumor angiogenesis and macrophage infiltration in colorectal cancer. *Cancer Lett* 128: 55–63

76 Nagaoka H, Iino Y, Takei H, Morishita Y (1998) Platelet-derived endothelial cell growth factor/thymidine phosphorylase expression in macrophages correlates with tumor angiogenesis and prognosis in invasive breast cancer. *Int J Oncol* 13: 449–454

77 Yao Y, Kubota T, Sato K, Kitai R (2001) Macrophage infiltration-associated thymidine phosphorylase expression correlates with increased microvessel density and poor prognosis in astrocytic tumors. *Clin Cancer Res* 7: 4021–4026

78 Tanaka Y, Kobayashi H, Suzuki M, Kanayama N, Terao T (2002) Thymidine phosphorylase expression in tumor-infiltrating macrophages may be correlated with poor prognosis in uterine endometrial cancer. *Hum Pathol* 33: 1105–1113

79 Dinarello CA (1996) Biologic basis for interleukin-1 in disease. *Blood* 87: 2095–2147

80 Saijo Y, Tanaka M, Miki M, Usui K, Suzuki T, Maemondo M, Hong X, Tazawa R, Kikuchi T, Matsushima K et al (2002) Proinflammatory cytokine IL-1 beta promotes tumor growth of Lewis lung carcinoma by induction of angiogenic factors: *in vivo* analysis of tumor-stromal interaction. *J Immunol* 169: 469–475

81 Chirivi RG, Chiodoni C, Musiani P, Garofalo A, Bernasconi S, Colombo MP, Giavazzi

R (1996) IL-1alpha gene-transfected human melanoma cells increase tumor-cell adhesion to endothelial cells and their retention in the lung of nude mice. *Int J Cancer* 67: 856–863

82 Voronov E, Shouval DS, Krelin Y, Cagnano E, Benharroch D, Iwakura Y, Dinarello CA, Apte RN (2003) IL-1 is required for tumor invasiveness and angiogenesis. *Proc Natl Acad Sci USA* 100: 2645–2650

83 Toi M, Harris AL, Bicknell R (1991) Interleukin-4 is a potent mitogen for capillary endothelium. *Biochem Biophys Res Commun* 174: 1287–1293

84 Fukushi J, Morisaki T, Shono T, Nishie A, Torisu H, Ono M, Kuwano M (1998) Novel biological functions of interleukin-4: formation of tube-like structures by vascular endothelial cells *in vitro* and angiogenesis *in vivo*. *Biochem Biophys Res Commun* 250: 444–448

85 Yao L, Pan J, Setiadi H, Patel KD, McEver RP (1996) Interleukin 4 or oncostatin M induces a prolonged increase in P-selectin mRNA and protein in human endothelial cells. *J Exp Med* 184: 81–92

86 Fukushi J, Ono M, Morikawa W, Iwamoto Y, Kuwano M (2000) The activity of soluble VCAM-1 in angiogenesis stimulated by IL-4 and IL-13. *J Immunol* 165: 2818–2823

87 Lee IY, Kim J, Ko EM, Jeoung EJ, Kwon YG, Choe J (2002) Interleukin-4 inhibits the vascular endothelial growth factor- and basic fibroblast growth factor-induced angiogenesis *in vitro*. *Mol Cells* 14: 115–121

88 Tartour E, Gey A, Sastre-Garau X, Pannetier C, Mosseri V, Kourilsky P, Fridman WH (1994) Analysis of interleukin 6 gene expression in cervical neoplasia using a quantitative polymerase chain reaction assay: evidence for enhanced interleukin 6 gene expression in invasive carcinoma. *Cancer Res* 54: 6243–6248

89 Wei LH, Kuo ML, Chen CA, Chou CH, Lai KB, Lee CN, Hsieh CY (2003) Interleukin-6 promotes cervical tumor growth by VEGF-dependent angiogenesis *via* a STAT3 pathway. *Oncogene* 22: 1517–1527

90 Kitadai Y, Takahashi Y, Haruma K, Naka K, Sumii K, Yokozaki H, Yasui W, Mukaida N, Ohmoto Y, Kajiyama G et al (1999) Transfection of interleukin-8 increases angiogenesis and tumorigenesis of human gastric carcinoma cells in nude mice. *Br J Cancer* 81: 647–653

91 Singh RK, Varney ML (2000) IL-8 expression in malignant melanoma: implications in growth and metastasis. *Histol Histopathol* 15: 843–849

92 Kitadai Y, Haruma K, Sumii K, Yamamoto S, Ue T, Yokozaki H, Yasui W, Ohmoto Y, Kajiyama G, Fidler IJ et al (1998) Expression of interleukin-8 correlates with vascularity in human gastric carcinomas. *Am J Pathol* 152: 93–100

93 Masuya D, Huang C, Liu D, Kameyama K, Hayashi E, Yamauchi A, Kobayashi S, Haba R, Yokomise H (2001) The intratumoral expression of vascular endothelial growth factor and interleukin-8 associated with angiogenesis in nonsmall cell lung carcinoma patients. *Cancer* 92: 2628–2638

94 Singh RK, Varney ML, Bucana CD, Johansson SL (1999) Expression of interleukin-8 in primary and metastatic malignant melanoma of the skin. *Melanoma Res* 9: 383–387

95 Eisma RJ, Spiro JD, Kreutzer DL (1999) Role of angiogenic factors: coexpression of interleukin-8 and vascular endothelial growth factor in patients with head and neck squamous carcinoma. *Laryngoscope* 109: 687–693
96 Vicari AP, Caux C (2002) Chemokines in cancer. *Cytokine Growth Factor Rev* 13: 143–154
97 Strieter RM, Polverini PJ, Kunkel SL, Arenberg DA, Burdick MD, Kasper J, Dzuiba J, Van Damme J, Walz A, Marriott D et al (1995) The functional role of the ELR motif in CXC chemokine-mediated angiogenesis. *J Biol Chem* 270: 27348–27357
98 Liss C, Fekete MJ, Hasina R, Lam CD, Lingen MW (2001) Paracrine angiogenic loop between head-and-neck squamous-cell carcinomas and macrophages. *Int J Cancer* 93: 781–785
99 Isik FF, Rand RP, Gruss JS, Benjamin D, Alpers CE (1996) Monocyte chemoattractant protein-1 mRNA expression in hemangiomas and vascular malformations. *J Surg Res* 61: 71–76
100 Salcedo R, Ponce ML, Young HA, Wasserman K, Ward JM, Kleinman HK, Oppenheim JJ, Murphy WJ (2000) Human endothelial cells express CCR2 and respond to MCP-1: direct role of MCP-1 in angiogenesis and tumor progression. *Blood* 96: 34–40
101 Belperio JA, Keane MP, Arenberg DA, Addison CL, Ehlert JE, Burdick MD, Strieter RM (2000) CXC chemokines in angiogenesis. *J Leukoc Biol* 68: 1–8
102 Fett JW, Strydom DJ, Lobb RR, Alderman EM, Bethune JL, Riordan JF, Vallee BL (1985) Isolation and characterization of angiogenin, an angiogenic protein from human carcinoma cells. *Biochemistry* 24: 5480–5486
103 Hu GF, Riordan JF, Vallee BL (1997) A putative angiogenin receptor in angiogenin-responsive human endothelial cells. *Proc Natl Acad Sci USA* 94: 2204–2209
104 Hu G, Riordan JF, Vallee BL (1994) Angiogenin promotes invasiveness of cultured endothelial cells by stimulation of cell-associated proteolytic activities. *Proc Natl Acad Sci USA* 91: 12096–12100
105 Etoh T, Shibuta K, Barnard GF, Kitano S, Mori M (2000) Angiogenin expression in human colorectal cancer: the role of focal macrophage infiltration. *Clin Cancer Res* 6: 3545–3551
106 Chopra V, Dinh TV, Hannigan EV (1997) Serum levels of interleukins, growth factors and angiogenin in patients with endometrial cancer. *J Cancer Res Clin Oncol* 123: 167–172
107 Chopra VV, Dinh TV, Hannigan EV (1996) Angiogenin, interleukins, and growth-factor levels in serum of patients with ovarian cancer: correlation with angiogenesis. *Cancer J Sci Am* 2: 279
108 Coussens LM, Tinkle CL, Hanahan D, Werb Z (2000) MMP-9 supplied by bone marrow-derived cells contributes to skin carcinogenesis. *Cell* 103: 481–490
109 Lewis CE, Leek R, Harris A, McGee JO (1995) Cytokine regulation of angiogenesis in breast cancer: the role of tumor-associated macrophages. *J Leukoc Biol* 57: 747–751
110 Pyke C, Graem N, Ralfkiaer E, Ronne E, Hoyer-Hansen G, Brunner N, Dano K (1993)

Receptor for urokinase is present in tumor-associated macrophages in ductal breast carcinoma. *Cancer Res* 53: 1911–1915

111 Vlodavsky I, Eldor A, Haimovitz-Friedman A, Matzner Y, Ishai-Michaeli R, Lider O, Naparstek Y, Cohen IR, Fuks Z (1992) Expression of heparanase by platelets and circulating cells of the immune system: possible involvement in diapedesis and extravasation. *Invasion Metastasis* 12: 112–127

112 Vlodavsky I, Korner G, Ishai-Michaeli R, Bashkin P, Bar-Shavit R, Fuks Z (1990) Extracellular matrix-resident growth factors and enzymes: possible involvement in tumor metastasis and angiogenesis. *Cancer Metastasis Rev* 9: 203–226

113 Thompson WD, Smith EB, Stirk CM, Marshall FI, Stout AJ, Kocchar A (1992) Angiogenic activity of fibrin degradation products is located in fibrin fragment E. *J Pathol* 168: 47–53

114 Eliceiri BP, Cheresh DA (1999) The role of alphav integrins during angiogenesis: insights into potential mechanisms of action and clinical development. *J Clin Invest* 103: 1227–1230.

115 Bischoff J (1997) Cell adhesion and angiogenesis. *J Clin Invest* 100: S37–S39

116 Brooks PC, Stromblad S, Sanders LC, von Schalscha TL, Aimes RT, Stetler-Stevenson WG, Quigley JP, Cheresh DA (1996) Localization of matrix metalloproteinase MMP-2 to the surface of invasive cells by interaction with integrin alpha v beta 3. *Cell* 85: 683–693

117 Stromblad S, Becker JC, Yebra M, Brooks PC, Cheresh DA (1996) Suppression of p53 activity and p21WAF1/CIP1 expression by vascular cell integrin alphaVbeta3 during angiogenesis. *J Clin Invest* 98: 426–433

118 Petitclerc E, Stromblad S, von Schalscha TL, Mitjans F, Piulats J, Montgomery AM, Cheresh DA, Brooks PC (1999) Integrin alpha(v)beta3 promotes M21 melanoma growth in human skin by regulating tumor cell survival. *Cancer Res* 59: 2724–2730

119 Friedlander M, Brooks PC, Shaffer RW, Kincaid CM, Varner JA, Cheresh DA (1995) Definition of two angiogenic pathways by distinct alpha v integrins. *Science* 270: 1500–1502

120 Trikha M, Zhou Z, Nemeth JA, Chen Q, Sharp C, Emmell E, Giles-Komar J, Nakada MT (2004) CNTO 95, a fully human monoclonal antibody that inhibits alphav integrins, has antitumor and antiangiogenic activity *in vivo*. *Int J Cancer* 110: 326–335

121 Carmeliet P, Lampugnani MG, Moons L, Breviario F, Compernolle V, Bono F, Balconi G, Spagnuolo R, Oostuyse B, Dewerchin M et al (1999) Targeted deficiency or cytosolic truncation of the VE-cadherin gene in mice impairs VEGF-mediated endothelial survival and angiogenesis. *Cell* 98: 147–157

122 Brooks PC (1996) Cell adhesion molecules in angiogenesis. *Cancer Metastasis Rev* 15: 187–194

123 Koch AE, Halloran MM, Haskell CJ, Shah MR, Polverini PJ (1995) Angiogenesis mediated by soluble forms of E-selectin and vascular cell adhesion molecule-1. *Nature* 376: 517–519

124 Nguyen M, Strubel NA, Bischoff J (1993) A role for sialyl Lewis-X/A glycoconjugates in capillary morphogenesis. *Nature* 365: 267–269
125 Labow MA, Norton CR, Rumberger JM, Lombard-Gillooly KM, Shuster DJ, Hubbard J, Bertko R, Knaack PA, Terry RW, Harbison ML et al (1994) Characterization of E-selectin-deficient mice: demonstration of overlapping function of the endothelial selectins. *Immunity* 1: 709–720
126 Williams CS, Mann M, DuBois RN (1999) The role of cyclooxygenases in inflammation, cancer, and development. *Oncogene* 18: 7908–7916
127 Langman MJ, Cheng KK, Gilman EA, Lancashire RJ (2000) Effect of anti-inflammatory drugs on overall risk of common cancer: case-control study in general practice research database. *BMJ* 320: 1642–1646
128 Balkwill F (2002) Tumor necrosis factor or tumor promoting factor? *Cytokine Growth Factor Rev* 13: 135–141
129 Singhal S, Mehta J, Desikan R, Ayers D, Roberson P, Eddlemon P, Munshi N, Anaissie E, Wilson C, Dhodapkar M et al (1999) Antitumor activity of thalidomide in refractory multiple myeloma. *N Engl J Med* 341: 1565–1571
130 Fine HA, Figg WD, Jaeckle K, Wen PY, Kyritsis AP, Loeffler JS, Levin VA, Black PM, Kaplan R, Pluda JM et al (2000) Phase II trial of the antiangiogenic agent thalidomide in patients with recurrent high-grade gliomas. *J Clin Oncol* 18: 708–715
131 Hurwitz H, Fehrenbacher L, Cartwright T, Hainsworth J, Heim W, Berlin J, Griffing S, Novotny W, Holmgren E, Kabbinavar F (2003) Bevacizumab (a monoclonal antibody to vascular endothelial growth factor) prolongs survival in first-line colorectal cancer (CRC): Results of a phase III trial of bevacizumab in combination with bolus IFL (irinotecan, 5-fluorouracil, leucovorin) as first-line therapy in subest with metastatic CRC. *Proc Am Soc Clin Oncol* 22: Late breaking news
132 Falcone DJ, Khan KM, Layne T, Fernandes L (1998) Macrophage formation of angiostatin during inflammation. A byproduct of the activation of plasminogen. *J Biol Chem* 273: 31480–31485
133 Scapini P, Nesi L, Morini M, Tanghetti E, Belleri M, Noonan D, Presta M, Albini A, Cassatella MA (2002) Generation of biologically active angiostatin kringle 1–3 by activated human neutrophils. *J Immunol* 168: 5798–5804

Apoptotic responses common to cancer and inflammation

Barbara Fingleton[1] *and Howard C. Crawford*[2]

[1]Department of Cancer Biology, Vanderbilt University Medical Center, Nashville TN 37232-6840, USA; [2]Department of Pharmacological Sciences, SUNY, Stony Brook, NY, USA

Introduction – Basic apoptotic mechanisms

The pathobiology of chronic inflammation and of cancer share many common attributes. Both can be considered "nonhealing wounds" due to the loss of normal tissue integrity. Both show evidence of dysregulated proliferation of particular cell types and consequently both are associated with hyperplasias. In addition, both chronic inflammation and cancer are also dependent on subverting the process of programmed cell death. The term "apoptosis" was first coined over 30 years ago to describe the morphological phenomenon known as programmed cell death [1]. In that time, many researchers have teased out the intricate pathways responsible for generating apoptotic responses in various cell types and in different contexts. We can now broadly divide apoptotic responses into two main types, extrinsic and intrinsic, although these are not mutually exclusive.

The extrinsic or receptor-mediated pathway occurs when a cell-surface receptor such as CD95/Fas/Apo1 or other tumor necrosis factor receptor (TNFr) superfamily member is bound by its cognate ligand e.g. Fas ligand (FasL)/CD95L/Apo1L or tumor necrosis factor α (TNFα) [2]. Ligand binding causes the receptor to trimerize, and to recruit a death domain-containing protein such as Fas-associated death domain (FADD), which in turn recruits procaspase-8 through interactions of death effector domains on both the proenzyme and FADD (Fig. 1). This complex containing FADD and procaspase-8, when recruited to the cytoplasmic tail of a death receptor, is termed a death-induced signaling complex or DISC. Procaspase-8 autocatalytically activates, probably through proximity interactions [3], and this starts a caspase-activation cascade ultimately leading to activation of effector caspases, e.g. caspase-3 and -6. These caspases are responsible for the proteolysis of various cellular proteins associated with apoptosis, for instance lamin, as well as activation of CAD, the caspase-activated DNase that generates the characteristic nucleosomal fragments [4].

The intrinsic or mitochondrial pathway is dependent on changes in mitochondrial permeability, mediated through Bcl family proteins, such as Bax, and the release

Cancer and Inflammation, edited by Douglas W. Morgan, Ulf J. Forssmann and Marian T. Nakada

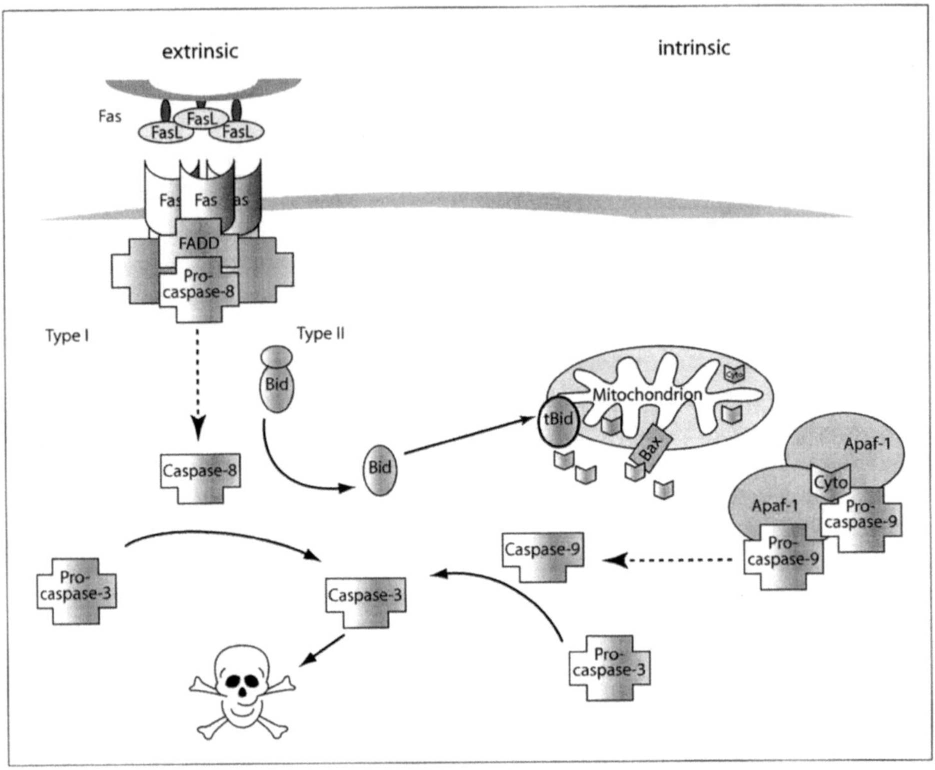

Figure 1
Extrinsic and intrinsic pathways of apoptosis. See text for explanation.
Cyt c, cytochrome C; FasL, Fas ligand; Apaf-1, apoptotic protease-activating factor 1.

of cytochrome C [5]. A complex called the apoptosome is formed consisting of released cytochrome C, apoptotic protease-activating factor 1 (Apaf-1) and procaspase-9 (Fig. 1). Oligomerization of Apaf-1, occurring after complex formation with cytochrome C, allows multiple procaspase-9 molecules to associate and activate by proximity interactions [6]. Processing of the procaspase occurs and a resultant caspase cascade leads to activation of effector caspases. As one of the examples of cross-talk between the two pathways, in some cell types caspase-8 not only results in direct activation of effector caspases but can also process another Bcl-2 proapoptotic family member Bid to the smaller tBid form that causes mitochondrial permeability and thus activation of the intrinsic pathway [7, 8].

Cells that use the receptor-mediated pathway have been subdivided into two categories, Type I and Type II [9, 10]. Type I cells are characterized by strong DISC formation in response to CD95 ligation with no cytochrome C release and, therefore, in these cells apoptosis cannot be inhibited by Bcl-2 or similar family members. Type I cells include thymocytes or fibroblasts, which have been shown to die in response to treatment with anti-Fas antibodies even in *Bid*-null mice [11]. Type II cells, on the other hand, use both receptor and mitochondrial pathways when a death receptor is activated. In these cells, receptor ligation results only in a weak procaspase-8 activation so amplification of the signal occurs through processing of Bid and consequent activation of the mitochondrial pathway. When this is the case, *Bcl-2* expression can block apoptosis induced by either extrinsic or intrinsic pathways. For example, hepatocytes exhibit massive cell death in response to anti-Fas antibody; however, those from *Bid*-null mice [11] or animals in which *Bcl-2* is overexpressed are protected [12, 13].

Another consequence of the activation of either apoptotic pathway is the translocation of phosphatidylserine to the outer cell membrane [14, 15]. This allows recognition of apoptotic cells by macrophages and their subsequent removal without generating an inflammatory response, one of the key hallmarks of the apoptotic process.

Apoptosis in cancer

Necessity for apoptosis

In their seminal review describing the process of tumorigenesis, Hanahan and Weinberg listed resistance to apoptosis as one of six necessary attributes for a tumor to develop [16]. Lessons learned from transgenic and knockout mice underscore the importance of apoptotic resistance in cancer development [17, 18]. Innate suicide mechanisms have evolved as safeguards against inappropriate accumulation of cells. Regulated growth is a balance between proliferative and death processes [19]. In tumors, both processes occur although the balance is frequently altered in favor of increased proliferation. As a mechanism of maintaining the appropriate balance, many proliferative signals can also induce cell death. A classic example is the E1A viral oncogenic protein. E1A induces proliferation *via* inactivation of the retinoblastoma (Rb) tumor suppressor. This leads to increased cell-cycle progression and thus proliferation. Loss of Rb function however also results in deregulated E2F transcription factor activity that directly induces p19ARF, an inducer of the pleiotropic signaling molecule p53, one function of which is to induce apoptosis. For E1A to successfully transform cells without triggering cell suicide, the p53 protective pathway must be bypassed [20]. Adenovirus can achieve this by co-expression with E1A of another viral gene E1B that acts to suppress apoptosis [21]. Hence E1A expression leads to both proliferative and apoptotic signals; however, the apoptotic signals can be selectively blocked by co-expression of E1B [22]. By studying the mechanisms through which E1B confers apoptotic repression, a number of pro- and anti-apoptotic molecules become apparent. p53 is one such pro-apoptotic molecule that often becomes mutated or lost in tumor cells, thus bypassing an innate suicide trigger. In fact, *TP53* (the gene that encodes p53) is the most commonly mutated gene in tumors [23].

Selection

What causes these protective mechanisms to be overcome? Is it a signal inherent to oncogenic signaling? As can be seen from the example with E1A, it is not necessarily the case that an oncogene will also confer apoptotic resistance. In fact, the opposite is often true. Due to effects on the cell cycle, some oncogenes actually promote apoptosis as a consequence of pushing toward proliferation, and triggering the apoptotic failsafe [24]. In a normal cell this would lead to cell death. In transformed cells where DNA mutations have arisen, some cells evolve mechanisms to counteract the death signal. For example, *TP53* may be mutated although this is frequently a late-stage mutation in many cancers. In some cells it is not the suicide signals from within but environmental pressures from without that force evolution of resistance. For example, we have shown that constant exposure to the death protein FasL of cells with functional components of the Fas pathway can select for a group of cells with the ability to evade that signal [25, 26]. The FasL may be from infiltrating immune cells or, in its solubilized version as generated by metalloproteinase activity, from cells adjacent to the nascent tumor. Another common selective pressure is loss of contact with extracellular matrix (ECM). Binding of cells to constituents of the ECM *via* cellular integrins is known to transmit survival signals and loss of these signals leads to a form of apoptosis known as anoikis [27, 28]. As tumors divide and lose their polarity, integrin binding and the attendant survival signals are frequently lost, forcing tumor cells to develop other methods of resisting cell death [29]. Hypoxia is another common feature of the tumor microenvironment. Low oxygen levels often cause cellular apoptosis through stress protein-mediated mitochondrial pathway activation. Tumor cells that can overcome these signals thus have a survival advantage; therefore, hypoxia acts as a selective pressure for cells with apoptotic resistance mechanisms [30].

Examples of resistance mechanisms

There are a myriad of ways in which tumor cells can evade a death signal. Here we discuss several of them.

The *Bcl-2* proto-oncogene was initially discovered associated with the breakpoint of a chromosomal translocation t(14:18) in B cell follicular lymphomas [31]. Further studies demonstrated that Bcl-2 was frequently overexpressed in tumors of

Table 1 - Mammalian members of the Bcl-2 family, subdivided into those that have been shown to act to inhibit apoptosis (anti-apoptotic) and those that induce it (pro-apoptotic).

Anti-apoptotic	**Pro-apoptotic**
Bcl-2	Bcl-X_S
Bcl-X_L	Bad
Bcl-w	Bid
A1	Bax
Mcl-1	Bok
	Bak
	Bik
	Bim
	Blk
	Mtd
	Nix
	Hrk

diverse origins [32]. Most importantly, it was the first oncogene discovered to function through a death-repressing rather than proliferation-promoting activity. This was established through studies in which overexpressed *Bcl-2* resulted in cell survival even in the face of potent death signals, e.g. growth factor withdrawal or γ-radiation. Conversely, downregulation of *Bcl-2* expression by antisense oligonucleotides led to cell death [33].

There are now known to be multiple Bcl-2 family members that can be divided into two distinct subgroups – those that promote and those that inhibit apoptosis (Tab. 1) [32]. Bcl family members interact by dimerization (both homo- and hetero-) and it is this process that controls whether pro- or anti-apoptotic signals are dominant. A number of animal studies have illustrated the advantages for a tumor of altering levels of specific Bcl-2 proteins. For example, overexpression of the oncogene *myc* leads to cellular transformation and tumor development; however, when combined with overexpression of the anti-apoptotic molecule Bcl-2, tumorigenesis is accelerated [34, 35]. Conversely, reduced levels of the pro-apoptotic protein *Bax* could accelerate mammary tumorigenesis in C3-SV40-TAg mice [36]. In this model, haploinsufficiency of Bax was sufficient to observe the effect. Also, it has been shown that survival signals from ECM are mediated through increased Bcl-2 or Bcl-X_L levels [37]. Perturbation of the integrin survival signal results in changes in subcellular localization of the pro-apoptotic protein Bax and subsequent cell death [38]. In tumor cells however, the levels of anti-apoptotic proteins do not fall and nor do pro-apoptotic Bcl proteins increase, with the end result being survival in the face of a normally potent death signal [39].

It has now become apparent that the Bcl-2 protein family can be controlled at multiple levels: transcriptional and post-transcriptional control of expression, protein turnover, conformation changes, proteolytic processing, and protein phosphorylation [32, 40]. Tumor cells have been shown to exploit all of these mechanisms to effect apoptotic resistance.

Expression of proteins known as inhibitors of apoptosis (IAPs) has recently gained prominence as a common resistance mechanism in cancers. IAPs were originally identified in baculovirus and found in many organisms from *Caenorhabditis elegans*, to *Drosophila* and mammals, indicating an ancient lineage [41] . There are eight known human IAPs: NAIP, cIAP1/HIAP-2, cIAP2/HIAP-1, XIAP, Livin, MLIAP, survivin and BRUCE, identified by the presence of one or more baculoviral IAP repeat (BIR) domain. These proteins act as inhibitors of the caspases, the proteolytic effectors of apoptosis. Survivin is one of the best-studied IAPs in human malignancies. Its expression appears to be mediated by at least two oncogenic pathways – p53 and the WNT/β-catenin pathway [42]. Survivin expression has been reported to be low in most adult human tissues; however, it is frequently overexpressed in many cancers and has been correlated with poor prognosis and survival of certain patient groups [43–47]. Targeted overexpression of survivin in mouse skin protects against ultraviolet radiation-induced apoptosis [48]. Conversely, livers from mice heterozygous for survivin demonstrated spontaneous apoptosis and increased susceptibility to Fas-induced cell death [49]. In addition, administration of antagonists of survivin was shown to suppress *in vivo* tumor growth. Homozygous deletion of survivin did not result in viable embryos due to defects in cell division, another role for this protein [50]. While survivin, like other IAPs, binds to caspases, it is thought that its principal mechanism of apoptosis inhibition is through modulation of the mitochondrial pathway.

The nuclear factor κB (NF-κB) family is another multi-protein family [51]. The most commonly expressed version consists of a heterodimer of Rel and p50, which is maintained in the cytoplasm in an inactive state through binding of inhibitory proteins of the inhibitor of κB (IκB) family. Specific cellular signals result in activity of kinases that phosphorylate IκB on particular serine residues. This phosphorylation event triggers ubiquitination and subsequent degradation by the proteasome of the inhibitor. Loss of the IκB protein frees the NF-κB dimer and it translocates to the nucleus where it can influence transcription of a variety of genes through binding to specific promoter elements. Many human cancer cell lines and samples from primary tumors have been shown to have constitutive NF-κB activity that may contribute to apoptotic resistance. This can be mediated through increased Bcl-2 expression, increased survivin expression or other molecules that directly interfere with various components of the apoptotic machinery. It is important to note however, that NF-κB is a multifunctional molecule and there are targets of this pathway that are pro-apoptotic, e.g. IEX-1 [52]. As with many molecules in cancer biology, the context i.e. the specific cell type and the other signals manifested concurrently, ultimately determines whether the dominant role of NF-κB activity is pro- or anti-apoptotic.

FADD-like IL-1β-converting enzyme (FLICE) inibitory protein (FLIP), a direct inhibitor of FasL signaling, is a molecule that binds to FADD and prevents procaspase-8 activation [53]. It is therefore a specific inhibitor of the extrinsic pathway [54] and is one of the mechanisms used to evade immune cell targeting of tumors. This was specifically demonstrated in a study using murine lymphoma cells transplanted into syngeneic mice [55]. Tumor cells expressing high levels of FLIP were significantly more tumorigenic than those with low levels and this occurred in mice wild-type or null for perforin, another molecule thought, like Fas, to be important for immune-mediated killing of tumor cells. In human patients, overexpression of FLIP has been reported in melanomas [54].

Apoptosis in immune cell control and inflammation

Much of what we know about apoptotic mechanisms has come from studies with immune cells. This is partly due to the ease with which immune cells, from both experimental animals and humans, can be obtained but also because the immune system is a prime example of the necessity for cell-death mechanisms to maintain homeostasis. When a foreign antigen is detected, immune responses ensure a rapid and, ideally, overwhelming targeting of the foreign material through expansion of B and T cells that specifically recognize that target. This is achieved through a complex network of cellular signaling mechanisms. One of the most important elements of the immune response is its rapid downregulation once the target has been neutralized. Dampening of the immune response is necessary as otherwise there would be an ever-increasing number of lymphocytes and effector cells capable of causing massive tissue destruction. Activation-induced cell death (AICD) is the predominant mechanism for maintenance of immune-system homeostasis. In AICD, lymphocytes use the Fas/FasL pathway to commit cellular suicide when they are no longer required [56]. Mice with mutations in either FasL (*gld* animals) or Fas (*lpr* animals) show very similar phenotypes, a general lymphoproliferative disorder that results in an excessive expansion of the lymphoid organs, e.g. thymus and spleen, and premature death of the animal [57, 58]. Humans with mutations or deletions of these genes also show lymphoproliferative and autoimmune symptoms [59, 60]. In addition, removal of self-reactive T and B lymphocytes necessary for immunological tolerance has been shown to require activation of Fas [61]. Resistance to Fas-mediated apoptosis in immune cells can therefore lead to serious pathological conditions such as autoimmunity, chronic inflammation or hematological cancers [62]. In most cases it is not defects in Fas or FasL but aberrant expression of signaling molecules downstream of the receptor that is responsible for resistance. These include many of the molecules already mentioned as being important in tumor development such as members of the Bcl family, NF-κB, and FLIP.

In response to damage caused by microbial pathogens or physical injury, the body exerts an inflammatory response. The purpose of the response is two-fold – to remove any extraneous pathogens and to induce tissue repair. Nearly 2000 years ago, the four hallmarks of inflammation were defined by the Roman scientist Celsus as "rubor, calor, dolor, tumor" that is redness, heat, pain, and swelling [63]. These are the symptoms of the chemical signals prostaglandins and cytokines, released by immune cells quickly recruited to the area of damage. Although uncomfortable these symptoms are a sign of an active repair process by the body. Chronic inflammatory states occur when this damage-control process is not appropriately downregulated.

The first sensors of injury are tissue-resident cells [64]. These can be macrophages (e.g. Kupffer cells of the liver or alveolar macrophages in the lung) or mast cells. Damaged tissue or microbial organisms release chemical signals detected by these sensor cells which in turn release their own set of signals – histamines, eicosonoids, and inflammatory cytokines such as TNFα. Dilation of nearby blood vessels and release of fluids from the vessels occurs as a result of these signals so allowing recruitment of additional inflammatory cells to the site. These physical changes manifest as the symptoms of inflammation described by Celsus. Neutrophils are activated through a combination of signals leading to the respiratory burst, degranulation, and hence release of a range of molecules including proteases (elastase, matrix metalloproteinase-8 (MMP-8), MMP-9), oxidants, and anti-bacterial proteins. Chemokines produced by mast cells, macrophages and neutrophils also serve to recruit lymphocytes. Cytotoxic T lymphocytes can kill infected or damaged cells by inducing apoptosis through Fas ligation or by using the perforin/granzyme system, which can activate the mitochondrial pathway [65]. Changes in the membranes of dying cells allow them to be recognized and engulfed by macrophages. Similarly, neutrophils that have performed their function are also cleared by macrophages. An inflammatory site therefore contains a variety of cell types and mix of proteases, reactive oxygen species, nitric oxide (NO) produced by inducible nitric oxide synthase (iNOS), an enzyme induced by inflammatory cells, and other chemicals, all with the task of removing terminally damaged tissue, remodeling the area of tissue damage and promoting tissue healing. Normally the process is tightly controlled and, upon resolution, immune cell activity and number are downregulated. However, in some cases resolution never occurs and a cycle of immune-mediated tissue destruction begins. In some cases, the persistent inflammatory state is related to autoimmune reactions where particular tissue antigens are viewed as foreign and thus provoke constant immune responses. This occurs for example in multiple sclerosis [66]. In other pathologies the etiology is not completely understood although autoimmune reactions may play a role, e.g. in inflammatory bowel diseases (IBDs) [67].

Apoptosis-resistant phenotypes have been described in a number of inflammatory diseases and efforts made to identify precisely the mechanisms associated with the resistance. For example, in clinically active multiple sclerosis, overexpression of the FLIP protein was observed in T cells and this correlated with the resistance of these cells to cell death [68]. IBDs can be divided into two subcategories – those that are Th1-associated such as Crohn's disease and those that evidence features of a Th2-mediated response such as ulcerative colitis [67]. In both types, the gut T cells involved demonstrate much-reduced sensitivity to apoptosis. This is both Fas-dependent (as used in AICD) and mitochondrially associated, illustrated by a resistance to lymphokine deficiency-induced apoptosis. Changes in expression of various Bcl family proteins have been detected in IBD patient samples and again correlated with apoptotic resistance [69–71]. In rheumatoid arthritis, several apoptosis-resistance mechanisms have been identified in both the inflammatory cells and the synovial fibroblasts that constitute the disease lesions [72].

Implications of apoptotic resistance: Inflammation as a cancer risk factor

Recently, the general concept that chronic inflammation is a risk factor for tumor formation has gained considerable momentum. Epidemiological studies have uncovered strong connections between chronic inflammation and carcinoma in the same tissue, particularly in the gastrointestinal and female reproductive tracts [73–80]. Chronic inflammation can arise from the persistence of a causative stimulus of acute inflammation or as a *de novo* response, with no apparent acute component. The chronic nature can be a result of infectious organisms resistant to immune response (e.g. *Helicobacter pylori* in the gastric mucosa, hepatitis virus in the liver, papilloma virus in the cervix), physical perturbations (e.g. ductal blockage in the pancreas or acid-reflux damage in Barrett's esophagus), or an autoimmune response (IBD). No matter the method of initiation, the persistence of inflammation assaults the target tissue with a morass of conflicting signals. As with an acute response, immune cells damage cells of the inflamed tissue and, in later stages, stimulate the target tissue to proliferate and heal. But in the chronic situation, with the inflammatory response unresolved, the tissue undergoes a constant cycle of destruction and healing; of death and proliferation. While the connection between chronic inflammation and cancer is certainly complex, there is some evidence that the constant bombardment of the target tissue with pro-apoptotic signals plays a significant role in the transition of chronic inflammation to neoplasia.

A number of groups have noted that persistent exposure of cells in culture to pro-apoptotic signals leads to cells resistant to apoptosis in general [25, 26, 81–83]. If this sort of selective process were to happen *in vivo*, by itself, it would be of little consequence. However, in the larger context of chronic inflammation, where the process is also promoting angiogenesis, proliferation, and genetic aberration, there is the very serious potential for full-blown apoptosis-resistant neoplastic transformation. Of course, the progression from chronic inflammation to neoplasia takes place gradually, and as such we can begin to dissect some of the cell-biological and molecular changes associated with chronic inflammation and early tumor progression. Not surprisingly, a number of these changes reflect alterations in the susceptibility of cells to apoptosis.

A pathological change common to tissues with chronic inflammation and early neoplasia is the presence of epithelial metaplasia, the apparent replacement of one predominant epithelial cell type with another. Metaplasia is most clearly recognized and documented in Barrett's esophagus, where the normal esophageal epithelium is replaced by what appears to be intestinal epithelium [84]. Similarly atrophic gastritis is frequently marked by intestinal metaplasia [85]. In the colon, a fairly common Paneth cell metaplasia is associated with ulcerative colitis [86]. In chronic pancreatitis, there is an apparent acinar-to-ductal-cell metaplasia [87]. Most importantly, in each case, the nearby normal epithelium is undergoing apoptosis whereas the metaplastic cells are recalcitrant to the death-inducing signals affecting their neighbors.

In pathology, the frequency with which metaplasia is found associated with cancer has led to the hypothesis that metaplasia is a potential cancer precursor. This is an attractive hypothesis considering the apparent plasticity of differentiation that metaplasia represents. However, it is also clear that these metaplastic cells are either not susceptible to or are able to actively escape the pro-apoptotic environment of the chronically inflamed state. Similar to the mechanisms that some cancers use to evade apoptosis, the majority of evidence suggests that metaplastic cells have activated anti-apoptotic pathways. The most commonly described mechanism of apoptotic resistance in metaplasia is expression of Bcl-2. The metaplastic atrophic gastritis [88], Barrett's esophagus [89], and chronic pancreatitis [90] have each been shown to express this anti-apoptotic factor. Expression of NF-κB is also commonly observed in the metaplastic epithelium of gastritis [91], hepatitis [92], and IBD [93, 94]. It is likely that other protective pathways commonly found in cancerous tissue are also active, but have yet to be examined.

Expression of anti-apoptotic molecules in metaplastic epithelium has serious implications for cancer risk. However, simple apoptotic resistance is not sufficient to give rise to a tumor. The proliferative nature of metaplastic epithelium certainly lends concomitant apoptotic resistance more weight, but even so, according to this model, enhanced expression of anti-apoptotic proteins is likely to disappear if the selective pressure of the inflammation can be resolved. Much more ominous is the recent association of iNOS activity with inactivating p53 mutations in colon cancer [95]. This is particularly interesting considering that iNOS is the predominant NOS expressed at sites of both inflammation and cancer and that the resulting overproduction of the free radical nitric oxide has been shown to lead to DNA damage and mutagenesis, primarily *via* reaction with molecular oxygen to form peroxynitrite. Intriguingly, low levels of NOS activity can itself protect from apoptosis in a p53-dependent manner, whereas high levels induce apoptosis also in a p53-dependent manner [96]. In chronic inflammation, where iNOS is the predominant NOS activity, NO levels tend to be high and, as such, contribute significantly to tissue destruction. It is tempting to speculate that the presumably random mutagenic activity of peroxynitrite should appear to more precisely target p53 inactivation, a phenomenon consistent with p53 mutation being a selective means to escape from NOS-induced apoptosis and form a more direct link between chronic inflammation and tumorigenesis. Consistent with this, a high proportion of ulcerative colitis samples have been shown to carry inactivating p53 mutations [95].

It is not obvious why metaplasia is associated with chronic inflammation. We have assumed that the metaplastic epithelia are not susceptible or are actively resistant to apoptosis, otherwise they would not be evident at all. However, with the multitude of signals provided by chronic inflammation, it is not yet known whether pro- or anti-apoptotic signals are required for the metaplastic transition. We have shown that genetic ablation of pro-apoptotic MMP-7 or FasL activities severely limited acinar-to-ductal metaplasia in chronic pancreatitis [26]. Similarly, diminishing apoptosis by inducing pancreatitis in a p53-null background also reduces ductal metaplasia [90]. While it is possible that these molecules have other signaling roles that influence metaplasia, it is intriguing to speculate that apoptotic resistance is intrinsic to these potential preneoplastic lesions and that upsetting the balance of either pro-apoptotic (selective pressure) or anti-apoptotic (protective signal) molecules would negatively influence their formation. Whatever the precise mechanisms involved, it is clear that the response of glandular tissue to chronic inflammation includes the genesis of cells, usually proliferative, that are resistant to apoptosis and frequently associated with early tumor progression.

Overcoming apoptotic resistance as a therapeutic approach

Selective resistance to apoptosis was first recognized as a major health-related problem with the recurrence of cancer following chemotherapy. Far too often the re-emergent tumor was unresponsive to the treatment protocol that appeared effective in prior attempts. It is now recognized that the majority of chemotherapeutic agents act by inducing apoptosis in their cellular targets [97, 98]. As the molecular pathways of apoptosis are better understood, it has become clear that the effects of selective pressure on a genetically unstable, rapidly dividing group of cells was usually temporary relief of the tumor burden, followed by the outgrowth of a subpopulation that carried advantageous resistant mutations. This is most evident with therapeutic agents that act through DNA damage (γ-radiation, 5-fluorouracil (5-FU), cisplatin, etc.), the apoptotic response normally being p53-dependent. Not surprisingly, tumors, especially late-stage tumors, initially resistant to these agents were found to have a high prevalence of inactivating p53 mutations [99]. Similarly, recurrence of resistant cancers from tumors initially responsive to these agents also were frequently found to have p53 mutations [100]. Over the years, evidence has accumulated to suggest that various other molecules responsible for resistance to apoptosis can be activated in chemoresistant tumors and other diseases [101–104]. Investigating methods that could modulate the function of these critical molecules has become a major activity in translational research and has resulted in some novel therapies currently being tested in the clinic.

As discussed previously, the pathology of IBD is related to excessive T cell activity in the gut. Investigative treatments for IBD include blocking particular pro-inflammatory cytokine pathways such as those mediated by interleukin-6 (IL-6) [105] or IL-12 [106, 107]. Blocking either of these pathways increases T cell apoptosis and ultimately results in attenuation of the inflammatory state. IL-12 blockade appears to influence Fas-dependent apoptosis through a pathway independent of Bcl-2 proteins whereas IL-6 blockade induces upregulation of pro-apoptotic Bcl-2 family members and thus promotes the mitochondrial pathway of apoptosis [108].

Inhibition of NF-κB has been demonstrated in a number of animal models to be an effective method of overcoming apoptotic resistance. In many cases this has been achieved by overexpression of a so-called "super-repressor" form of IκBα, which lacks the serine residues necessary for phosphorylation and therefore subsequent ubiquitination, thus preventing NF-κB translocation to the nucleus [101]. Additionally, non-steroidal anti-inflammatory drugs (NSAIDs) have been shown to act, at least in part, through modulation of NF-κB. For example, sulindac treatment can cause apoptotic cell death in colon cancer cells deficient in cyclo-oxygenase activity, the recognized target of this drug [109]. This is thought to be a result of inhibiting IκB kinase (IKK), the enzyme required to phosphorylate the repressor IκB. Proteasome inhibitors are another way of inhibiting NF-κB activity as proteasome-dependent degradation of IκB is necessary for release of the active NF-κB signaling molecule [110]. Velcade, previously known as PS-341, from Millennium Pharmaceuticals Inc. was recently approved by the US Food and Drug Administration (FDA) for use in relapsed and refractory multiple myeloma. It is the first proteasome inhibitor to receive FDA approval. Velcade is being tested in a number of ongoing clinical trials for a variety of indications, both as a single agent and in combination with chemotherapy [111]. As a general proteasome inhibitor, however, the effects of velcade are not limited to downregulation of NF-κB signaling and this non-specificity may be an issue with this agent or others like it. Another drug, PS-1145, has been identified as a potent NF-κB inhibitor through inhibition of IKK. Further development of this agent may allow specific inhibition of NF-κB to be achieved pharmacologically for the benefit of patients with cancers or inflammatory diseases.

Antisense strategies are also being therapeutically explored [112]. Both Bcl-2 and survivin have been targeted and molecules directed against each of them arc in clinical trials. Bcl-2 antisense, developed by Genta Inc. and known as Oblimersen/Genasense/G3139, has been tested clinically both as a single agent and in combination with chemotherapeutic agents [113]. The agent is tolerable with no dose-limiting toxicities reported in a phase I trial in patients with acute leukemia [114]. Preliminary indications are that it shows some efficacy on its own but it has significant value when used in combination. Importantly, clinical specimens from patients treated with this drug indicate successful down-modulation of the target *bcl-2* [115]. There are currently three different phase III trials recruiting patients in which chemotherapy alone *versus* chemotherapy plus antisense will be compared in patients with multiple myeloma, chronic lymphocytic leukemia, or small-cell lung cancer [116]. A further modification of the *bcl-2* antisense approach is the development of a bispecific antisense molecule that targets both *bcl-2* and $bcl\text{-}X_L$ [117]. This has been tested against a range of cell lines *in vitro* and against breast and colorectal tumor xenografts where it significantly inhibited tumor growth while reducing Bcl-2 and Bcl-X_L protein levels.

Survivin is upregulated early in the tumorigenic process and its expression correlated with poorer prognosis. Additionally, there is very limited expression in normal adult tissues – limited to thymocytes, bone marrow stem cells, and basal colonic epithelium – making it an attractive "tumor-specific" target [118]. There are several strategies to target survivin: (i) an immune-based mechanism using survivin peptides to generate a cytolytic T cell response targeting tumor cells; (ii) molecular antagonists including survivin-specific antisense and ribozymes to abrogate expression or dominant-negative mutants that abrogate survivin activity; and (iii) pharmacological approaches that target a specific phosphorylation event required for function e.g. use of flavopiridol [119]. The vaccine approach is supported by the demonstration that cytolytic T cells against survivin peptides can be found in patients with various cancers [120, 121]. All of these approaches have shown their potential usefulness in pre-clinical animal studies [119].

TNF-related apoptosis-inducing ligand (TRAIL) is, like FasL, a member of the TNF family of death-inducing ligands. TRAIL binds to two death receptors competent for signaling, DR4 and DR5, and also to several decoy receptors [2]. DR4 and DR5 are not expressed in normal tissues but are considerably overexpressed in a number of cancers. This suggests the use of TRAIL as an apoptosis-inducing agent specific for cancer cells [122]. Recombinant TRAIL was being explored as a therapeutic approach by Genentech and Immunex although its current status is unknown. Some doubts were raised as to whether this was a safe approach when it was shown that normal human hepatocytes were exquisitely sensitive to TRAIL exposure [123, 124].

The lipid kinase phosphoinositide 3-kinase and its downstream effector the serine/threonine kinase Akt, also known as protein kinase B, are activated as a result of many oncogenic pathways for example, Ras [125, 126]. One of the upstream inhibitors of this pathway, *PTEN* [127], is a gene frequently lost in early tumor development. The functions of this pathway are myriad and include effects on cell cycle, glucose metabolism, transcription, and cell motility [126]. Apoptosis and cell survival are also significantly affected. One way in which Akt signaling has been shown to downregulate apoptosis in tumor cells is through phosphorylation of pro-apoptotic Bcl family members thus blocking their function in increasing mitochondrial permeability. Another target is MDM-2, which when phosphorylated moves to the nucleus where it modulates the function of p53 [128]. Several agents in clinical trials (e.g. geldanamycin, UCN-01) have been shown to affect Akt and other specific inhibitors are being developed for use both as single agents and for use in combination with chemotherapy.

As stated earlier, *TP53* is a gene frequently mutated in cancers. One of its many functions is to promote apoptosis through the mitochondrial pathway. Restoration of normal p53 activity may therefore be expected to facilitate death signaling in cancer cells. Both biological and chemical approaches have been explored as ways to restore wild-type p53 signaling in tumors [129]. Biological methods include p53 gene therapy i.e. deliverance of a functional *TP53* gene into tumor cells that have lost it [130], and selective deletion of cells carrying mutant protein using genetically engineered virus [131] or by a vaccine-stimulated immune system [132]. There are currently a number of clinical trials sponsored by Introgen Therapeutics examining the effects of an adenovirus carrying wild-type p53 in patients with head and neck cancers and, in trials sponsored by the U.S. National Cancer Institute, in patients with lung cancers [116]. In addition a vaccine approach, where peptides specifically representing mutant p53 protein are injected into patients to stimulate an immune response against tumor cells, is being tested against ovarian cancer and other solid malignancies. Chemicals that can stabilize or activate the mutant p53 or modulate its interaction with other proteins are also in development [133, 134].

There are a number of other therapeutic avenues currently being explored which would lead to reinstatement of intact apoptotic signaling, although by means of indirect targets. Examples include inhibitors of histone deacetylase, heat-shock proteins or 3-hydroxy-3-methylglutaryl-CoA (HMG-CoA) reductase. For more information on these targets, the reader is referred to an excellent review discussing modulators of apoptosis as therapeutic agents for cancer [113].

In conclusion, apoptosis is an essential mechanism for control of cell number in many tissues and in the cells of the immune system. Mechanisms to inhibit apoptosis have evolved to allow fine control of the process and these have been subverted in the pathological states of chronic inflammation and tumor progression. Our increased understanding of the various molecules involved in the cell-death process and its inhibition has led to the rational design of therapeutic approaches to restore normal death-pathway signaling. Further refinement of these strategies combined with profiling of the particular pathways affected in individual patients will lead to effective methods of overcoming a whole range of pathological conditions and even chemoprevention approaches for patients at risk for tumor development following chronic inflammation.

References

1 Kerr JF, Wyllie AH, Currie AR (1972) Apoptosis: a basic biological phenomenon with wide-ranging implications in tissue kinetics. *Br J Cancer* 26: 239–257

2 Ashkenazi A, Dixit VM (1999) Apoptosis control by death and decoy receptors. *Curr Opin Cell Biol* 11: 255–260

3 Salvesen GS, Dixit VM (1999) Caspase activation: the induced-proximity model. *Proc Natl Acad Sci USA* 96: 10964–10967

4 Nagata S (2000) Apoptotic DNA fragmentation. *Exp Cell Res* 256: 12–18

5 Green DR, Reed JC (1998) Mitochondria and apoptosis. *Science* 281: 1309–1312

6 Saleh A, Srinivasula SM, Acharya S, Fishel R, Alnemri ES (1999) Cytochrome c and dATP-mediated oligomerization of Apaf-1 is a prerequisite for procaspase-9 activation. *J Biol Chem* 274: 17941–17945

7 Luo X, Budihardjo I, Zou H, Slaughter C, Wang X (1998) Bid, a Bcl2 interacting protein, mediates cytochrome c release from mitochondria in response to activation of cell surface death receptors. *Cell* 94: 481–490

8 Li H, Zhu H, Xu CJ, Yuan J (1998) Cleavage of BID by caspase 8 mediates the mitochondrial damage in the Fas pathway of apoptosis. *Cell* 94: 491–501

9 Scaffidi C, Fulda S, Srinivasan A, Friesen C, Li F, Tomaselli KJ, Debatin KM, Krammer PH, Peter ME (1998) Two CD95 (APO-1/Fas) signaling pathways. *EMBO J* 17: 1675–1687

10 Scaffidi C, Schmitz I, Zha J, Korsmeyer SJ, Krammer PH, Peter ME (1999) Differential modulation of apoptosis sensitivity in CD95 type I and type II cells. *J Biol Chem* 274: 22532–22538

11 Yin XM, Wang K, Gross A, Zhao Y, Zinkel S, Klocke B, Roth KA, Korsmeyer SJ (1999) Bid-deficient mice are resistant to Fas-induced hepatocellular apoptosis. *Nature* 400: 886–891

12 Lacronique V, Mignon A, Fabre M, Viollet B, Rouquet N, Molina T, Porteu A, Henrion A, Bouscary D, Varlet P et al (1996) Bcl-2 protects from lethal hepatic apoptosis induced by an anti-Fas antibody in mice. *Nat Med* 2: 80–86

13 Rodriguez I, Matsuura K, Khatib K, Reed JC, Nagata S, Vassalli P (1996) A bcl-2 transgene expressed in hepatocytes protects mice from fulminant liver destruction but not from rapid death induced by anti-Fas antibody injection. *J Exp Med* 183: 1031–1036

14 Krahling S, Callahan MK, Williamson P, Schlegel RA (1999) Exposure of phosphatidylserine is a general feature in the phagocytosis of apoptotic lymphocytes by macrophages. *Cell Death Differ* 6: 183–189

15 Williamson P, van den Eijnde S, Schlegel RA (2001) Phosphatidylserine exposure and phagocytosis of apoptotic cells. *Methods Cell Biol* 66: 339–364

16 Hanahan D, Weinberg RA (2000) The hallmarks of cancer. *Cell* 100: 57–70

17 Strasser A, O'Connor L, Huang DC, O'Reilly LA, Stanley ML, Bath ML, Adams JM,

Cory S, Harris AW (1996) Lessons from bcl-2 transgenic mice for immunology, cancer biology and cell death research. *Behring Inst Mitt* 101–117
18 Lyons SK, Clarke AR (1997) Apoptosis and carcinogenesis. *Br Med Bull* 53: 554–569
19 Jaklevic B, Su TT (2003) Cell turnover: flexible coupling meets the needs of development. *Curr Biol* 13: R805–R807
20 Lowe SW, Lin AW (2000) Apoptosis in cancer. *Carcinogenesis* 21: 485–495
21 Rao L, Debbas M, Sabbatini P, Hockenbery D, Korsmeyer S, White E (1992) The adenovirus E1A proteins induce apoptosis, which is inhibited by the E1B 19-kDa and Bcl-2 proteins. *Proc Natl Acad Sci USA* 89: 7742–7746
22 Debbas M, White E (1993) Wild-type p53 mediates apoptosis by E1A, which is inhibited by E1B. *Genes Dev* 7: 546–554
23 Knudson AG (2002) Cancer genetics. *Am J Med Genet* 111: 96–102
24 Guo M, Hay BA (1999) Cell proliferation and apoptosis. *Curr Opin Cell Biol* 11: 745–752
25 Fingleton B, Vargo-Gogola T, Crawford HC, Matrisian LM (2001) Matrilysin expression selects for cells with reduced sensitivity to apoptosis. *Neoplasia* 3: 459–468
26 Crawford HC, Scoggins CR, Washington MK, Matrisian LM, Leach SD (2002) Matrix metalloproteinase-7 is expressed by pancreatic cancer precursors and regulates acinar-to-ductal metaplasia in exocrine pancreas. *J Clin Invest* 109: 1437–1444
27 Frisch SM, Francis H (1994) Disruption of epithelial cell-matrix interactions induces apoptosis. *J Cell Biol* 124 : 619–626
28 Frisch SM, Ruoslahti E (1997) Integrins and anoikis. *Curr Opin Cell Biol* 9: 701–706
29 Weaver VM, Lelievre S, Lakins JN, Chrenek MA, Jones JC, Giancotti F, Werb Z, Bissell MJ (2002) beta4 Integrin-dependent formation of polarized three-dimensional architecture confers resistance to apoptosis in normal and malignant mammary epithelium. *Cancer Cell* 2: 205–216
30 Graeber TG, Osmanian C, Jacks T, Housman DE, Koch CJ, Lowe SW, Giaccia AJ (1996) Hypoxia-mediated selection of cells with diminished apoptotic potential in solid tumours. *Nature* 379: 88–91
31 Tsujimoto Y, Cossman J, Jaffe E, Croce CM (1985) Involvement of the bcl-2 gene in human follicular lymphoma. *Science* 228: 1440–1443
32 Reed JC (1998) Bcl-2 family proteins. *Oncogene* 17: 3225–3236
33 Schlagbauer-Wadl H, Klosner G, Heere-Ress E, Waltering S, Moll I, Wolff K, Pehamberger H, Jansen B (2000) Bcl-2 antisense oligonucleotides (G3139) inhibit Merkel cell carcinoma growth in SCID mice. *J Invest Dermatol* 114: 725–730
34 Strasser A, Harris AW, Bath ML, Cory S (1990) Novel primitive lymphoid tumours induced in transgenic mice by cooperation between myc and bcl-2. *Nature* 348: 331–333
35 Cory S, Vaux DL, Strasser A, Harris AW, Adams JM (1999) Insights from Bcl-2 and

Myc: malignancy involves abrogation of apoptosis as well as sustained proliferation. *Cancer Res* 59: 1685s–1692s
36 Shibata MA, Liu ML, Knudson MC, Shibata E, Yoshidome K, Bandey T, Korsmeyer SJ, Green JE (1999) Haploid loss of bax leads to accelerated mammary tumor development in C3(1)/SV40-TAg transgenic mice: reduction in protective apoptotic response at the preneoplastic stage. *EMBO J* 18: 2692–2701
37 Rosen K, Rak J, Leung T, Dean NM, Kerbel RS, Filmus J (2000) Activated Ras prevents downregulation of Bcl-X(L) triggered by detachment from the extracellular matrix. A mechanism of Ras-induced resistance to anoikis in intestinal epithelial cells. *J Cell Biol* 149: 447–456
38 Gilmore AP, Metcalfe AD, Romer LH, Streuli CH (2000) Integrin-mediated survival signals regulate the apoptotic function of Bax through its conformation and subcellular localization. *J Cell Biol* 149: 431–446
39 Rosen K, Rak J, Leung T, Dean NM, Kerbel RS, Filmus J (2000) Activated Ras prevents downregulation of Bcl-X(L) triggered by detachment from the extracellular matrix. A mechanism of Ras-induced resistance to anoikis in intestinal epithelial cells. *J Cell Biol* 149: 447–456
40 Antonsson B, Martinou JC (2000) The Bcl-2 protein family. *Exp Cell Res* 256: 50–57
41 Deveraux QL, Reed JC (1999) IAP family proteins – suppressors of apoptosis. *Genes Dev* 13: 239–52
42 Altieri DC (2003) Survivin and apoptosis control. *Adv Cancer Res* 88: 31–52
43 Kappler M, Kotzsch M, Bartel F, Fussel S, Lautenschlager C, Schmidt U, Wurl P, Bache M, Schmidt H, Taubert H et al (2003) Elevated expression level of survivin protein in soft-tissue sarcomas is a strong independent predictor of survival. *Clin Cancer Res* 9: 1098–1104
44 Kennedy SM, O'Driscoll L, Purcell R, Fitz-Simons N, McDermott EW, Hill AD, O'Higgins NJ, Parkinson M, Linehan R, Clynes M (2003) Prognostic importance of survivin in breast cancer. *Br J Cancer* 88: 1077–1083
45 Kajiwara Y, Yamasaki F, Hama S, Yahara K, Yoshioka H, Sugiyama K, Arita K, Kurisu K (2003) Expression of survivin in astrocytic tumors: correlation with malignant grade and prognosis. *Cancer* 97: 1077–1083
46 Grabowski P, Kuhnel T, Muhr-Wilkenshoff F, Heine B, Stein H, Hopfner M, Germer CT, Scherubl H (2003) Prognostic value of nuclear survivin expression in oesophageal squamous cell carcinoma. *Br J Cancer* 88: 115–119
47 Nakayama K, Kamihira S (2002) Survivin an important determinant for prognosis in adult T-cell leukemia: a novel biomarker in practical hemato-oncology. *Leuk Lymphoma* 43: 2249–2255
48 Grossman D, Kim PJ, Blanc-Brude OP, Brash DE, Tognin S, Marchisio PC, Altieri DC (2001) Transgenic expression of survivin in keratinocytes counteracts UVB-induced apoptosis and cooperates with loss of p53. *J Clin Invest* 108: 991–999
49 Conway EM, Pollefeyt S, Steiner-Mosonyi M, Luo W, Devriese A, Lupu F, Bono F, Leducq N, Dol F, Schaeffer P et al (2002) Deficiency of survivin in transgenic mice

exacerbates Fas-induced apoptosis *via* mitochondrial pathways. *Gastroenterology* 123: 619–631

50 Uren AG, Wong L, Pakusch M, Fowler KJ, Burrows FJ, Vaux DL, Choo KH (2000) Survivin and the inner centromere protein INCENP show similar cell- cycle localization and gene knockout phenotype. *Curr Biol* 10: 1319–1328

51 Barkett M, Gilmore TD (1999) Control of apoptosis by Rel/NF-kappaB transcription factors. *Oncogene* 18: 6910–6924

52 Arlt A, Grobe O, Sieke A, Kruse ML, Folsch UR, Schmidt WE, Schafer H (2001) Expression of the NF-kappa B target gene IEX-1 (p22/PRG1) does not prevent cell death but instead triggers apoptosis in Hela cells. *Oncogene* 20: 69–76

53 Kataoka T, Schroter M, Hahne M, Schneider P, Irmler M, Thome M, Froelich CJ, Tschopp J (1998) FLIP prevents apoptosis induced by death receptors but not by perforin/granzyme B, chemotherapeutic drugs, and gamma irradiation. *J Immunol* 161: 3936–3942

54 Irmler M, Thome M, Hahne M, Schneider P, Hofmann K, Steiner V, Bodmer JL, Schroter M, Burns K, Mattmann C et al (1997) Inhibition of death receptor signals by cellular FLIP. *Nature* 388: 190–195

55 Medema JP, de Jong J, van Hall T, Melief CJ, Offringa R (1999) Immune escape of tumors *in vivo* by expression of cellular FLICE- inhibitory protein. *J Exp Med* 190: 1033–1038

56 Hildeman DA, Zhu Y, Mitchell TC, Kappler J, Marrack P (2002) Molecular mechanisms of activated T cell death *in vivo*. *Curr Opin Immunol* 14: 354–359

57 Nagata S, Suda T (1995) Fas and Fas ligand: lpr and gld mutations. *Immunol Today* 16: 39–43

58 Cohen PL, Eisenberg RA (1991) Lpr and gld: single gene models of systemic autoimmunity and lymphoproliferative disease. *Annu Rev Immunol* 9: 243–269

59 Sneller MC, Wang J, Dale JK, Strober W, Middelton LA, Choi Y, Fleisher TA, Lim MS, Jaffe ES, Puck JM et al (1997) Clincial, immunologic, and genetic features of an autoimmune lymphoproliferative syndrome associated with abnormal lymphocyte apoptosis. *Blood* 89: 1341–1348

60 Fisher GH, Rosenberg FJ, Straus SE, Dale JK, Middleton LA, Lin AY, Strober W, Lenardo MJ, Puck JM (1995) Dominant interfering Fas gene mutations impair apoptosis in a human autoimmune lymphoproliferative syndrome. *Cell* 81: 935–946

61 Van Parijs L, Abbas AK (1996) Role of Fas-mediated cell death in the regulation of immune responses. *Curr Opin Immunol* 8: 355–361

62 Straus SE, Jaffe ES, Puck JM, Dale JK, Elkon KB, Rosen-Wolff A, Peters AM, Sneller MC, Hallahan CW, Wang J et al (2001) The development of lymphomas in families with autoimmune lymphoproliferative syndrome with germline Fas mutations and defective lymphocyte apoptosis. *Blood* 98: 194–200

63 Celsus AC (1938) *De Medicina Book III*. Loeb Classical Library, Harvard University Press, Cambridge

64 Nathan C (2002) Points of control in inflammation. *Nature* 420: 846–852

65 Trapani JA, Smyth MJ (2002) Functional significance of the perforin/granzyme cell death pathway. *Nat Rev Immunol* 2: 735–747
66 Chitnis T, Khoury SJ (2003) 20. Immunologic neuromuscular disorders. *J Allergy Clin Immunol* 111: S659–S668
67 Fiocchi C (1998) Inflammatory bowel disease: etiology and pathogenesis. *Gastroenterology* 115: 182–205
68 Semra YK, Seidi OA, Sharief MK (2001) Overexpression of the apoptosis inhibitor FLIP in T cells correlates with disease activity in multiple sclerosis. *J Neuroimmunol* 113: 268–274
69 Bu P, Keshavarzian A, Stone DD, Liu J, Le PT, Fisher S, Qiao L (2001) Apoptosis: one of the mechanisms that maintains unresponsiveness of the intestinal mucosal immune system. *J Immunol* 166: 6399–6403
70 Itoh J, de La Motte C, Strong SA, Levine AD, Fiocchi C (2001) Decreased Bax expression by mucosal T cells favours resistance to apoptosis in Crohn's disease. *Gut* 49: 35–41
71 Di Sabatino A, Corazza GR (2001) Surviving too long in Crohn's disease. *Gut* 49: 6–8
72 Baier A, Meineckel I, Gay S, Pap T (2003) Apoptosis in rheumatoid arthritis. *Curr Opin Rheumatol* 15: 274–279
73 Lowenfels AB, Maisonneuve P, Cavallini G, Ammann RW, Lankisch PG, Andersen JR, Dimagno EP, Andren-Sandberg A, Domellof L (1993) Pancreatitis and the risk of pancreatic cancer. International Pancreatitis Study Group. *N Engl J Med* 328: 1433–1437
74 Lowenfels AB, Maisonneuve P, Whitcomb DC (2000) Risk factors for cancer in hereditary pancreatitis. International Hereditary Pancreatitis Study Group. *Med Clin North Am* 84: 565–573
75 Uemura N, Okamoto S, Yamamoto S, Matsumura N, Yamaguchi S, Yamakido M, Taniyama K, Sasaki N, Schlemper RJ (2001) *Helicobacter pylori* infection and the development of gastric cancer. *N Engl J Med* 345: 784–789
76 Fox JG, Wang TC (2001) *Helicobacter pylori* – not a good bug after all! *N Engl J Med* 345: 829–832
77 Eaden JA, Abrams KR, Mayberry JF (2001) The risk of colorectal cancer in ulcerative colitis: a meta-analysis. *Gut* 48: 526–535
78 Jankowski JA, Harrison RF, Perry I, Balkwill F, Tselepis C (2000) Barrett's metaplasia. *Lancet* 356: 2079–2085
79 Nissen NN, Martin P (2002) Hepatocellular carcinoma: the high-risk patient. *J Clin Gastroenterol* 35: S79–S85
80 Cox JT (1995) Epidemiology of cervical intraepithelial neoplasia: the role of human papillomavirus. *Baillieres Clin Obstet Gynaecol* 9: 1–37
81 Kitada S, Zapata JM, Andreeff M, Reed JC (1999) Bryostatin and CD40-ligand enhance apoptosis resistance and induce expression of cell survival genes in B-cell chronic lymphocytic leukaemia. *Br J Haematol* 106: 995–1004

82 Kakihara T, Fukuda T, Kamishima T, Naito M, Tanaka A, Uchiyama M, Kishi K (1997) Resistance to apoptosis induced by serum depletion and all-trans retinoic acid in drug-resistant leukemic cell lines. *Leuk Lymphoma* 26: 369–376
83 Landowski TH, Gleason-Guzman MC, Dalton WS (1997) Selection for drug resistance results in resistance to Fas-mediated apoptosis. *Blood* 89: 1854–1861
84 Falk GW (2002) Barrett's esophagus. *Gastroenterology* 122: 1569–1591
85 Sipponen P (2002) Gastric cancer: pathogenesis, risks, and prevention. *J Gastroenterol* 37 (Suppl 13): 39–44
86 Tanaka M, Saito H, Kusumi T, Fukuda S, Shimoyama T, Sasaki Y, Suto K, Munakata A, Kudo H (2001) Spatial distribution and histogenesis of colorectal Paneth cell metaplasia in idiopathic inflammatory bowel disease. *J Gastroenterol Hepatol* 16: 1353– 1359
87 Luttges J, Kloppel G (2000) Precancerous conditions of pancreatic carcinoma. *J Hepatobiliary Pancreat Surg* 7: 568–574
88 Lauwers GY, Scott GV, Hendricks J (1994) Immunohistochemical evidence of aberrant bcl-2 protein expression in gastric epithelial dysplasia. *Cancer* 73: 2900–2904
89 Lauwers GY, Kandemir O, Kubilis PS, Scott GV (1997) Cellular kinetics in Barrett's epithelium carcinogenic sequence: roles of apoptosis, bcl-2 protein, and cellular proliferation. *Mod Pathol* 10: 1201–1208
90 Scoggins CR, Meszoely IM, Wada M, Means AL, Yang L, Leach SD (2000) p53-dependent acinar cell apoptosis triggers epithelial proliferation in duct-ligated murine pancreas. *Am J Physiol Gastrointest Liver Physiol* 279: G827–G836
91 Keates S, Hitti YS, Upton M, Kelly CP (1997) *Helicobacter pylori* infection activates NF-kappa B in gastric epithelial cells. *Gastroenterology* 113: 1099–1109
92 Boya P, Larrea E, Sola I, Majano PL, Jimenez C, Civeira MP, Prieto J (2001) Nuclear factor-kappa B in the liver of patients with chronic hepatitis C: decreased RelA expression is associated with enhanced fibrosis progression. *Hepatology* 34: 1041–1048
93 Neurath MF, Pettersson S, Meyer zum Buschenfelde KH, Strober W (1996) Local administration of antisense phosphorothioate oligonucleotides to the p65 subunit of NF-kappa B abrogates established experimental colitis in mice. *Nat Med* 2: 998–1004
94 Schreiber S, Nikolaus S, Hampe J (1998) Activation of nuclear factor kappa B inflammatory bowel disease. *Gut* 42: 477–484
95 Hussain SP, Amstad P, Raja K, Ambs S, Nagashima M, Bennett WP, Shields PG, Ham AJ, Swenberg JA, Marrogi AJ et al (2000) Increased p53 mutation load in noncancerous colon tissue from ulcerative colitis: a cancer-prone chronic inflammatory disease. *Cancer Res* 60: 3333–3337
96 Lala PK, Chakraborty C (2001) Role of nitric oxide in carcinogenesis and tumour progression. *Lancet Oncol* 2: 149–156
97 Kerr JF, Winterford CM, Harmon BV (1994) Apoptosis. Its significance in cancer and cancer therapy. *Cancer* 73: 2013–2026

98 Fisher DE (1994) Apoptosis in cancer therapy: crossing the threshold. *Cell* 78: 539–542
99 Weinstein JN, Myers TG, O'Connor PM, Friend SH, Fornace AJ Jr, Kohn KW, Fojo T, Bates SE, Rubinstein LV, Anderson NL et al (1997) An information-intensive approach to the molecular pharmacology of cancer. *Science* 275: 343–349
100 Lowe SW, Bodis S, McClatchey A, Remington L, Ruley HE, Fisher DE, Housman DE, Jacks T (1994) p53 status and the efficacy of cancer therapy *in vivo*. *Science* 266: 807–810
101 Yamamoto Y, Gaynor RB (2001) Therapeutic potential of inhibition of the NF-kappaB pathway in the treatment of inflammation and cancer. *J Clin Invest* 107: 135–142
102 Wang CY, Cusack JC Jr, Liu R, Baldwin AS Jr (1999) Control of inducible chemoresistance: enhanced anti-tumor therapy through increased apoptosis by inhibition of NF-kappaB. *Nat Med* 5: 412–417
103 O'Gorman DM, Cotter TG (2001) Molecular signals in anti-apoptotic survival pathways. *Leukemia* 15: 21–34
104 Reed JC (2002) Apoptosis-based therapies. *Nat Rev Drug Disc* 1: 111–121
105 Atreya R, Mudter J, Finotto S, Mullberg J, Jostock T, Wirtz S, Schutz M, Bartsch B, Holtmann M, Becker C et al (2000) Blockade of interleukin 6 trans signaling suppresses T-cell resistance against apoptosis in chronic intestinal inflammation: evidence in crohn disease and experimental colitis *in vivo*. *Nat Med* 6: 583–588
106 Fuss IJ, Marth T, Neurath MF, Pearlstein GR, Jain A, Strober W (1999) Anti-interleukin 12 treatment regulates apoptosis of Th1 T cells in experimental colitis in mice. *Gastroenterology* 117: 1078–1088
107 Neurath MF, Fuss I, Kelsall BL, Stuber E, Strober W (1995) Antibodies to interleukin 12 abrogate established experimental colitis in mice. *J Exp Med* 182: 1281–1290
108 Neurath MF, Finotto S, Fuss I, Boirivant M, Galle PR, Strober W (2001) Regulation of T-cell apoptosis in inflammatory bowel disease: to die or not to die, that is the mucosal question. *Trends Immunol* 22: 21–26
109 Yamamoto Y, Yin MJ, Lin KM, Gaynor RB (1999) Sulindac inhibits activation of the NF-kappaB pathway. *J Biol Chem* 274: 27307–27314
110 Hideshima T, Chauhan D, Richardson P, Mitsiades C, Mitsiades N, Hayashi T, Munshi N, Dang L, Castro A, Palombella V et al (2002) NF-kappa B as a therapeutic target in multiple myeloma. *J Biol Chem* 277: 16639–16647
111 Adams J (2003) Potential for proteasome inhibition in the treatment of cancer. *Drug Discov Today* 8: 307–315
112 Dias N, Stein CA (2002) Potential roles of antisense oligonucleotides in cancer therapy. The example of Bcl-2 antisense oligonucleotides. *Eur J Pharm Biopharm* 54: 263–269
113 Penn LZ (2001) Apoptosis modulators as cancer therapeutics. *Curr Opin Invest Drugs* 2: 684–92
114 Marcucci G, Byrd JC, Dai G, Klisovic MI, Kourlas PJ, Young DC, Cataland SR, Fish-

er DB, Lucas D, Chan KK et al (2003) Phase 1 and pharmacodynamic studies of G3139, a Bcl-2 antisense oligonucleotide, in combination with chemotherapy in refractory or relapsed acute leukemia. *Blood* 101: 425–432

115 Rudin CM, Otterson GA, Mauer AM, Villalona-Calero MA, Tomek R, Prange B, George CM, Szeto L, Vokes EE (2002) A pilot trial of G3139, a bcl-2 antisense oligonucleotide, and paclitaxel in patients with chemorefractory small-cell lung cancer. *Ann Oncol* 13: 539–545

116 National Institutes of Health/ National Library of Medicine (Clinical Trials web page) http://clinicaltrials.gov

117 Gautschi O, Tschopp S, Olie RA, Leech SH, Simoes-Wust AP, Ziegler A, Baumann B, Odermatt B, Hall J, Stahel RA et al (2001) Activity of a novel bcl-2/bcl-xL-bispecific antisense oligonucleotide against tumors of diverse histologic origins. *J Natl Cancer Inst* 93: 463–471

118 Altieri DC (2003) Survivin and apoptosis control. *Adv Cancer Res* 88: 31–52

119 Altieri DC (2003) Validating survivin as a cancer therapeutic target. *Nat Rev Cancer* 3: 46–54

120 Andersen MH, Pedersen LO, Capeller B, Brocker EB, Becker JC, thor Straten P (2001) Spontaneous cytotoxic T-cell responses against survivin-derived MHC class I-restricted T-cell epitopes *in situ* as well as *ex vivo* in cancer patients. *Cancer Res* 61: 5964–5968

121 Andersen MH, Pedersen LO, Becker JC, Straten PT (2001) Identification of a cytotoxic T lymphocyte response to the apoptosis inhibitor protein survivin in cancer patients. *Cancer Res* 61: 869–872

122 Ashkenazi A (2002) Targeting death and decoy receptors of the tumour-necrosis factor superfamily. *Nat Rev Cancer* 2: 420–430

123 Jo M, Kim TH, Seol DW, Esplen JE, Dorko K, Billiar TR, Strom SC (2000) Apoptosis induced in normal human hepatocytes by tumor necrosis factor- related apoptosis-inducing ligand. *Nat Med* 6: 564–567

124 Nagata S (2000) Steering anti-cancer drugs away from the TRAIL. Nat Med 6: 502–503

125 Kandel ES, Hay N (1999) The regulation and activities of the multifunctional serine/threonine kinase Akt/PKB. *Exp Cell Res* 253: 210–229

126 Chang F, Lee JT, Navolanic PM, Steelman LS, Shelton JG, Blalock WL, Franklin RA, McCubrey JA (2003) Involvement of PI3K/Akt pathway in cell cycle progression, apoptosis, and neoplastic transformation: a target for cancer chemotherapy. *Leukemia* 17: 590–603

127 Stambolic V, Suzuki A, de la Pompa JL, Brothers GM, Mirtsos C, Sasaki T, Ruland J, Penninger JM, Siderovski DP, Mak TW (1998) Negative regulation of PKB/Akt-dependent cell survival by the tumor suppressor PTEN. *Cell* 95: 29–39

128 Zheleva DI, Lane DP, Fischer PM (2003) The p53-Mdm2 pathway: targets for the development of new anticancer therapeutics. *Mini Rev Med Chem* 3: 257–270

129 Chene P (2001) Targeting p53 in cancer. *Curr Med Chem Anti-Canc Agents* 1: 151–161
130 Shimada H, Matsubara H, Ochiai T (2002) p53 gene therapy for esophageal cancer. *J Gastroenterol* 37 (Suppl 14): 87–91
131 Post LE (2002) Selectively replicating adenoviruses for cancer therapy: an update on clinical development. *Curr Opin Invest Drugs* 3: 1768–1772
132 Chada S, Mhashilkar A, Roth JA, Gabrilovich D (2003) Development of vaccines against self-antigens: the p53 paradigm. *Curr Opin Drug Disc Dev* 6: 169–173
133 Foster BA, Coffey HA, Morin MJ, Rastinejad F (1999) Pharmacological rescue of mutant p53 conformation and function. *Science* 286: 2507–2510
134 Chene P (2003) Inhibiting the p53-MDM2 interaction: an important target for cancer therapy. *Nat Rev Cancer* 3: 102–109

Cyclooxygenase activity in gastrointestinal cancer development and progression: prospects as a therapeutic target

John P. Lynch[1] *and Gary R. Lichtenstein*[2]

[1]Division of Gastroenterology, Department of Medicine, University of Pennsylvania, Philadelphia, PA 19104, USA; [2]Hospital of the University of Pennsylvania, Division of Gastroenterology, Department of Medicine, University of Pennsylvania, Philadelphia, PA 19104, USA

Introduction

Gastrointestinal malignancies are a leading cause of morbidity and mortality worldwide. The Global Burden of Disease study estimated that in 1990 cancers of the gastrointestinal tract were responsible for more than 40% of all cancer deaths, nearly 2.2 million people [1, 2]. Interestingly, the incidence of these cancers can vary considerably between regions. This is most likely due to a variety of factors including environmental exposures, diet, social habits, and genetic backgrounds. Given the enormity of the problem, it has been the focus of intense research for many years. A great deal has been learned about the mechanisms governing the development and progression of human cancers. Research over the last decade has established that the progression from normal tissue to neoplasia is in every case a stepwise process [3–5]. Genetic and epigenetic instability appears fundamentally important to this process.

An observation that has emerged from these and other studies is that cancer often arises in the setting of chronic inflammation [6–11]. Inflammation in this setting can act as both the initiator and promoter of carcinogenesis. Additionally, even in the absence of a chronic inflammatory setting, tumors themselves often elicit an inflammatory response that can enhance tumor growth and metastasis [10]. Insights gained into the role of inflammation in carcinogenesis and tumor progression have provided a rational basis for primary prevention [12–15] and have begun to affect the management of patients with cancer [16–18]. This review will attempt to summarize the current concepts regarding the role of cyclooxygenases (COXs) in gastrointestinal cancer development and progression, as well as emerging prospects for COX inhibitors in gastrointestinal cancer chemoprevention and therapy.

Cancer and Inflammation, edited by Douglas W. Morgan, Ulf J. Forssmann and Marian T. Nakada

Role of inflammation in gastrointestinal cancer development

Chronic gastrointestinal inflammatory conditions are associated with neoplasia

The causes of chronic inflammation in gastrointestinal tissues are quite varied and are reviewed elsewhere in this volume (see chapter by Nam and Murthy). They include bacterial infections like *Helicobacter pylori*, a cause of chronic gastritis, and the chronic viral hepatidities B and C. Recurrent acute chemical or enzymatic injuries, as occur with gastro-esophageal reflux (GERD) or recurrent acute pancreatitis, can precipitate chronic changes in these tissues as they respond to the repeated injuries. Lastly, autoimmune processes, as is classically seen in the small intestine and colon with inflammatory bowel diseases (IBDs), can be a source of chronic inflammation as well. Despite the diversity of the causes, these chronic inflammatory conditions have all been associated with increased risks for the development of cancer [6–10].

There are a number of mechanisms that have been proposed to explain this association between inflammation and cancer. Inflammatory cells, when activated, induce and express enzymes like NADPH oxidase, xanthine oxidase, and inducible nitric oxide synthase (iNOS) that generate high levels of free radicals and oxidants. These highly reactive oxygen and nitrogen species can in turn react with and damage DNA, RNA, lipids, and proteins, causing mutations and altered functions, and thus lead to neoplastic transformation [19, 20]. Cytokines, like tumor necrosis factor α (TNFα) and IL-10, and chemokines like macrophage migration inhibitory factor (MIF) and macrophage-inflammatory protein-1β (MIP-1β), are secreted by inflammatory cells and in many studies appear to promote the growth and metastasis of tumors [21–25]. Often these cytokines and chemokines are also secreted by cancer cells themselves. Their cellular targets as well as their actions are quite diverse. These secreted factors can act in both a paracrine and an autocrine fashion to induce cancer cell proliferation and inhibit apoptosis, as well as enhance tumor cell migration through the surrounding stroma. They can also induce new blood-vessel growth (angiogenesis) to further support tumor growth. Lastly, tumor-derived cytokines and chemokines can modulate the immune response to inhibit normal surveillance mechanisms that target neoplastic cells. These factors promote leukocyte infiltration, which leads to degradation of stromal elements, thereby enhancing neoplastic cell migration and metastasis [10, 21, 24, 25].

Inflammation and inflammatory cells also release eicosanoids, oxygenated lipids produced by arachidonic acid metabolism [17, 26, 27]. Eicosanoids include the prostanoids (prostaglandins and thromboxane) and leukotrienes. Much like the cytokines and chemokines, eicosanoids have been associated with promoting transformation by enhancing cell proliferation and motility while reducing apoptosis [28–31]. Eicosanoids also induce angiogenesis [32] and suppress normal immune surveillance mechanisms [33–36]. This further supports tumor growth. Lastly, eicosanoids can also induce cytokine and chemokine synthesis and release, thereby further potentiating the inflammatory response [37-39]. Due to these many beneficial effects on tumor growth and survival, increased eicosanoid biosynthesis, particularly of prostaglandins, can frequently be seen in many cancers.

Given the importance of chronic inflammation in the development and progression of many gastrointestinal cancers, reversal of the inflammatory condition has been a therapeutic focus for several years. Treatment and resolution of chronic hepatitis B or C with interferon therapy, mesalamine therapy for ulcerative colitis, clearance of *H. pylori* colonization, and acid suppression for GERD patients are considered to be standards of care. Several of these therapies have been reported in clinical trials to reduce the risk for cancer [40–43]. However, not all patients respond to these therapies with a resolution of the inflammatory condition. In others, precancerous changes or frank carcinoma have already occurred. Efforts for these patients have focused instead on inhibiting the production of the inflammatory mediators by both normal and neoplastic cells. Inhibitors of prostaglandin biosynthesis, which block the activity of the enzyme COX, may prove particularly useful in this regard.

Mechanisms of prostaglandin biosynthesis

The COX enzyme catalyzes the rate-limiting step in prostaglandin biosynthesis

The eicosanoids have been under scrutiny for more than 70 years [17, 27, 44]. Eicosanoids are known as mediators of the primary symptoms of inflammation including pain, swelling, erythema, and warmth. In the 1990s, the techniques of molecular biology were employed to define and understand this important biosynthetic pathway. Many of the important enzymes were cloned, their expression patterns and regulation explored, and their three-dimensional structures solved [17, 27].

The first step in eicosanoid biosynthesis involves the release of arachidonic acid from phospholipid membranes (Fig. 1) [17, 27]. This step is catalyzed by phospholipase activity, primarily by one of the many forms of phospholipase A_2 (PLA_2). In general, the PLA_2 forms can be categorized into two groups, secreted and cytosolic. The secreted forms ($sPLA_2$) are smaller (14 kDa) and extensively disulfide linked. They are expressed and secreted when cells are stimulated by pro-inflammatory cytokines like TNFα and interleukin-1 (IL-1). The cytosolic forms ($cPLA_2$) are larger (85 kDa) and are translocated to phospholipid membranes when activated [27]. $cPLA_2$ primarily localizes to nuclear envelope and endoplasmic reticulum (ER) membranes when activated. Mitogens and cytokines can induce both cytosolic and secreted PLA_2 gene transcription, and glucocorticoids may actively suppress their expression.

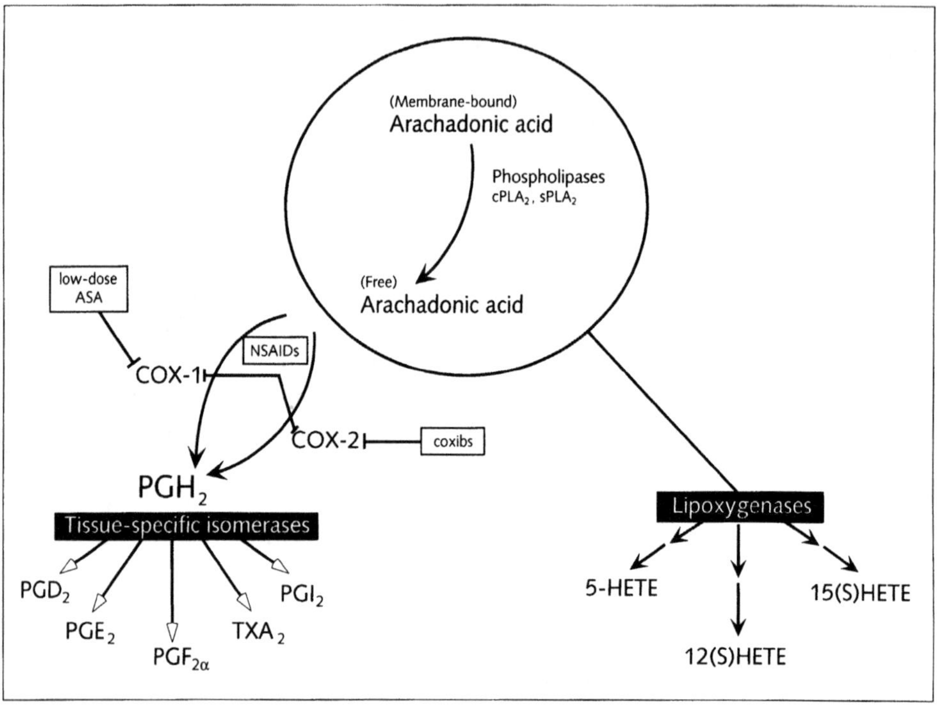

Figure 1
Eicosanoid biosynthetic pathway [17, 27].
Arachidonic acid is released from nuclear and endoplasmic reticulum phospholipid membranes by phospholipase activity, primarily by phospholipase A_2. Free arachidonic acid is shunted toward prostanoid or leukotriene production by the actions of the enzymes COX-1 or COX-2, or lipoxygenase, respectively. COX activity produces prostaglandin H_2 (PGH_2), which is then converted to the final prostenoid product by the actions of tissue-specific isomerases. PGH_2 production from arachidonic acid by COX is the rate-limiting step in prostanoid biosynthesis.
$cPLA_2$, cytosolic phospholipase A_2; $sPLA_2$, secreted phospholipase A_2; PG, prostaglandin; TXA_2, thromboxane; HETE, hydroxyeicosatetraenoic acid.

Next, free arachidonic acid is shunted toward prostanoid or leukotriene production by the actions of the enzymes COX or lipoxygenase, respectively (Fig. 1) [27]. There are two forms of the COX enzyme, COX-1 and COX-2. Both forms are integral membrane proteins located in the nuclear and ER membranes. Therefore, $cPLA_2$ activation and translocation to the nuclear and ER membranes colocalizes arachidonic acid production with the COX enzymes, thereby further enhancing prostanoid synthesis. Prostaglandin H_2 (PGH_2) is then converted to the final prostenoid product by the actions of tissue-specific isomerases (Fig. 1). In the central nervous system this yields PGD_2. PGE_2 and PGI_2 are synthesized largely in vascular beds and gastrointestinal epithelium. $PGF_{2\alpha}$ is produced in smooth muscle, and thromboxane (TXA_2) in platelets [17]. PGH_2 production from arachidonic acid by COX is the rate-limiting step in prostanoid biosynthesis. This is why the COX enzymes are frequently targeted therapeutically to reduce or inhibit the inflammatory response.

Although COX-1 and COX-2 are structurally and functionally similar, their biologic roles are distinctive due to different patterns of expression. The *COX-1* gene is stably and continuously expressed in a number of tissues and has primary roles in regulating platelet aggregation, renal blood flow, and gastric mucosa cytoprotection [27]. COX-1 mRNA and protein levels are not highly inducible and do not significantly respond to growth factor and cytokine signaling. The *COX-2* gene is the inducible isoform, responding to inflammatory signals and injury to promote tissue repair and regeneration [27]. COX-2 has other physiologic roles in the brain, vas deferens, islet cells, and kidneys. Signaling from growth factors and cytokines enhances *COX-2* gene transcription, which elevates COX-2 mRNA and protein levels. These same signals can also increase COX-2 mRNA stability, further amplifying COX-2 mRNA and protein levels.

Mechanisms of COX-2 induction in inflammation and neoplasia

COX-2 gene expression is regulated by both transcriptional and post-transcriptional mechanisms. Investigators interested in studying these processes isolated the *COX-2* gene (also known as PGHS-2 synthase) from diverse mammalian species including humans, mice, rats, horses, and cows [45–48]. Analysis of the promoter sequences revealed a classic-promoter structure, with a canonical TATA-box sequence just upstream of the transcription initiation site. Putative binding sites for a great many transcription factors were noted, including ubiquitous factors like SP-1 and CCAAT/enhancer-binding protein (C/EBP), immediate-early response factors like activator protein-1 (AP-1), activating transcription factor/cAMP-response element (ATF/CRE), and myocyte-specific enhancer factor 2 (MEF2), and the inducible factors nuclear factor κB (NF-κB), polyoma enhancer activator-3 (PEA-3), and glucocorticoid receptor [45–48]. Also noted were AU-rich sequences in the 3' untranslated region (UTR) of the COX-2 mRNA, which are similar to elements within the 3'UTR of many cytokine and proto-oncogenes [27]. These sequences typically provide an additional level to regulate expression by acting as mRNA instability determinants.

Numerous *in vitro* and a few *in vivo* studies have begun to dissect these promoters to discern the relative importance of these elements in the induction of COX-2 gene expression [49, 50–62, 64]. The mitogen-activated protein kinase (MAPK) signaling pathway is commonly activated by growth factors, cytokines, and oncogenes [63]. It is therefore not surprising that the MAPKs, including extracellular-signal-regulated kinase (ERK) 1/2, p38^{MAPK}, c-Jun N-terminal kinase (JNK), and ERK5, are likely critical regulators of *COX-2* gene expression with inflammation or neoplastic transformation. Gastrin, basic fibroblast growth factor (bFGF), and IL-1β and IL-17, among other factors, have been reported to induce COX-2 expression through activation of the MAPK cascade [52, 54, 56, 62]. Oncogenic Ras and *H. pylori* bacterial virulence factors also reportedly increase COX-2 expression *via* ERK1/2 activation [57, 64]. *H. pylori* may also enhance COX-2 expression *via* NF-κB and AP-1 activation [53]. Thus, the MAPK pathway can respond to a diverse set of signals and stimuli to induce *COX-2* gene expression.

Other transcription factors and signaling pathways have been reported to regulate *COX-2* gene expression, including some that may be disease-specific. Interferon-γ induces COX-2 expression in macrophages *via* Janus kinase/signal transduction and activators of transcription (JAK/STAT), interferon-regulatory factors 1 and 2 [51]. COX-2 induction by IL-1β and TNFα requires NF-κB activation and nuclear translocation [58, 62]. Hypertonic stress can induce COX-2 expression in medullary epithelial cells of the kidney, and this effect is dependent upon epidermal growth factor (EGF) receptor activation [55]. Steroid-hormone nuclear receptors peroxisome proliferator-activated receptor δ (PPARδ) and PPARγ appear to have opposing effects on COX-2 transcription, with PPARδ activating and PPARg inhibiting expression [59, 60]. The hepatitis B virus X-protein has been reported to increase COX-2 promoter activity in an nuclear factor of activated T cells (NF-AT)-dependent manner [65]. Lastly, COX-2 expression in colon cancer cells is dependent upon Wnt/β-catenin/T cell factor transcriptional activity [59].

COX-2 mRNA instability is an important constituent of COX-2 regulation in most cells [66–70]. The AU-rich sequences in the 3'UTR confers mRNA instability under basal conditions or in the presence of glucocorticoids [67, 68, 70], while IL-1 treatment or oncogenic Ras expression promote mRNA stability [50, 64]. In addition to enhancing COX-2 gene transcription, p38^{MAPK} or p42/44^{MAPK} MAPK activation also induces COX-2 mRNA stability, and this effect can be blocked by phosphoinositide 3-kinase (PI3K) activity [64, 66, 69]. The RNA-binding protein HuR binds the AU-rich sequences and is required for COX-2 mRNA stabilization [66] in one cell line; however, its role in MAPK-mediated mRNA stabilization across broad cell and tissue types is at present unknown.

COX-2 in gastrointestinal cancer

COX-2 expression in preneoplastic and neoplastic conditions of the gastrointestinal tract

The epithelium of the gastrointestinal tract is exposed to a noxious environment. Some of this exposure is by individual choice (i.e. tobacco, alcohol), and some is the nature of the digestive process where enzymes and chemicals (i.e. HCl, bile acids) are secreted to reduce ingested materials into absorbable components. These same reagents would digest gastrointestinal epithelia equally well if there were not protective measures in place. Investigators have examined COX expression in gastrointestinal tissues. Based on these studies, constitutive COX-1 expression by gastrointestinal epithelia appears to provide a cytoprotective role by inducing defensive mechanisms and reducing epithelial cell apoptosis [71–74]. COX-2 is generally undetectable in these normal tissues; however, COX-2 mRNA and protein levels are greatly increased with disease states like inflammation and neoplasia [71–76]. Perhaps most significantly clinically, elevations of COX-2 mRNA and protein have been detected in pre-neoplastic conditions as well as the earliest stages of many different cancers.

Esophageal squamous cell and adenocarcinoma

Esophageal squamous cell carcinoma (ESCC) is the more common of the two esophageal malignancies worldwide [8, 26]. In the USA, ESCC occurs more frequently in African-American males than any other subgroup, and heavy tobacco and alcohol consumption are recognized risk factors. Multiple studies have concluded COX-2 levels were elevated considerably in ESCC [77–79]. The frequency of elevated COX-2 expression in ESCC was about 90% across several studies. Squamous epithelial dysplasia of the esophagus is a precancerous lesion that predisposes to ESCC development. Increased levels of COX-2 protein and mRNA have been detected in these early precancerous lesions [78–80]. In one recent study, moderate elevations of COX-2 protein were detected in 35 of 47 (74%) esophageal squamous dysplasias [79]. COX-2 staining intensity and frequency increased further in the ESCC examined. Some 86% (74 of 86) were positive for COX-2. RNA and protein were isolated from a subset of these lesions, and reverse transcriptase-PCR and immunoblotting studies confirmed the immunohistochemical findings. Elevations in COX-2 expression correlated with increased proliferating-cell nuclear antigen (PCNA) staining, a marker for increased proliferation [78, 79]. Similar rates of COX-2 elevations have been reported in studies of head and neck squamous cell cancers (HNSCCs) and precancerous dysplasia. Given the epidemiologic and biologic similarities between ESCC and HNSCC, these findings further emphasize the critical role of enhanced COX-2 expression in the development and progression of squamous cell cancers of the gastrointestinal tract.

Esophageal adenocarcinoma (EAC), although less common than ESCC, has been the fastest rising malignancy among white males in the USA over the last three decades, and in this subgroup EAC is more prevalent than ESCC [8, 26]. Several factors and conditions are known to increase the risk for the development of EAC, including obesity, smoking, diet, chronic gastro-esophageal reflux disease (GERD), and perhaps most significantly Barrett's esophagus (BE). BE occurs at the gastro-esophageal junction and is the replacement of normal squamous esophageal mucosa with an intestinalized columnar epithelium. Chronic GERD is the single greatest risk factor for the development of BE; approximately 10% of these patients will acquire intestinal metaplasia at the gastro-esophageal junction. BE is considered to be a pre-malignant lesion, even in the absence of dysplasia, as the risk for EAC is increased considerably over the general population. Induction of COX-2 expression is a common and early event in the sequence of BE metaplasia to dysplasia to EAC [75, 77, 81–83]. Several studies have reported increased COX-2 mRNA and protein expression in 40–80% of BE cases [75, 81–83]. In EAC, these frequencies increased to between 80 and 100% [77, 81–83]. Elevated COX-2 expression in EAC was associated with increased rates of local and distant metastasis, as well as reduced 5-year survival [84]. Two studies reported finding increasing COX-2 expression in the progression from BE to low-grade dysplasia to high-grade dysplasia to EAC [82, 83]. Furthermore, gastric and bile acids further enhanced COX-2 levels in both normal squamous as well as Barrett's mucosa, but the response was greater in the BE tissues [82, 85]. For all of these reasons, increased COX-2 expression is an important feature in the development and progression of esophageal adenocarcinoma.

Gastric cancer

Gastric cancer is a common malignancy worldwide, and a leading cause of cancer mortality in several countries in Eastern Asia [6, 26]. The incidence of gastric cancer is declining in the United States, although each year there are an estimated 22 000 new cases diagnosed. The only curative approach is surgical resection; unfortunately the majority of new diagnoses are made at advanced stages of the disease that often preclude curative therapy. Gastric cancers arise from a complex interplay of factors like diet, genetic predisposition, and environmental exposures, including *H. pylori* infection. In fact, the strong epidemiologic association of *H. pylori* infection with gastric adenocarcinoma prompted the World Health Organization to classify *H. pylori* as a carcinogen [6]. The chronic gastritis associated with persistent *H. pylori* infection begins with chronic inflammation and often later progresses to glandular atrophy and intestinal metaplasia [6]. This inflammatory environment, as well as *H. pylori* virulence factors, induce genetic mutations and stimulate the release of growth factors that together serve to enhance gastric carcinogenesis. In support of this hypothesis, *H. pylori* infection has been associated with greater proliferative rates in non-cancer tissues and alterations in apoptotic rates [86]. COX-2 expression is likely to have an important role in this process [26, 87]. Chronic *H. pylori* gastritis was associated with elevated COX-2 levels when compared with uninfected or *H. pylori*-eradicated controls [88, 89].

This expression was further increased in gastric tissues with intestinal metaplasia [89, 90]. In studies of gastric neoplasia, COX-2 mRNA and protein levels are significantly increased in 60–80% of gastric adenocarcinomas when compared with paired normal mucosa [91–94]. However, this induction was observed only in the intestinal-type gastric cancer, not the diffuse type [90, 94, 95]. Overexpression of COX-2 by gastric carcinomas was associated with tissue invasion and metastasis [96–98]. Finally, COX-2 levels were increased in 20–40% of gastric adenomas or gastric dysplasias [94, 98], suggesting that COX-2 expression increases in the progression from metaplasia to dysplasia to carcinoma in the stomach. In summary, COX-2 expression is likely an important promoter of intestinal-type gastric carcinogenesis, particularly carcinogenesis that is associated with *H. pylori* chronic infection.

Pancreatic neoplasias

Pancreatic ductal carcinoma (PDC) remains one of the more lethal malignancies despite intensive surgical and oncologic therapy and research. There are approximately 25 000 new cases of PDC diagnosed in the USA each year, with only 3–5% of these patients surviving 5 years [11, 99, 100]. In the last decade, significant advances have been made in understanding the preneoplastic and genetic lesions that promote the acquisition and progression of this deadly disease. Chronic pancreatitis, from all of its causes (tropical, cystic fibrosis, hereditary, and alcoholic) is now recognized as a significant risk factor for the development of PDC [10, 11]. The inflammation from the pancreatitis is associated with inducing gene mutations that promote PDC, especially mutations in K-*ras*. The inflammation as well as the activating K-*ras* mutations may serve to induce COX-2 expression. COX-2 expression was elevated in 80–90% of patients with chronic pancreatitis, and this appeared to correlate with the frequency of attacks [101]. COX-2 mRNA and protein levels were reportedly increased in 60–90% of PDCs examined across multiple studies, with a single study reporting a frequency as low as 40% [99, 100, 102–104]. Many pancreatic adenocarcinoma cell lines likewise express COX-2 at elevated levels. In many of these studies COX-2 elevations correlated with increased proliferative rates, as determined by Ki-67 or PCNA staining. COX-2 levels in the preneoplastic lesions for PDC (pancreatic intraepithelial neoplasia) increased from normal pancreatic ducts to pancreatic intraepithelial neoplasia to adenocarcinoma [105]. Studies with the less-aggressive intraductal papillary-mucinous tumors (IPMT) also suggested COX-2 expression is increased in the progression from IPMT hyperplasia (10%) to adenoma and carcinoma (60–70%) [103, 106]. Finally, COX-2 levels in pancreatic neuroendocrine tumors correlated strongly with a more aggressive and faster-growing phenotype. COX-2 is continuously expressed in pancreatic islet cells; however, those endocrine neoplasms with high levels of COX-2 expression were more frequently metastatic, grew to larger sizes, and had higher rates of mitotic activity and angiogenic invasion [107]. In summary, COX-2 expression was frequently elevated in the majority of pancreatic neoplasms and was associated with a more aggressive and proliferative cancer.

Hepatocellular carcinoma (HCC)

HCC is the most common form of primary liver tumor, the incidence of which has been increasing in the USA over the past 30 years [108]. This increasing incidence is thought to be largely due to the rising prevalence of hepatitis C infection during the same time period. Hepatic cirrhosis from any cause is considered to be a predisposing condition for the development of HCC, although virus-induced cirrhosis may be a more potent etiology. The prognosis for patients with HCC remains poor, with 5-year survival rates only 5% [108], in part because HCC often occurs in the setting of cirrhosis, limiting surgical options. COX expression is barely detectable in histologically normal liver. However, prostaglandins and the cyclooxygenase enzymes are essential for the normal proliferative response to partial hepatectomy, and during liver regeneration [30]. It is not surprising then that hepatic COX-2 mRNA and protein levels are increased in the setting of chronic hepatitis or cirrhosis [7, 9, 109–112]. More importantly, the frequency of COX-2 expression increases from 30% in chronic hepatitis to 80% in cirrhosis to nearly 90% in the presence of dysplasia [110]. In well-differentiated HCC, the frequency of COX-2 expression is reported to approach 100% [7, 9, 109–112]. Surprisingly, COX-2 expression is increased in less than 20% of poorly differentiated HCCs [7, 9, 109], suggesting COX-2 overexpression may not be necessary in the late stages of HCC progression [9]. Thus, COX-2 overexpression appears to be a critical factor in the development of dysplasia and HCC in the setting of chronic hepatitis and cirrhosis, but this requirement is lost when the cancer progresses to an advanced, poorly differentiated stage.

Colon cancer and colitis-associated cancer

The association of COX-2 expression with sporadic and familial forms of colon cancer has been well studied and is reviewed elsewhere in this volume (chapter by Maurer and Kessler). To summarize these findings very briefly, COX-2 protein and mRNA were noted to be elevated in a high percentage of colon adenomas and carcinomas examined. Several mechanisms have been proposed to explain this enhanced expression, including adenomatous polyposis coli (APC) mutations leading to dysregulated β-catenin/T cell factor [61], oncogenic Ras [57, 64], and stimulation by growth-factors and cytokines including gastrin [52, 54, 56]. COX-2 activity is absolutely necessary for adenoma formation in a murine model of familial adenomatosis polyposis [113]. Clinical studies support the hypothesis that COX-2 is an important agent in the progression of colon carcinogenesis. In prospective randomized clinical trials, the non-steroidal anti-inflammatory drug (NSAID) sulindac and the COX-2-specific inhibitor celecoxib significantly regressed polyp formation in patients with familial adenomatosis polyposis [12–15]. COX-2 expression likely plays a significant role in another form of colon carcinogenesis, colitis associated carcinogenesis. Expression of COX-2 is markedly increased in the intestinal epithelium of Crohn's and ulcerative colitis patients with active colitis [43, 76, 114]. In addition, overexpression of COX-2 mRNA and protein in ulcerative colitis-associated neoplasia has been reported [115]. Moreover, multiple studies have shown that the aspirin-derivative compound mesalamine may have anti-cancer effects for ulcerative colitis patients [42, 43]. Thus, COX-2 expression and activity appear to be centrally important for the development and progression of the principle forms of colon cancer including familial, sporadic, and colitis-associated cancer.

Inhibition of COX-2 activity and its effects on gastrointestinal cancer

While there is considerable circumstantial evidence linking COX-2 overexpression with carcinogenesis in gastrointestinal tissues, the clinical and mechanistic studies remain incomplete. Here we will review briefly some of the clinical/epidemiologic, animal-model, and *in vitro* studies that investigate COX-2's role in non-colonic gastrointestinal tumorigenesis.

Clinical/epidemiologic studies

Except for two studies in the colon [12, 13], there have been no randomized, placebo-controlled trials of COX-2-specific inhibitors and the prevention of non-colonic gastrointestinal malignancies. Population-based case-controlled studies have, however, suggested there may be a link. Several studies from the USA and Europe have seemed to confirm that frequent users of aspirin or non-specific NSAIDS have reduced rates of esophageal and gastric cancer [116–120]. Moreover, results from two studies suggested that treatment with COX-2 inhibitors reduced proliferation in BE epithelial cells, further bolstering the epidemiologic studies [121, 122]. The data for pancreatic cancer are less certain, with some studies suggesting a benefit with aspirin and NSAID use [116–118], one study suggesting no effect [123], and one study suggesting instead an increased risk of cancer [120]. A recent meta-analysis concluded that regular aspirin or NSAID use may be chemoprotective for gastric and esophageal cancers [116]. Additional case-controlled studies of aspirin and NSAID use in patients with pancreatic cancer and HCC would be helpful.

Animal models of non-colonic carcinogenesis

A limited number of studies have been reported regarding the effectiveness of COX-2 inhibitors in reducing the incidence of cancer in animal models for esophageal, gastric, and pancreatic cancer. Two reports using a rat model for BE and esophageal adenocarcinoma found that treatment with COX inhibitors significantly reduced reflux-associated inflammation and the relative risk of developing esophageal adenocarcinoma [124, 125]. Surprisingly, the treatment did not reduce the incidence of BE in these animals. In another study, the NSAID piroxicam (more selective for COX-1) was ineffective at inhibiting N-nitrosomethylbenzylamine (NMBA)-induced esophageal adenocarcinoma [126]. The COX-2-specific inhibitor nimesulide effectively decreased the incidence of gastric cancer in a murine model for *H. pylori*-associated gastric carcinogenesis [127]. COX-2-specific and non-specific inhibitors reduced the incidence of pancreatic adenocarcinoma, as well as hepatic metastases, in several hamster models of pancreatic cancer [128–130]. Lastly, in a recent study using a rat model for hepatic fibrosis and carcinogenesis, a COX-2-specific inhibitor significantly inhibited fibrosis in a dose-dependent manner, as well as completely blocking the progression to cirrhosis and HCC [131]. Though limited in number, these studies of COX-2 inhibition in animal models of carcinogenesis are encouraging.

In vitro studies

There is a wealth of *in vitro* data concerning the effects of COX-2-specific inhibitors on the proliferation and viability of esophageal squamous [132] and adenocarcinoma cells [133], as well as gastric [134], pancreatic [135–137] and hepatocellular carcinoma [109]. These studies nearly uniformly demonstrate the effectiveness of COX-2 inhibitors at reducing proliferation and inducing apoptosis *in vitro*. Several of these studies examined the consequences of COX-2 inhibition on the growth of human cancer xenografts in nude mice. Once again, treatment with COX-2 inhibitors suppressed the growth of these xenografts [132, 134, 136], bolstering these *in vitro* findings with *in vivo* correlates. One important aspect of this *in vitro* work has been the study of the mechanisms by which the COX-2 inhibitors achieve their potent anti-cancer effects.

Mechanisms by which COX-2 inhibitors suppress gastrointestinal cancer development and progression

Numerous *in vitro* and *in vivo* studies have suggested increased COX-2 activity promotes carcinogenesis, and a number of mechanisms have been proposed (Fig. 2). In one study, overexpression of COX-2 was sufficient to induce metastatic mammary carcinogenesis [138], marking COX-2 as a potent oncogene. While the production

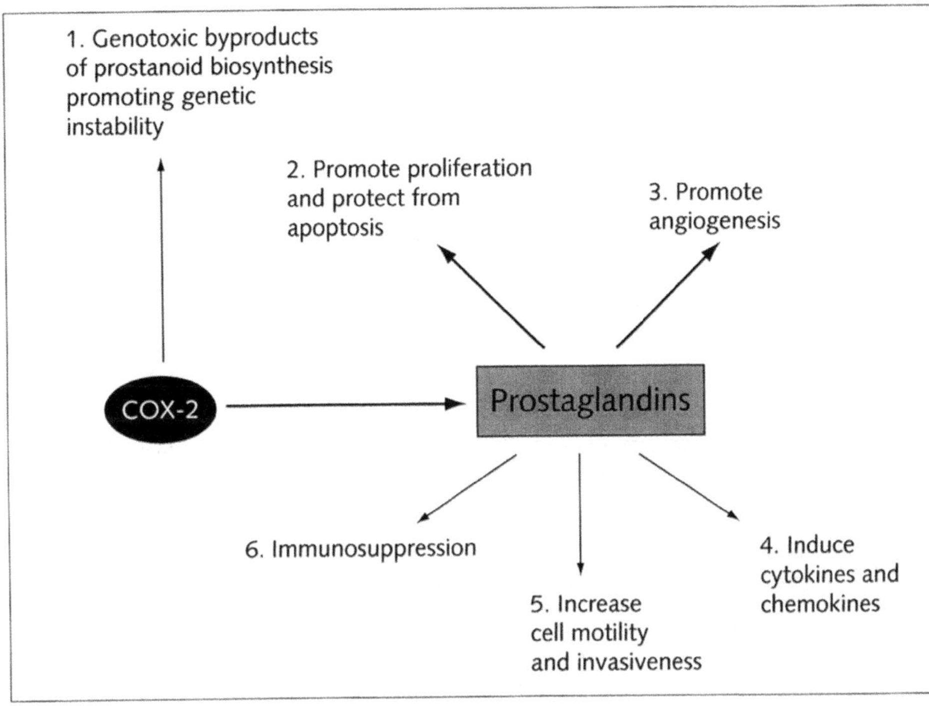

Figure 2
COX-2 activity promotes gastrointestinal cancer development and progression.
Chronic COX-2 enzymatic activity can induce and promote carcinogenesis due to the effects of prostenoid biosynthesis. Eicosanoid biosynthesis produces genotoxic byproducts like organic free radicals and reactive oxygen species that are highly mutagenic. This would induce genetic instability and could lead to cancer formation. The prostenoids that COX-2 activity helps to synthesize mediate many of the effects of COX-2 overexpression. Prostaglandins have been associated with promoting transformation by enhancing cell proliferation and motility while reducing apoptosis. They also support angiogenesis and suppress the normal immune surveillance mechanisms. This further supports tumor growth. Lastly, prostanoids can also induce cytokine and chemokine synthesis and release. These factors can have similar effects on proliferation, apoptosis, motility, angiogenesis, and immune suppression and therefore can synergize with the prostaglandins to enhance tumor progression.

of prostenoids is believed to be one of the main mechanisms by which COX-2 activity enhances tumorigenesis, COX-2 activity may in itself be carcinogenic [20]. Genotoxic byproducts of eicosanoid biosynthesis, like organic free-radicals and reactive oxygen species, are mutagenic and may induce the genetic instability that is a cardinal feature of cancer [20]. Therefore, COX-2 overexpression as the result of chronic inflammation may both induce and support neoplastic transformation and tumorigenesis.

The prostenoids that COX-2 activity helps to synthesize mediate many of the effects of COX-2 overexpression. Perhaps their most significant effect is the regulation of cellular proliferation and apoptosis. Prostenoids have long been known for their trophic effects on gastrointestinal epithelium [28, 29]. Recently it has been demonstrated that they are also required for proliferation during liver regeneration [30]. Cancer cells frequently retain this proliferative response to prostaglandins, which is perhaps why COX-2 is frequently over expressed in many cancers. This dependence upon prostaglandins may prove to be a weakness, however, as treatment of these cancers with COX-2 inhibitors reduces proliferation and limits tumor growth *in vitro* and *in vivo* [109, 131–135]. The mechanism for this effect is unknown. Several reports have suggested COX-2 inhibitors induce a G_1 cell-cycle arrest by enhancing the expression of the G_1 cyclin-dependent kinase inhibitors $p21^{waf1}$ and p27 [136, 139, 140]. This G_1 arrest may be mediated by enhanced nuclear localization of p53, a potent p21waf1 transcriptional activator. Prostenoids are able to sequester the tumor suppressor p53 in the cytoplasm, effectively inactivating it. COX-2 inhibitors reverse this effect, allowing p53 to translocate to the nucleus and alter gene expression [141]. Alternatively, PPARδ and PPARγ members of the nuclear hormone superfamily have been implicated in COX-dependent and -independent regulation of proliferation [49, 142–144]. Much work needs to be done to improve our understanding of this critical mechanism.

Another important feature of prostaglandins is that they protect cells from normal apoptotic mechanisms. While this is a beneficial effect when utilized by normal cells [145, 146], it is disastrous when it protects neoplastic cells from normal apoptotic cell death. As with proliferation, COX-2 inhibition provoked an apoptotic response in a broad range of cancers *in vitro* and *in vivo* [133–135], and this effect was dose-dependent. COX-2 inhibitors appeared to promote apoptosis through differing mechanisms, including up regulation of the pro-apoptotic protein Bax [80] or reducing the expression of anti-apoptotic proteins Bcl-2 [147], Bcl-X_L [148], or Mcl-1 [149]. Although a definitive mechanism has not been determined, the well-established pro-apoptotic features of COX-2 inhibitors make them attractive agents for cancer chemoprevention and therapy.

The growth of a tumor beyond a few millimeters in size depends upon the ability of the cancer cells to recruit a supportive vascular structure by normal endothelial cells. This process is known as angiogenesis [32]. Cardinal features of angiogenesis include the elaboration of vascular growth factors, migration of endothelial cells through the stromal matrix, and lastly the formation of tubular networks by the endothelial cells [32]. The prostaglandins synthesized by increased COX-2 activity enhance neovascularization by directly stimulating endothelial cell migration, as well as promoting the release of additional proangiogenic factors like bFGF, transforming growth-factor β, and vascular endothelial growth factor [32, 137,

150–152]. This is supported by *in vitro* studies in which endothelial cells are cocultured with cancer cells [32, 137, 151–153]. Furthermore, *in vivo* studies examining the effects of COX-2 inhibitors on human cancer xenografts reported that significant reductions in tumor growth were strongly associated with diminished microvascular density in the growing cancer [154, 155]. The prominent anti-angiogenic properties of the COX-2 inhibitors are an important reason why these agents are being tested as both a chemopreventative and a sensitizing agent in the treatment of established cancers.

Prostenoids likely mediate other significant effects of COX-2 on cancer progression. PGE_2 stimulates cytokine and growth factor production [37–39]. These factors can induce cancer cell proliferation, promote angiogenesis and cancer cell metastases, and suppress normal anti-tumor immune surveillance mechanisms, among other effects. Moreover, PGE_2 itself is a potent immune modulator [33–36]. Direct effects of PGE_2 include the inhibition of lymphocyte-activated killer (LAK) cell proliferation and the enhancement of IL-10 expression, both of which protect the tumor from destruction by the immune system [34–36]. Finally, prostenoids promote motility and tissue invasion by a variety of normal cell types including dendritic and vascular endothelial cells [31]. Unfortunately, they have similar effects on cancer cells [156, 157], which can lead to cancer metastasis. COX-2 activity and PGE2 production enhance cancer cell production of matrix metalloproteases [157]. This enables the cancer to break down stromal elements and basement membranes to permit tissue invasion. Cellular motility is similarly increased [31, 156, 157]. Together these characteristics permit cancer cells to freely migrate and metastasize.

Lastly, there is a growing consensus that COX-2 inhibitors and NSAIDs like sulindac may provide anti-cancer effects that are independent of the COX-2 enzyme [9, 158]. This is based on observations of the effects of COX inhibitors in cells without cyclooxygenase enzymes [159–161]. In addition, some NSAID derivatives without appreciable COX inhibitory activity still retain anti-cancer effects *in vitro* and *in vivo* [162–164]. Several mechanisms for this COX-independent effect have been proposed, including alterations of the NF-κB [165], Akt/proteinkinase B [166], and proteinkinase C-β1 [167] signaling pathways. PPARδ and PPARγ have been identified by several groups as potential mediators of this COX-independent anti-cancer effect [49, 142–144]. While it remains to be seen if these COX-independent effects are clinically relevant [158], they suggest the possibility that alternative therapeutic targets might exist.

The use of COX-2 inhibitors as an adjuvant or sensitizing agent for cancer chemotherapy and radiation therapy

The COX-2 enzyme provides cancer cells with survival advantages over non-transformed cells, including the enhancement of angiogenesis, proliferation, and metastasis and the suppression of apoptosis and anti-tumor immune surveillance. Given these broad effects, investigators have been interested in employing COX-2 inhibitors in therapies targeting established cancers [16–18]. Preliminary *in vitro* and *in vivo* studies have been encouraging and suggested there may be synergy between the anticancer effects of chemotherapeutic agents and COX-2 inhibitors [168–170]. Moreover, early clinical trials have suggested COX-2 inhibitors may increase response rates of patients treated with chemotherapy [171] or chemoradiotherapy [18, 172] compared with historical controls. However, the combined therapy has been reported to increase patient toxicity [172, 173], and in one study was ineffective [173]. The utility of combining chemo- and radiotherapies with COX-2 inhibitors is at present an area of great hope. It will undoubtedly be a focus for clinical researchers in the coming years as clinicians struggle to determine the optimum dosing and timing for these inhibitors in their well-studied therapeutic regimens.

Considerations regarding the use of COX-2 inhibitors as chemopreventatives

The development and use of phyto- and chemopreventatives to prevent the development of cancer is certainly an area of great promise and excitement [174]. It is hoped that in the future it will be possible to considerably reduce an individual's risk for developing cancer simply by the daily use of well-tolerated dietary supplements (i.e. vitamin E, folate, Ca^{2+}) or medications (i.e. aspirin) [174]. Rather than treating cancers as they arise with invasive procedures and toxic medications, we will intervene in the neoplastic process to prevent its completion. However, there are serious considerations regarding the implementation of this preventative therapy.

First, these agents must be safe and well tolerated [17]. Very little toxicity will be acceptable if treating otherwise healthy patients with low risk for developing cancer, particularly if it requires daily treatment for many years. Second, the agents must have proven efficacy by prospective, placebo-controlled studies. Lastly, the therapy must be cost-effective. Given the potentially large numbers of people to be treated, the agent will need to be inexpensive. In view of these constraints, what are the prospects for COX inhibitors as chemopreventatives?

As we have seen, COX-2 activity appears to be critical for the development and progression of a number of gastrointestinal cancers. Moreover, COX-2 expression is increased in preneoplastic conditions as well as early cancers, suggesting COX-2 inhibition may prevent carcinogenic progression at several stages. Non-specific COX inhibitors like aspirin and NSAIDs have the advantage of being inexpensive; however, their chronic use is associated with significant side effects including gastrointestinal ulceration and bleeding, as well as renal dysfunction [17, 71]. These side effects are thought to be due to inhibition of COX-1 and loss of its cytoprotective activity. COX-2-specific inhibitors ("coxibs") are relatively new agents that inhibit the COX-2 enzyme and have little effect on COX-1. They therefore have virtually none of the toxic effects associated with the NSAIDs [71]. At present they are costly, but in time this will change. There are two prospective, randomized placebo-controlled studies demonstrating efficacy of celecoxib in reducing the number of polyps formed in familial adenomatosis polyopsis patients [12, 13]. There are a far greater number of *in vitro* and animal studies that strongly support a role for coxibs as a potent chemopreventative. For this reason, a number of clinical trials involving coxibs in the prevention or treatment of gastrointestinal neoplasia have been initiated or planned [7, 9, 17, 18, 26, 175].

Summary and perspectives

Gastrointestinal malignancies frequently arise in the setting of chronic inflammation. Research from many groups worldwide has shown us that COX-2 levels and activity are frequently elevated in chronic inflammation. Moreover, in the progression to cancer, these levels climb higher still. The COX-2 enzyme is an oncogene. Overexpression of this enzyme's activity, either by chronic inflammation or during neoplastic transformation, yields a broad array of effects which can initiate neoplastic transformation, as well as support tumor progression. It is because of the breadth of its effects that COX-2 is an interesting target for chemopreventative and chemotherapeutic strategies. With the advent of effective, well-tolerated inhibitors (coxibs), clinical interest in this enzyme as a therapeutic target has blossomed. Although incomplete, our new understanding of the role of COX-2 in gastrointestinal carcinogenesis has already significantly impacted on patient care, and will continue to do so for the foreseeable future. Increasingly rapid research developments and technological advances will transform the way we prevent, diagnose, and treat these common and deadly forms of cancer.

References

1 Parkin DM, Pisani P, Ferlay J (1999) Global cancer statistics. *CA Cancer J Clin* 49 (1): 33–64

2 Parkin DM, Bray F, Ferlay J, Pisani P (2001) Estimating the world cancer burden: Globocan 2000. *Int J Cancer* 94 (2): 153–156

3 Lynch JP, Hoops TC (2002) The genetic pathogenesis of colorectal cancer. *Hematol Oncology Clinics of North America* 16 (4): 1–36

4 Fearon ER, Vogelstein B (1990) A genetic model for colorectal tumorigenesis. *Cell* 61 (5): 759–767

5 Kinzler KW, Vogelstein B (1996) Lessons from hereditary colorectal cancer. *Cell* 87 (2): 159–170

6 Sepulveda AR, Graham DY (2002) Role of Helicobacter pylori in gastric carcinogenesis. *Gastroenterol Clin North Am* 31 (2): 517–535
7 Hu KQ (2002) Rationale and feasibility of chemoprovention of hepatocellular carcinoma by cyclooxygenase-2 inhibitors. *J Lab Clin Med* 139 (4): 234–243
8 el-Serag HB (2002) The epidemic of esophageal adenocarcinoma. *Gastroenterol Clin North Am* 31 (2): 421–440
9 Koga H (2003) Hepatocellular carcinoma: is there a potential for chemoprevention using cyclooxygenase-2 inhibitors? *Cancer* 98 (4): 661–667
10 Farrow B, Evers BM (2002) Inflammation and the development of pancreatic cancer. *Surg Oncol* 10 (4): 153–169
11 Whitcomb DC, Pogue-Geile K (2002) Pancreatitis as a risk for pancreatic cancer. *Gastroenterol Clin North Am* 31 (2): 663–678
12 Steinbach G, Lynch PM, Phillips RK, Wallace MH, Hawk E, Gordon GB, Wakabayashi N, Saunders B, Shen Y, Fujimura T et al (2000) The effect of celecoxib, a cyclooxygenase-2 inhibitor, in familial adenomatous polyposis. *N Engl J Med* 342 (26): 1946–1952
13 Phillips RK, Wallace MH, Lynch PM, Hawk E, Gordon GB, Saunders BP, Wakabayashi N, Shen Y, Zimmerman S, Godio L et al (2002) A randomised, double blind, placebo controlled study of celecoxib, a selective cyclooxygenase 2 inhibitor, on duodenal polyposis in familial adenomatous polyposis. *Gut* 50 (6): 857–860
14 Giardiello FM, Hamilton SR, Krush AJ, Piantadosi S, Hylind LM, Celano P, Booker SV, Robinson CR, Offerhaus GJ (1993) Treatment of colonic and rectal adenomas with sulindac in familial adenomatous polyposis. *N Engl J Med* 328 (18): 1313–1316
15 Cruz-Correa M, Hylind LM, Romans KE, Booker SV, Giardiello FM (2002) Long-term treatment with sulindac in familial adenomatous polyposis: a prospective cohort study. *Gastroenterology* 122 (3): 641–645
16 Milas L, Mason KA, Crane CH, Liao Z, Masferrer J (2003) Improvement of radiotherapy or chemoradiotherapy by targeting COX-2 enzyme. *Oncology (Huntingt)* 17 (5 Suppl 5): 15–24
17 Thun MJ, Henley SJ, Patrono C (2002) Nonsteroidal anti-inflammatory drugs as anticancer agents: mechanistic, pharmacologic, and clinical issues. *J Natl Cancer Inst* 94 (4): 252–266
18 Choy H, Milas L (2003) Enhancing radiotherapy with cyclooxygenase-2 enzyme inhibitors: a rational advance? *J Natl Cancer Inst* 95 (19): 1440–1452
19 Ohshima H, Tatemichi M, Sawa T (2003) Chemical basis of inflammation-induced carcinogenesis. *Arch Biochem Biophys* 417 (1): 3–11
20 Marks F, Furstenberger G (2000) Cancer chemoprevention through interruption of multistage carcinogenesis. The lessons learnt by comparing mouse skin carcinogenesis and human large bowel cancer. *Eur J Cancer* 36 (3): 314–329
21 Mocellin S, Wang E, Marincola FM (2001) Cytokines and immune response in the tumor microenvironment. *J Immunother* 24 (5): 392–407

22 Saito S, Kitayama J, Jin ZX, Tsuno N, Kaisaki S, Seto Y, Nagawa H (2003) Beta-chemokine, macrophage inflammatory protein-1beta (MIP-1beta), is highly expressed in diffuse type human gastric cancers. *J Exp Clin Cancer Res* 22 (3): 453–459

23 Salcedo R, Oppenheim JJ (2003) Role of chemokines in angiogenesis: CXCL12/SDF-1 and CXCR4 interaction, a key regulator of endothelial cell responses. *Microcirculation* 10 (3–4): 359–370

24 White ES, Strieter RM, Arenberg DA (2002) Chemokines as therapeutic targets in non-small cell lung cancer. *Curr Med Chem Anti-Canc Agents* 2 (3): 403–417

25 Balkwill F (2002) Tumor necrosis factor or tumor promoting factor? *Cytokine Growth Factor Rev* 13 (2): 135–141

26 Krishnan K, Brenner DE (2001) Prostaglandin inhibitors and the chemoprevention of noncolonic malignancy. *Gastroenterol Clin North Am* 30 (4): 981–1000

27 Crofford LJ (2001) Prostaglandin biology. *Gastroenterol Clin North Am* 30 (4): 863–876

28 Goodlad RA, Lee CY, Levin S, Wright NA (1991) Effects of the prostaglandin analogue misoprostol on cell proliferation in the canine small intestine. *Exp Physiol* 76 (4): 561–566

29 Goodlad RA, Madgwick AJ, Moffatt MR, Levin S, Allen JL, Wright NA (1990) The effects of the prostaglandin analogue, misoprostol, on cell proliferation and cell migration in the canine stomach. *Digestion* 46 (Suppl 2): 182–187

30 Rudnick DA, Perlmutter DH, Muglia LJ (2001) Prostaglandins are required for CREB activation and cellular proliferation during liver regeneration. *Proc Natl Acad Sci USA* 98 (15): 8885–8890

31 Dormond O, Foletti A, Paroz C, Ruegg C (2001) NSAIDs inhibit alpha V beta 3 integrin-mediated and Cdc42/Rac-dependent endothelial-cell spreading, migration and angiogenesis. *Nat Med* 7 (9): 1041–1047

32 Fosslien E (2001) Review: molecular pathology of cyclooxygenase-2 in cancer-induced angiogenesis. *Ann Clin Lab Sci* 31 (4): 325–348

33 Roper RL, Phipps RP (1994) Prostaglandin E2 regulation of the immune response. *Adv Prostaglandin Thromboxane Leukot Res* 22: 101–111

34 Kucharzik T, Lugering N, Winde G, Domschke W, Stoll R (1997) Colon carcinoma cell lines stimulate monocytes and lamina propria mononuclear cells to produce IL-10. *Clin Exp Immunol* 110 (2): 296–302

35 Kambayashi T, Alexander HR, Fong M, Strassmann G (1995) Potential involvement of IL-10 in suppressing tumor-associated macrophages. Colon-26-derived prostaglandin E2 inhibits TNF-alpha release *via* a mechanism involving IL-10. *J Immunol* 154 (7): 3383–3390

36 Wang Z, Chen Y, Zheng R, Qin D, Chen X, Wang Y, Liu G (1997) *in vitro* effects of prostaglandin E2 or indomethacin on the proliferation of lymphokine-activated killer cells and their cytotoxicity against bladder tumor cells in patients with bladder cancer. *Prostaglandins* 54 (5): 769–779

37 Hilkens CM, Snijders A, Snijdewint FG, Wierenga EA, Kapsenberg ML (1996) Modu-

lation of T-cell cytokine secretion by accessory cell-derived products. *Eur Respir J Suppl* 22: 90s–94s

38 Marcinkiewicz J (1997) Regulation of cytokine production by eicosanoids and nitric oxide. *Arch Immunol Ther Exp (Warsz)* 45 (2–3): 163–167

39 Shao J, Lee SB, Guo H, Evers BM, Sheng H (2003) Prostaglandin E2 stimulates the growth of colon cancer cells *via* induction of amphiregulin. *Cancer Res* 63 (17): 5218–5223

40 Okuno M, Kojima S, Moriwaki H (2001) Chemoprevention of hepatocellular carcinoma: concept, progress and perspectives. *J Gastroenterol Hepatol* 16 (12): 1329–1335

41 Ahmad A, Govil Y, Frank BB (2003) Gastric mucosa-associated lymphoid tissue lymphoma. *Am J Gastroenterol* 98 (5): 975–986

42 Allgayer H (2003) Review article: mechanisms of action of mesalazine in preventing colorectal carcinoma in inflammatory bowel disease. *Aliment Pharmacol Ther* 18 (Suppl 2): 10–14

43 Itzkowitz SH (2002) Cancer prevention in patients with inflammatory bowel disease. *Gastroenterol Clin North Am* 31 (4): 1133–1144

44 Robinson DR (1997) Regulation of prostaglandin synthesis by antiinflammatory drugs. *J Rheumatol* (Suppl) 47: 32–39

45 Tazawa R, Xu XM, Wu KK, Wang LH (1994) Characterization of the genomic structure, chromosomal location and promoter of human prostaglandin H synthase-2 gene. *Biochem Biophys Res Commun* 203 (1): 190–199

46 Kraemer SA, Arthur KA, Denison MS, Smith WL, DeWitt DL (1996) Regulation of prostaglandin endoperoxide H synthase-2 expression by 2,3,7,8,-tetrachlorodibenzo-p-dioxin. *Arch Biochem Biophys* 330 (2): 319–328

47 Sirois J, Levy LO, Simmons DL, Richards JS (1993) Characterization and hormonal regulation of the promoter of the rat prostaglandin endoperoxide synthase 2 gene in granulosa cells. Identification of functional and protein-binding regions. *J Biol Chem* 268 (16): 12199–12206

48 Liu J, Antaya M, Boerboom D, Lussier JG, Silversides DW, Sirois J (1999) The delayed activation of the prostaglandin G/H synthase-2 promoter in bovine granulosa cells is associated with down-regulation of truncated upstream stimulatory factor-2. *J Biol Chem* 274 (49): 35037–35045

49 Trifan OC, Hla T (2003) Cyclooxygenase-2 modulates cellular growth and promotes tumorigenesis. *J Cell Mol Med* 7 (3): 207–222

50 Sheng H, Shao J, Dubois RN (2001) K-Ras-mediated increase in cyclooxygenase 2 mRNA stability involves activation of the protein kinase B1. *Cancer Res* 61 (6): 2670–2675

51 Blanco JC, Contursi C, Salkowski CA, DeWitt DL, Ozato K, Vogel SN (2000) Interferon regulatory factor (IRF)-1 and IRF-2 regulate interferon gamma-dependent cyclooxygenase 2 expression. *J Exp Med* 191(12): 2131–2144

52 Guo YS, Cheng JZ, Jin GF, Gutkind JS, Hellmich MR, Townsend CM Jr (2002) Gastrin stimulates cyclooxygenase-2 expression in intestinal epithelial cells through multiple sig-

naling pathways. Evidence for involvement of ERK5 kinase and transactivation of the epidermal growth factor receptor. *J Biol Chem* 277 (50): 48755–48763

53 Seo JH, Kim H, Kim KH (2002) Cyclooxygenase-2 expression by transcription factors in Helicobacter pylori-infected gastric epithelial cells: comparison between HP 99 and NCTC 11637. *Ann NY Acad Sci* 973: 477–480

54 Tessner TG, Muhale F, Schloemann S, Cohn SM, Morrison A, Stenson WF (2003) Basic fibroblast growth factor upregulates cyclooxygenase-2 in I407 cells through p38 MAP kinase. *Am J Physiol Gastrointest Liver Physiol* 284 (2): G269–G279

55 Zhao H, Tian W, Tai C, Cohen DM (2003) Hypertonic induction of COX-2 expression in renal medullary epithelial cells requires transactivation of the EGFR. *Am J Physiol Renal Physiol* 285 (2): F281–F288

56 Faour WH, Mancini A, He QW, Di Battista JA (2003) T-cell-derived interleukin-17 regulates the level and stability of cyclooxygenase-2 (COX-2) mRNA through restricted activation of the p38 mitogen-activated protein kinase cascade: role of distal sequences in the 3'-untranslated region of COX-2 mRNA. *J Biol Chem* 278 (29): 26897–26907

57 Juttner S, Cramer T, Wessler S, Walduck A, Gao F, Schmitz F, Wunder C, Weber M, Fischer SM, Schmidt WE et al (2003) Helicobacter pylori stimulates host cyclooxygenase-2 gene transcription: critical importance of MEK/ERK-dependent activation of USF1/-2 and CREB transcription factors. *Cell Microbiol* 5 (11): 821–834

58 Huang WC, Chen JJ, Inoue H, Chen CC (2003) Tyrosine phosphorylation of I-kappa B kinase alpha/beta by protein kinase C-dependent c-Src activation is involved in TNF-alpha-induced cyclooxygenase-2 expression. *J Immunol* 170 (9): 4767–4775

59 Glinghammar B, Skogsberg J, Hamsten A, Ehrenborg E (2003) PPARdelta activation induces COX-2 gene expression and cell proliferation in human hepatocellular carcinoma cells. *Biochem Biophys Res Commun* 308 (2): 361–368

60 Han S, Inoue H, Flowers LC, Sidell N (2003) Control of COX-2 gene expression through peroxisome proliferator-activated receptor gamma in human cervical cancer cells. *Clin Cancer Res* 9 (12): 4627–4635

61 Araki Y, Okamura S, Hussain SP, Nagashima M, He P, Shiseki M, Miura K, Harris CC (2003) Regulation of cyclooxygenase-2 expression by the Wnt and ras pathways. *Cancer Res* 63 (3): 728–734

62 Newton R, Kuitert LM, Bergmann M, Adcock IM, Barnes PJ (1997) Evidence for involvement of NF-kappaB in the transcriptional control of COX-2 gene expression by IL-1beta. *Biochem Biophys Res Commun* 237 (1): 28–32

63 Johnson GL, Lapadat R (2002) Mitogen-activated protein kinase pathways mediated by ERK, JNK, and p38 protein kinases. *Science* 298 (5600): 1911–1912

64 Sheng H, Williams CS, Shao J, Liang P, DuBois RN, Beauchamp RD (1998) Induction of cyclooxygenase-2 by activated Ha-ras oncogene in Rat-1 fibroblasts and the role of mitogen-activated protein kinase pathway. *J Biol Chem* 273 (34): 22120–22127

65 Lara-Pezzi E, Gomez-Gaviro MV, Galvez BG, Mira E, Iniguez MA, Fresno M, Martinez AC, Arroyo AG, Lopez-Cabrera M (2002) The hepatitis B virus X protein promotes

tumor cell invasion by inducing membrane-type matrix metalloproteinase-1 and cyclooxygenase-2 expression. *J Clin Invest* 110(12): 1831–1838
66 Sengupta S, Jang BC, Wu MT, Paik JH, Furneaux H, Hla T (2003) The RNA-binding protein HuR regulates the expression of cyclooxygenase-2. *J Biol Chem* 278 (27): 25227–25233
67 Gou Q, Liu CH, Ben-Av P, Hla T (1998) Dissociation of basal turnover and cytokine-induced transcript stabilization of the human cyclooxygenase-2 mRNA by mutagenesis of the 3'-untranslated region. *Biochem Biophys Res Commun* 242 (3): 508–512
68 Ristimaki A, Narko K, Hla T (1996) Down-regulation of cytokine-induced cyclo-oxygenase-2 transcript isoforms by dexamethasone: evidence for post-transcriptional regulation. *Biochem J* 318 (Pt 1): 325–331
69 Monick MM, Robeff PK, Butler NS, Flaherty DM, Carter AB, Peterson MW, Hunninghake GW (2002) Phosphatidylinositol 3-kinase activity negatively regulates stability of cyclooxygenase 2 mRNA. *J Biol Chem* 277 (36): 32992–33000
70 Dixon DA, Kaplan CD, McIntyre TM, Zimmerman GA, Prescott SM (2000) Post-transcriptional control of cyclooxygenase-2 gene expression. The role of the 3'-untranslated region. *J Biol Chem* 275 (16): 11750–11757
71 Hawkey CJ, Jones JI (2001) Gastrointestinal safety of COX-2 specific inhibitors. *Gastroenterol Clin North Am* 30 (4): 921–936
72 Cohn SM, Schloemann S, Tessner T, Seibert K, Stenson WF (1997) Crypt stem cell survival in the mouse intestinal epithelium is regulated by prostaglandins synthesized through cyclooxygenase-1. *J Clin Invest* 99 (6): 1367–1379
73 Houchen CW, Stenson WF, Cohn SM (2000) Disruption of cyclooxygenase-1 gene results in an impaired response to radiation injury. *Am J Physiol Gastrointest Liver Physiol* 279 (5): G858–865
74 Cryer B (2001) Mucosal defense and repair. Role of prostaglandins in the stomach and duodenum. *Gastroenterol Clin North Am* 30 (4): 877–894
75 Kandil HM, Tanner G, Smalley W, Halter S, Radhika A, Dubois RN (2001) Cyclooxygenase-2 expression in Barrett's esophagus. *Dig Dis Sci* 46 (4): 785–789
76 Singer II, Kawka DW, Schloemann S, Tessner T, Riehl T, Stenson WF (1998) Cyclooxygenase 2 is induced in colonic epithelial cells in inflammatory bowel disease. *Gastroenterology* 115 (2): 297–306
77 Zimmermann KC, Sarbia M, Weber AA, Borchard F, Gabbert HE, Schror K (1999) Cyclooxygenase-2 expression in human esophageal carcinoma. *Cancer Res* 59 (1): 198–204
78 Shamma A, Yamamoto H, Doki Y, Okami J, Kondo M, Fujiwara Y, Yano M, Inoue M, Matsuura N, Shiozaki H et al (2000) Up-regulation of cyclooxygenase-2 in squamous carcinogenesis of the esophagus. *Clin Cancer Res* 6 (4): 1229–1238
79 Yu HP, Xu SQ, Liu L, Shi LY, Cai XK, Lu WH, Lu B, Su YH, Li YY (2003) Cyclooxygenase-2 expression in squamous dysplasia and squamous cell carcinoma of the esophagus. *Cancer Lett* 198 (2): 193–201
80 Aggarwal S, Taneja N, Lin L, Orringer MB, Rehemtulla A, Beer DG (2000) Indo-

methacin-induced apoptosis in esophageal adenocarcinoma cells involves upregulation of Bax and translocation of mitochondrial cytochrome C independent of COX-2 expression. *Neoplasia* 2 (4): 346–356

81 Wilson KT, Fu S, Ramanujam KS, Meltzer SJ (1998) Increased expression of inducible nitric oxide synthase and cyclooxygenase-2 in Barrett's esophagus and associated adenocarcinomas. *Cancer Res* 58 (14): 2929–2934

82 Shirvani VN, Ouatu-Lascar R, Kaur BS, Omary MB, Triadafilopoulos G (2000) Cyclooxygenase 2 expression in Barrett's esophagus and adenocarcinoma: *Ex vivo* induction by bile salts and acid exposure. *Gastroenterology* 118 (3): 487–496

83 Morris CD, Armstrong GR, Bigley G, Green H, Attwood SE (2001) Cyclooxygenase-2 expression in the Barrett's metaplasia-dysplasia-adenocarcinoma sequence. *Am J Gastroenterol* 96 (4): 990–996

84 Buskens CJ, Van Rees BP, Sivula A, Reitsma JB, Haglund C, Bosma PJ, Offerhaus GJ, Van Lanschot JJ, Ristimaki A (2002) Prognostic significance of elevated cyclooxygenase 2 expression in patients with adenocarcinoma of the esophagus. *Gastroenterology* 122 (7): 1800–1807

85 Kaur BS, Triadafilopoulos G (2002) Acid- and bile-induced PGE(2) release and hyperproliferation in Barrett's esophagus are COX-2 and PKC-epsilon dependent. *Am J Physiol Gastrointest Liver Physiol* 283 (2): G327–334

86 Wambura C, Aoyama N, Shirasaka D, Sakai T, Ikemura T, Sakashita M, Maekawa S, Kuroda K, Inoue T, Ebara S et al (2002) Effect of *Helicobacter pylori*-induced cyclooxygenase-2 on gastric epithelial cell kinetics: implication for gastric carcinogenesis. *Helicobacter* 7(2): 129–138

87 Jiang XH, Wong BC (2003) Cyclooxygenase-2 inhibition and gastric cancer. *Curr Pharm Des* 9 (27): 2281–2288

88 Konturek PC, Hartwich A, Zuchowicz M, Labza H, Pierzchalski P, Karczewska E, Bielanski W, Hahn EG, Konturek SJ (2000) Helicobacter pylori, gastrin and cyclooxygenases in gastric cancer. *J Physiol Pharmacol* 51 (4 Pt 1): 737–749

89 Sung JJ, Leung WK, Go MY, To KF, Cheng AS, Ng EK, Chan FK (2000) Cyclooxygenase-2 expression in Helicobacter pylori-associated premalignant and malignant gastric lesions. *Am J Pathol* 157 (3): 729–735

90 Walker, MM (2002) Cyclooxygenase-2 expression in early gastric cancer, intestinal metaplasia and *Helicobacter pylori* infection. *Eur J Gastroenterol Hepatol* 14 (4): 347–349

91 Ristimaki A, Honkanen N, Jankala H, Sipponen P, Harkonen M (1997) Expression of cyclooxygenase-2 in human gastric carcinoma. *Cancer Res* 57 (7): 1276–1280

92 Uefuji K, Ichikura T, Mochizuki H, Shinomiya N (1998) Expression of cyclooxygenase-2 protein in gastric adenocarcinoma. *J Surg Oncol* 69 (3): 168–172

93 Ratnasinghe D, Tangrea JA, Roth MJ, Dawsey SM, Anver M, Kasprzak BA, Hu N, Wang QH, Taylor PR (1999) Expression of cyclooxygenase-2 in human adenocarcinomas of the gastric cardia and corpus. *Oncol Rep* 6 (5): 965–968

94 Saukkonen K, Nieminen O, van Rees B, Vilkki S, Harkonen M, Juhola M, Mecklin JP,

Sipponen P, Ristimaki A (2001) Expression of cyclooxygenase-2 in dysplasia of the stomach and in intestinal-type gastric adenocarcinoma. *Clin Cancer Res* 7 (7): 1923–1931

95 Yamagata R, Shimoyama T, Fukuda S, Yoshimura T, Tanaka M, Munakata A (2002) Cyclooxygenase-2 expression is increased in early intestinal-type gastric cancer and gastric mucosa with intestinal metaplasia. *Eur J Gastroenterol Hepatol* 14 (4): 359–363

96 Ohno R, Yoshinaga K, Fujita T, Hasegawa K, Iseki H, Tsunozaki H, Ichikawa W, Nihei Z, Sugihara K (2001) Depth of invasion parallels increased cyclooxygenase-2 levels in patients with gastric carcinoma. *Cancer* 91 (10): 1876–1881

97 Murata H, Kawano S, Tsuji S, Tsuji M, Sawaoka H, Kimura Y, Shiozaki H, Hori M (1999) Cyclooxygenase-2 overexpression enhances lymphatic invasion and metastasis in human gastric carcinoma. *Am J Gastroenterol* 94 (2): 451–455

98 Uefuji K, Ichikura T, Mochizuki H (2001) Expression of cyclooxygenase-2 in human gastric adenomas and adenocarcinomas. *J Surg Oncol* 76 (1): 26–30

99 Okami J, Yamamoto H, Fujiwara Y, Tsujie M, Kondo M, Noura S, Oshima S, Nagano H, Dono K, Umeshita K et al (1999) Overexpression of cyclooxygenase-2 in carcinoma of the pancreas. *Clin Cancer Res* 5 (8): 2018–2024

100 Tucker ON, Dannenberg AJ, Yang EK, Zhang F, Teng L, Daly JM, Soslow RA, Masferrer JL, Woerner BM, Koki AT et al (1999) Cyclooxygenase-2 expression is up-regulated in human pancreatic cancer. *Cancer Res* 59 (5): 987–990

101 Schlosser W, Schlosser S, Ramadani M, Gansauge F, Gansauge S, Beger HG (2002) Cyclooxygenase-2 is overexpressed in chronic pancreatitis. *Pancreas* 25 (1): 26–30

102 Molina MA, Sitja-Arnau M, Lemoine MG, Frazier ML, Sinicrope FA (1999) Increased cyclooxygenase-2 expression in human pancreatic carcinomas and cell lines: growth inhibition by nonsteroidal anti-inflammatory drugs. *Cancer Res* 59 (17): 4356–4362

103 Niijima M, Yamaguchi T, Ishihara T, Hara T, Kato K, Kondo F, Saisho H (2002) Immunohistochemical analysis and *in situ* hybridization of cyclooxygenase-2 expression in intraductal papillary-mucinous tumors of the pancreas. *Cancer* 94 (5): 1565–1573

104 Kong G, Kim EK, Kim WS, Lee KT, Lee YW, Lee JK, Paik SW, Rhee JC (2002) Role of cyclooxygenase-2 and inducible nitric oxide synthase in pancreatic cancer. *J Gastroenterol Hepatol* 17 (8): 914–921

105 Maitra A, Ashfaq R, Gunn CR, Rahman A, Yeo CJ, Sohn TA, Cameron JL, Hruban RH, Wilentz RE (2002) Cyclooxygenase 2 expression in pancreatic adenocarcinoma and pancreatic intraepithelial neoplasia: an immunohistochemical analysis with automated cellular imaging. *Am J Clin Pathol* 118 (2): 194–201

106 Kokawa A, Kondo H, Gotoda T, Ono H, Saito D, Nakadaira S, Kosuge T, Yoshida S (2001) Increased expression of cyclooxygenase-2 in human pancreatic neoplasms and potential for chemoprevention by cyclooxygenase inhibitors. *Cancer* 91 (2): 333–338

107 Ohike N, Morohoshi T (2001) Immunohistochemical analysis of cyclooxygenase (COX)-2 expression in pancreatic endocrine tumors: association with tumor progression and proliferation. *Pathol Int* 51 (10): 770–777

108 Bailey, MA, EM Brunt (2002) Hepatocellular carcinoma: predisposing conditions and precursor lesions. *Gastroenterol Clin North Am* 31(2): 641–662
109 Bae SH, Jung ES, Park YM, Kim BS, Kim BK, Kim DG, Ryu WS (2001) Expression of cyclooxygenase-2 (COX-2) in hepatocellular carcinoma and growth inhibition of hepatoma cell lines by a COX-2 inhibitor, NS-398. *Clin Cancer Res* 7 (5): 1410–1418
110 Kondo M, Yamamoto H, Nagano H, Okami J, Ito Y, Shimizu J, Eguchi H, Miyamoto A, Dono K, Umeshita K et al (1999) Increased expression of COX-2 in nontumor liver tissue is associated with shorter disease-free survival in patients with hepatocellular carcinoma. *Clin Cancer Res* 5 (12): 4005–4012
111 Koga H, Sakisaka S, Ohishi M, Kawaguchi T, Taniguchi E, Sasatomi K, Harada M, Kusaba T, Tanaka M, Kimura R et al (1999) Expression of cyclooxygenase-2 in human hepatocellular carcinoma: relevance to tumor dedifferentiation. *Hepatology* 29 (3): 688–696
112 Morinaga S, Yamamoto Y, Noguchi Y, Imada T, Rino Y, Akaike M, Sugimasa Y, Takemiya S, Kameda Y, Takanashi Y (2002) Cyclooxygenase-2 mRNA is up-regulated in cirrhotic or chronic hepatitis liver adjacent to hepatocellular carcinoma. *J Gastroenterol Hepatol* 17 (10): 1110–1116
113 Nakatsugi S, Fukutake M, Takahashi M, Fukuda K, Isoi T, Taniguchi Y, Sugimura T, Wakabayashi K (1997) Suppression of intestinal polyp development by nimesulide, a selective cyclooxygenase-2 inhibitor, in Min mice. *Jpn J Cancer Res* 88 (12): 1117–1120
114 Wallace JL (2001) Prostaglandin biology in inflammatory bowel disease. *Gastroenterol Clin North Am* 30 (4): 971–980
115 Agoff SN, Brentnall TA, Crispin DA, Taylor SL, Raaka S, Haggitt RC, Reed MW, Afonina IA, Rabinovitch PS, Stevens AC et al (2000) The role of cyclooxygenase 2 in ulcerative colitis-associated neoplasia. *Am J Pathol* 157 (3): 737–745
116 Gonzalez-Perez A, Garcia Rodriguez LA, Lopez-Ridaura R (2003) Effects of non-steroidal anti-inflammatory drugs on cancer sites other than the colon and rectum: a meta-analysis. *BMC Cancer* 3 (1): 28
117 Anderson KE, Johnson TW, Lazovich D, Folsom AR (2002) Association between nonsteroidal anti-inflammatory drug use and the incidence of pancreatic cancer. *J Natl Cancer Inst* 94 (15): 1168–1171
118 Coogan PF, Rosenberg L, Palmer JR, Strom BL, Zauber AG, Stolley PD, Shapiro S (2000) Nonsteroidal anti-inflammatory drugs and risk of digestive cancers at sites other than the large bowel. *Cancer Epidemiol Biomarkers Prev* 9 (1): 119–123
119 Akre K, Ekstrom AM, Signorello LB, Hansson LE, Nyren O (2001) Aspirin and risk for gastric cancer: a population-based case-control study in Sweden. *Br J Cancer* 84 (7): 965–968
120 Langman MJ, Cheng KK, Gilman EA, Lancashire RJ (2000) Effect of anti-inflammatory drugs on overall risk of common cancer: case-control study in general practice research database. *BMJ* 320 (7250): 1642–1646
121 Kaur BS, Khamnehei N, Iravani M, Namburu SS, Lin O, Triadafilopoulos G (2002)

Rofecoxib inhibits cyclooxygenase 2 expression and activity and reduces cell proliferation in Barrett's esophagus. *Gastroenterology* 123 (1): 60–67

122 Buttar NS, Wang KK, Anderson MA, Dierkhising RA, Pacifico RJ, Krishnadath KK, Lutzke LS (2002) The effect of selective cyclooxygenase-2 inhibition in Barrett's esophagus epithelium: an *in vitro* study. *J Natl Cancer Inst* 94 (6): 422–429

123 Menezes RJ, Huber KR, Mahoney MC, Moysich KB (2002) Regular use of aspirin and pancreatic cancer risk. *BMC Public Health* 2 (1): 18

124 Chen X, Li N, Wang S, Hong J, Fang M, Yousselfson J, Yang P, Newman RA, Lubet RA, Yang CS (2002) Aberrant arachidonic acid metabolism in esophageal adenocarcinogenesis, and the effects of sulindac, nordihydroguaiaretic acid, and alpha-difluoromethylornithine on tumorigenesis in a rat surgical model. *Carcinogenesis* 23(12): 2095–2102

125 Buttar NS, Wang KK, Leontovich O, Westcott JY, Pacifico RJ, Anderson MA, Krishnadath KK, Lutzke LS, Burgart LJ (2002) Chemoprevention of esophageal adenocarcinoma by COX-2 inhibitors in an animal model of Barrett's esophagus. *Gastroenterology* 122 (4): 1101–1112

126 Carlton PS, Gopalakrishnan R, Gupta A, Liston BW, Habib S, Morse MA, Stoner GD (2002) Piroxicam is an ineffective inhibitor of N-nitrosomethylbenzylamine-induced tumorigenesis in the rat esophagus. *Cancer Res* 62 (15): 4376–4382

127 Hahm KB, Song YJ, Oh TY, Lee JS, Surh YJ, Kim YB, Yoo BM, Kim JH, Han SU, Nahm KT et al (2003) Chemoprevention of *Helicobacter pylori*-associated gastric carcinogenesis in a mouse model: is it possible? *J Biochem Mol Biol* 36 (1): 82–94

128 Furukawa F, Nishikawa A, Lee IS, Kanki K, Umemura T, Okazaki K, Kawamori T, Wakabayashi K, Hirose M (2003) A cyclooxygenase-2 inhibitor, nimesulide, inhibits postinitiation phase of N-nitrosobis(2-oxopropyl)amine-induced pancreatic carcinogenesis in hamsters. *Int J Cancer* 104 (3): 269–273

129 Schuller HM, Zhang L, Weddle DL, Castonguay A, Walker K, Miller MS (2002) The cyclooxygenase inhibitor ibuprofen and the FLAP inhibitor MK886 inhibit pancreatic carcinogenesis induced in hamsters by transplacental exposure to ethanol and the tobacco carcinogen NNK. *J Cancer Res Clin Oncol* 128 (10): 525–532

130 Wenger FA, Kilian M, Bisevac M, Khodadayan C, von Seebach M, Schimke I, Guski H, Muller JM (2002) Effects of Celebrex and Zyflo on liver metastasis and lipidperoxidation in pancreatic cancer in Syrian hamsters. *Clin Exp Metastasis* 19 (8): 681–687

131 Yamamoto H, Kondo M, Nakamori S, Nagano H, Wakasa K, Sugita Y, Chang-De J, Kobayashi S, Damdinsuren B, Dono K et al (2003) JTE-522, a cyclooxygenase-2 inhibitor, is an effective chemopreventive agent against rat experimental liver fibrosis1. *Gastroenterology* 125 (2): 556–571

132 Nishimura G, Yanoma S, Mizuno H, Kawakami K, Tsukuda M (1999) A selective cyclooxygenase-2 inhibitor suppresses tumor growth in nude mouse xenografted with human head and neck squamous carcinoma cells. *Jpn J Cancer Res* 90 (10): 1152–1162

133 Souza RF, Shewmake K, Beer DG, Cryer B, Spechler SJ (2000) Selective inhibition of cyclooxygenase-2 suppresses growth and induces apoptosis in human esophageal adenocarcinoma cells. *Cancer Res* 60 (20): 5767–5772

134 Sawaoka H, Kawano S, Tsuji S, Tsujii M, Gunawan ES, Takei Y, Nagano K, Hori M (1998) Cyclooxygenase-2 inhibitors suppress the growth of gastric cancer xenografts *via* induction of apoptosis in nude mice. *Am J Physiol* 274 (6 Pt 1): G1061–1067
135 Ding XZ, Tong WG, Adrian TE (2000) Blockade of cyclooxygenase-2 inhibits proliferation and induces apoptosis in human pancreatic cancer cells. *Anticancer Res* 20(4): 2625–2631
136 Tseng WW, Deganutti A, Chen MN, Saxton RE, Liu CD (2002) Selective cyclooxygenase-2 inhibitor rofecoxib (Vioxx) induces expression of cell cycle arrest genes and slows tumor growth in human pancreatic cancer. *J Gastrointest Surg* 6(6): 838–843; discussion 844
137 Chu J, Lloyd FL, Trifan OC, Knapp B, Rizzo MT (2003) Potential involvement of the cyclooxygenase-2 pathway in the regulation of tumor-associated angiogenesis and growth in pancreatic cancer. *Mol Cancer Ther* 2(1): 1–7
138 Liu CH, Chang SH, Narko K, Trifan OC, Wu MT, Smith E, Haudenschild C, Lane TF, Hla T (2001) Overexpression of cyclooxygenase-2 is sufficient to induce tumorigenesis in transgenic mice. *J Biol Chem* 276 (21): 18563–18569
139 Makitie AA, Chau M, Lim S, Viani MA, Gilbert R, Lim MS, Jordan RC (2003) Selective inhibition of cyclooxygenase 2 induces p27kip1 and skp2 in oral squamous cell carcinoma. *J Otolaryngol* 32 (4): 226–229
140 Detjen KM, Welzel M, Wiedenmann B, Rosewicz S (2003) Nonsteroidal anti-inflammatory drugs inhibit growth of human neuroendocrine tumor cells *via* G1 cell-cycle arrest. *Int J Cancer* 107 (5): 844–853
141 Swamy MV, Herzog CR, Rao CV (2003) Inhibition of COX-2 in colon cancer cell lines by celecoxib increases the nuclear localization of active p53. *Cancer Res* 63 (17): 5239–5242
142 Nikitakis NG, Hebert C, Lopes MA, Reynolds MA, Sauk JJ (2002) PPARgamma-mediated antineoplastic effect of NSAID sulindac on human oral squamous carcinoma cells. *Int J Cancer* 98 (6): 817–823
143 Wick M, Hurteau G, Dessev C, Chan D, Geraci MW, Winn RA, Heasley LE, Nemenoff RA (2002) Peroxisome proliferator-activated receptor-gamma is a target of nonsteroidal anti-inflammatory drugs mediating cyclooxygenase-independent inhibition of lung cancer cell growth. *Mol Pharmacol* 62 (5): 1207–1214
144 He TC, Chan TA, Vogelstein B, Kinzler KW (1999) PPARdelta is an APC-regulated target of nonsteroidal anti-inflammatory drugs. *Cell* 99 (3): 335–345
145 Hoshino T, Tsutsumi S, Tomisato W, Hwang HJ, Tsuchiya T, Mizushima T (2003) Prostaglandin E2 protects gastric mucosal cells from apoptosis *via* EP2 and EP4 receptor activation. *J Biol Chem* 278 (15): 12752–12758
146 Yang H, Majno P, Morel P, Toso C, Triponez F, Oberholzer J, Mentha G, Lou J (2002) Prostaglandin E(1) protects human liver sinusoidal endothelial cell from apoptosis induced by hypoxia reoxygenation. *Microvasc Res* 64(1): 94–103
147 Sheng H, Shao J, Morrow JD, Beauchamp RD, DuBois RN (1998) Modulation of apoptosis and Bcl-2 expression by prostaglandin E2 in human colon cancer cells. *Cancer Res* 58 (2): 362–366

148 Zhang L, Yu J, Park BH, Kinzler KW, Vogelstein B (2000) Role of BAX in the apoptotic response to anticancer agents. *Science* 290 (5493): 989–992
149 Nzeako UC, Guicciardi ME, Yoon JH, Bronk SF, Gores GJ (2002) COX-2 inhibits Fas-mediated apoptosis in cholangiocarcinoma cells. *Hepatology* 35(3): 552–559
150 Gately S, Kerbel R (2003) Therapeutic potential of selective cyclooxygenase-2 inhibitors in the management of tumor angiogenesis. *Prog Exp Tumor Res* 37: 179–192
151 Ben-Av P, Crofford LJ, Wilder RL, Hla T (1995) Induction of vascular endothelial growth factor expression in synovial fibroblasts by prostaglandin E and interleukin-1: a potential mechanism for inflammatory angiogenesis. *FEBS Lett* 372 (1): 83–87
152 Leung WK, To KF, Go MY, Chan KK, Chan FK, Ng EK, Chung SC, Sung JJ (2003) Cyclooxygenase-2 upregulates vascular endothelial growth factor expression and angiogenesis in human gastric carcinoma. *Int J Oncol* 23 (5): 1317–1322
153 Jones MK, Szabo IL, Kawanaka H, Husain SS, Tarnawski AS (2002) von Hippel Lindau tumor suppressor and HIF-1alpha: new targets of NSAIDs inhibition of hypoxia-induced angiogenesis. *FASEB J* 16 (2): 264–266
154 Sawaoka H, Tsuji S, Tsujii M, Gunawan ES, Sasaki Y, Kawano S, Hori M (1999) Cyclooxygenase inhibitors suppress angiogenesis and reduce tumor growth *in vivo*. *Lab Invest* 79 (12): 1469–1477
155 Leahy KM, Ornberg RL, Wang Y, Zweifel BS, Koki AT, Masferrer JL (2002) Cyclooxygenase-2 inhibition by celecoxib reduces proliferation and induces apoptosis in angiogenic endothelial cells *in vivo*. *Cancer Res* 62 (3): 625–631
156 Sheng H, Shao J, Washington MK, DuBois RN (2001) Prostaglandin E2 increases growth and motility of colorectal carcinoma cells. *J Biol Chem* 276 (21): 18075–18081
157 Dohadwala M, Luo J, Zhu L, Lin Y, Dougherty GJ, Sharma S, Huang M, Pold M, Batra RK, Dubinett SM (2001) Non-small cell lung cancer cyclooxygenase-2-dependent invasion is mediated by CD44. *J Biol Chem* 276 (24): 20809–20812
158 Marx J (2001) Cancer research. Anti-inflammatories inhibit cancer growth – but how? *Science* 291(5504): 581–582
159 Zhang X, Morham SG, Langenbach R, Young DA (1999) Malignant transformation and antineoplastic actions of nonsteroidal antiinflammatory drugs (NSAIDs) on cyclooxygenase-null embryo fibroblasts. *J Exp Med* 190 (4): 451–459
160 Eibl G, Reber HA, Wente MN, Hines OJ (2003) The selective cyclooxygenase-2 inhibitor nimesulide induces apoptosis in pancreatic cancer cells independent of COX-2. *Pancreas* 26 (1): 33–41
161 Hanif R, Pittas A, Feng Y, Koutsos MI, Qiao L, Staiano-Coico L, Shiff SI, Rigas B (1996) Effects of nonsteroidal anti-inflammatory drugs on proliferation and on induction of apoptosis in colon cancer cells by a prostaglandin-independent pathway. *Biochem Pharmacol* 52 (2): 237–245
162 Rice PL, Kelloff J, Sullivan H, Driggers LJ, Beard KS, Kuwada S, Piazza G, Ahnen DJ (2003) Sulindac metabolites induce caspase- and proteasome-dependent degradation of beta-catenin protein in human colon cancer cells. *Mol Cancer Ther* 2 (9): 885–892
163 Piazza GA, Alberts DS, Hixson LJ, Paranka NS, Li H, Finn T, Bogert C, Guillen JM,

Brendel K, Gross PH et al (1997) Sulindac sulfone inhibits azoxymethane-induced colon carcinogenesis in rats without reducing prostaglandin levels. *Cancer Res* 57 (14): 2909–2915
164 Liu JJ, Wang JY, Hertervig E, Nilsson A, Duan RD (2002) Sulindac induces apoptosis, inhibits proliferation and activates caspase-3 in Hep G2 cells. *Anticancer Res* 22 (1A): 263–266
165 Yamamoto Y, Yin MJ, Lin KM, Gaynor RB (1999) Sulindac inhibits activation of the NF-kappaB pathway. *J Biol Chem* 274 (38): 27307–27314
166 Arico S, Pattingre S, Bauvy C, Gane P, Barbat A, Codogno P, Ogier-Denis E (2002) Celecoxib induces apoptosis by inhibiting 3-phosphoinositide-dependent protein kinase-1 activity in the human colon cancer HT-29 cell line. *J Biol Chem* 277 (31): 27613–27621
167 Jiang XH, Lam SK, Lin MC, Jiang SH, Kung HF, Slosberg ED, Soh JW, Weinstein IB, Wong BC (2002) Novel target for induction of apoptosis by cyclo-oxygenase-2 inhibitor SC-236 through a protein kinase C-beta(1)-dependent pathway. *Oncogene* 21 (39): 6113–6122
168 Hsueh CT, Chiu CF, Kelsen DP, Schwartz GK (2000) Selective inhibition of cyclooxygenase-2 enhances mitomycin-C-induced apoptosis. *Cancer Chemother Pharmacol* 45 (5): 389–396
169 Yip-Schneider MT, Sweeney CJ, Jung SH, Crowell PL, Marshall MS (2001) Cell cycle effects of nonsteroidal anti-inflammatory drugs and enhanced growth inhibition in combination with gemcitabine in pancreatic carcinoma cells. *J Pharmacol Exp Ther* 298 (3): 976–985
170 Sugiura T, Saikawa Y, Kubota T, Suganuma K, Otani Y, Watanabe M, Kumai K, Kitajima M (2003) Combination chemotherapy with JTE-522, a novel selective cyclooxygenase-2 inhibitor, and cisplatin against gastric cancer cell lines *in vitro* and *in vivo*. *In Vivo* 17 (3): 229–233
171 Altorki NK, Keresztes RS, Port JL, Libby DM, Korst RJ, Flieder DB, Ferrara CA, Yankelevitz DF, Subbaramaiah K, Pasmantier MW et al (2003) Celecoxib, a selective cyclo-oxygenase-2 inhibitor, enhances the response to preoperative paclitaxel and carboplatin in early-stage non-small-cell lung cancer. *J Clin Oncol* 21 (14): 2645–2650
172 Crane CH, Mason K, Janjan NA, Milas L (2003) Initial experience combining cyclooxygenase-2 inhibition with chemoradiation for locally advanced pancreatic cancer. *Am J Clin Oncol* 26 (4): S81–84
173 Becerra CR, Frenkel EP, Ashfaq R, Gaynor RB (2003) Increased toxicity and lack of efficacy of Rofecoxib in combination with chemotherapy for treatment of metastatic colorectal cancer: A phase II study. *Int J Cancer* 105 (6): 868–872
174 Turini ME, DuBois RN (2002) Primary prevention: phytoprevention and chemoprevention of colorectal cancer. *Hematol Oncol Clin North Am* 16 (4): 811–840
175 Fennerty MB (2002) Does chemoprevention of Barrett's esophagus using acid suppression and/or COX-2 inhibition prevent neoplastic progression? *Rev Gastroenterol Disord* 2 (Suppl 2): S30–S37

Effects of cyclooxygenase-2 (COX-2) inhibitors in colorectal cancer

Christoph A. Maurer and Katharina M. Kessler

Hospital of Liestal, Rheinstrasse 26, CH-4410 Liestal, Switzerland

Introduction

Colorectal cancer is one of the leading causes of cancer-related deaths in the western world [1, 2]. In the United States, colorectal cancer is the second most common form of malignant tumor [3]. Therefore, prevention of this disease has been more and more focused recently [4]. The use of colorectal cancer-screening programs has resulted in a decrease in the incidence and the mortality rates of colorectal cancer [5,6]. However, the acceptance of screening tests is low [7–9]. Thus, current screening and treatment strategies for colorectal cancer are not sufficiently effective [10]. Recently, some studies reported that cyclooxygenase (COX) inhibitors are able to reduce the incidence of colorectal adenoma and colorectal cancer and that the mortality rate from colorectal cancer may be improved by up to 65% [11–14]. Furthermore, the inhibition of COX-2 activity in patients with familial adenomatous polyposis (FAP) syndrome seems to be related to a reduced formation of colorectal polyps [15]. The following chapter discusses the mechanism of action and the role of COX-2 inhibitors in prevention of colorectal cancer, based on a broad literature search.

Natural source and function of COXs

Arachidonic acid metabolites circulate through the organism and show a wide spectrum of pharmacological effects, such as physiological stimuli that modulate and maintain homeostasis [16]. These metabolites are also produced during acute and chronic inflammatory processes, and it is generally accepted that they mediate many of the symptoms of inflammation such as edema and pain [17]. Multiple enzymatic steps are involved in the biosynthesis of prostanoids. The first step is the release of arachidonic acid from membrane phospholipids by phospholipases, including

Cancer and Inflammation, edited by Douglas W. Morgan, Ulf J. Forssmann and Marian T. Nakada

phospholipase A_2 [18]. Arachidonic acid is then converted to prostaglandin H_2 by prostaglandin H synthase which exhibits two distinct catalytic activities, COX and peroxidase [19]. Two COX isoforms were identified: the primarily expressed COX-1 and the inducible COX-2 [20]. Different biological functions are mediated by these two isoenzymes. COX-1 is constitutively expressed at a stable level in many tissues, e.g. platelets, gastrointestinal mucosa, and others, and produces prostanoic acids that predominantly regulate normal cellular processes such as regeneration of the gastrointestinal mucosa [21]. In contrast, the COX-2 gene is an immediate-early response gene and follows rapidly in response to mitogenic stimuli, tumor promoters, cytokines and growth factors [22]. Since non-steroidal anti-inflammatory drugs (NSAIDs) inhibit both COX-1 and COX-2, these drugs have the risk of severe side effects, exemplified by gastrointestinal ulcer formation and bleeding [23–26]. As a result of research that characterized the role of COX-2 in prostaglandin and prostanoic acid production [27], a class of anti-inflammatory and analgesic agents has been developed that primarily inhibit COX-2 while sparing COX-1 at therapeutic dosages [28, 29].

Carcinogenesis of colorectal cancer

More than 95% of human colorectal carcinomas develop from normal mucosa via adenomatous polyps to carcinomas, hence following the adenoma-carcinoma sequence. This statement is underlined by the fact that the epidemiology of adenomas is closely similar to the epidemiology of colorectal cancer itself [30, 31]. It is estimated that the progression from polyp to cancer occurs over 5–10 years [32]. Therefore, prevention of colorectal adenoma formation and removal of colorectal adenomas once detected are thought to result in a highly effective prevention from colorectal carcinoma [2].

About 90% of colorectal cancers occur sporadically and about 10% of colorectal cancers are hereditary, i.e. the FAP syndrome and the hereditary non-polyposis colorectal cancer syndrome, two dominantly inherited conditions with 100 and 80% life-time risks of developing colorectal cancer, respectively [33]. Patients with FAP have an inherited germ-line adenomatous polyposis coli (APC) mutation. The locus could be identified from chromosome 5q21 [34]. If FAP is left untreated, colorectal cancer is the unavoidable consequence [35]. The risk of cancer is generally related to the number of polyps and to the age of the patient [36]. This small collective of patients usually is in a routine screening program. For that reason, the adenomatous polyp formation serves as a practicable target in chemoprevention studies [32]. Indeed, the first clinical observations of a regression of pre-existing adenomas following continuous use of NSAIDs could be found in patients with FAP [37]. Meanwhile, there is accumulating evidence that NSAIDs can reduce the number and size of polyps in patients with FAP [38].

Table 1 - Evidence suggesting a crucial role of COX-2 expression in colorectal cancer

	Colorectal tumors	Normal intestinal mucosa
Prostaglandin levels in intestinal cells [39]	↑↑	↔
Proliferation rate due to prostaglandins [40]	↑↑	↑
Evidence of COX-1 [41]	↑	↑
Evidence of COX-2 [41]	↑↑↑	↑
Effects of NSAIDs in cell growth [32,42]	↓↓↓	↓
Risk for colorectal cancer by regular use of NSAIDs [43]		↓↓↓ (40–50%)

Preventive effectiveness of COX-2 inhibitors in colorectal cancer

Several lines of evidence suggest a crucial role of COX-2 expression in colorectal cancer (see Tab. 1) and propose specific COX-2 inhibitors as a chemopreventative tool.

Experimental data and animal studies

The role of COX-2 in colorectal tumorigenesis in mice was studied by Oshima et al. [44] to determine the effects of COX-2-gene-knockouts and a new COX-2 inhibitor. In the study, the heterozygous Apcdelta716-knockout mice, a mouse model of human FAP, were either crossed with COX-2-gene-knockout mice, or fed chow containing a COX-2-selective inhibitor. Apcdelta716 litter mates were used as positive controls, which developed 652 ± 198 (mean ± SD) polyps at 10 weeks. Both introduction of the *COX-2* gene mutation and feeding with the COX-2-selective inhibitor dramatically reduced the number and the size of intestinal polyps in Apcdelta716-knockout mice. These results provide direct genetic evidence that COX-2 plays a key role in tumorigenesis, and indicate that COX-2-selective inhibitors may be a new class of therapeutic agents for colorectal polyposis and cancer in mice.

Sheng et al. [45] selected two transformed human colon cancer cell lines for studies on the role of COX-2 in intestinal tumorigenesis. They evaluated HCA-7 cells which constitutively express high levels of COX-2 protein and HCT-116 cells which lack COX-2 protein. When nude mice implanted with HCA-7 cells were treated with a selective COX-2 inhibitor (SC-58125), tumor formation was reduced by 85–90%. SC-58125 also inhibited colony formation of cultured HCA-7 cells. Conversely, SC-58125 had no effect on HCT-116 implants in nude mice or colony formation in culture. These data provide evidence that there may be a direct link between selective inhibition of the COX-2 pathway and intestinal cancer growth.

In a further experiment, the highly selective COX-2 inhibitor SC-58635 administered to carcinogen-treated rats caused a 40% reduction in colonic aberrant crypt foci formation [46].

Several NSAIDs including indomethacin, piroxicam, ibuprofen, aspirin, and sulindac were tested in laboratory animals [47–52]. These studies showed that treatment with NSAIDs results in an impressive reduction in the size and number of intestinal tumors. These observations led to a series of human studies examining the relationship between NSAID use and colorectal neoplasia, as described below.

All of the NSAIDs examined reduced the proliferation and transformed the morphology of the cells in a time- and concentration-dependent manner. Cellular pathways leading to cell death might contribute to the anti-neoplastic effects of these compounds. Thus, NSAIDs might trigger cell death by apoptosis, a process that is involved in many biological events, such as tumorigenesis [42]. Nonetheless, NSAIDs can inhibit colon cancer cell growth by inhibiting cell cycle progression and inducing apoptotic cell death in a COX-independent fashion. For instance, structurally different NSAIDs have been demonstrated to reduce the levels of cell-cycle-regulatory proteins [42]. Furthermore, Santini et al. [53] explained that the highly selective COX-2 inhibitor L-745,337 and sodium salicylate, a weak inhibitor of COX isoenzymes, reduce colon cancer cell growth by a mechanism that may involve p53-independent induction of the tumor suppressor $p21^{WAF-1}$/cip1.

Clinical studies and comparison with other NSAID (Sulindac, Aspirin)

Due to the findings in these rodent models, several NSAIDs were tested in clinical studies to assess the relevance of these results in human colon cancer [54].

Levels of COX-1 and COX-2 could be determined from rodent tumor models as well as from human adenomatous and carcinomatous tissues [55–57]. A key question is whether the inhibitory effect of NSAIDs on colon carcinogenesis is mediated by inhibition of COX-1, COX-2 or both, or by inhibition of other cellular targets of NSAIDs. Summarizing the results, no change in COX-1 expression, but an upregulation of COX-2 in adenomas and adenocarcinomas was found [41, 58, 59]. In addition, COX-2 has been shown to alter cellular adhesion, apoptosis and angiogenesis, contributing to its neoplastic potential [60].

Aspirin, as the most widely known and used COX-2 inhibitor, has been the topic of many surveillance studies [61]. In a prospective randomized trial it has recently been shown that daily use of aspirin is associated with a significant reduction in the incidence of colorectal adenomas in patients with previous colorectal cancer [62]. Aspirin, taken regularly at a dosage of 325 mg per day, decreased the number of adenomas and the time of adenoma development. 325 mg of aspirin is a commonly used dosage for several indications, such as arteriosclerotic disease, but it increases the risk of bleeding [63, 64]. In another study, low-dose aspirin (81 mg) was proved to have a moderate chemopreventive effect on adenomas of the large bowel [65]. Further studies deal with dose-finding analyses of aspirin in the inhibition of prostaglandin E_2 from rectal muscosa [66, 67]. Other studies observed that the effect of NSAIDs, including aspirin, on colorectal neoplasia does not depend strongly on the dosage [68, 69]. Due to the well-known gastrointestinal toxicity of aspirin, focus has been placed on this adverse effect in assessing the cost-effectiveness of aspirin chemoprevention [1, 70]. Drugs with similar mechanisms but better safety profiles might offer superior chemoprevention.

Sulindac can cause regression in patients with FAP [37]. One of the retrospective studies was community-based [71], whereas the others were hospital-based [12, 14, 72–74]. A small study on patients with diffuse colonic polyposis evaluated sulindac at 200 mg twice daily [75]. A decrease in the number and size of colorectal polyps could be demonstrated. Following these results, a prospective randomized study was performed, using 150 mg of sulindac twice a day [38]. A reduction in the number and size of polyps was shown here as well. Several additional randomized clinical trials also present the reducing effect of sulindac on colorectal polyps [38, 76–78].

Of the COX-2 inhibitors, celecoxib, as one of the "new" generation NSAIDs with selective inhibition of COX-2, was the first to appear in a randomized trial. To determine whether the inhibition of COX could reduce the number of polyps in patients with FAP, the effect of celecoxib was assessed by Steinbach et al. [15]. Treatment with 400 mg of celecoxib twice daily for 6 months was associated with a significant reduction in the number of polyps from the baseline in comparison with the placebo group. The group receiving 100 mg twice a day did not show any significant change, although a reduction of 25% or more in the number of colorectal polyps was seen in 31% of the patients. Regression of polyps was observed in the rectum as well as in the left and right colon. Hence treatment with celecoxib is thought to be a useful adjunctive chemotherapy in addition to routine endoscopic surveillance and surgery [79].

Additive effects against human colon cancer could be demonstrated in a combination treatment of celecoxib and herceptin in assays *in vitro* and *in vivo* [80]. Furthermore, a combination therapy of a COX-2 inhibitor with a tyrosine kinase inhibitor such as IRESSA, a selective epidermal growth factor receptor-tyrosine kinase inhibitor, is also proposed to be evaluated *in vitro* and in patients with colorectal cancer [81].

Summary and conclusion

The importance of the COX pathway in human disease was recognized with the discovery that NSAIDs, a group of compounds that have been used in the treatment of various inflammatory disorders, can inhibit the activity of COX [32]. The two COX isoenzymes, COX-1 and COX-2, convert arachidonates into prostaglandins. An increased level of prostaglandins could be found in human colorectal tumours compared with normal intestinal mucosa [39,40]. To examine the role of COX in colorectal adenomas and adenocarcinomas, the levels of COX-1 and COX-2 were determined in these cells. The key points were little changed in COX-1 expression but increased levels of COX-2 in adenomas and adenocarcinomas [57]. These expression patterns suggested that NSAIDs could suppress tumor growth *via* an inhibition of COX-2.

All clinical studies were able to demonstrate that NSAIDs have a clear protective effect, although adenomas developed in some patients who were receiving treatment. Thus NSAIDs cannot be recommended as a replacement for surveillance colonoscopy. COX-2 inhibitors seem to have become the most interesting medical option in preventing colorectal cancer due to fewer side effects in comparison with conventional NSAIDs. However, clinical trials investigating the preventive effect of different NSAIDs for sporadic primary colorectal cancer would be desirable, but difficult to perform. Trials investigating the effects of NSAIDs on recurrent cancer and metachronous second primary cancers in patients with resected colorectal cancer appear more feasible.

References

1 Ladabaum U, Chopra CL, Huang G, Schelman JM, Chernew ME, Fendrick AM (2001) Aspirin as an adjunct to screening for prevention of sporadic colorectal cancer. A cost-effectiveness analysis. *Ann Intern Med* 135: 769–781

2 Winawer SJ, Zauber AG, O'Brien MJ, Gottlieb LS, Sternberg SS; Stewart ET, Bond JH, Schapiro M, Panish JF, Waye JD et al (1992) The National Polyp Study. Design, methods and characteristics of patients with newly diagnosed polyps. The National Polyp Study Workgroup. *Cancer* 70 (5 Suppl): 1236–1245

3 Landis SH, Murray T, Bolden S, Wingo PA (1999) Cancer statistics 1999. *CA Cancer J Clin* 49: 8–31

4 Dubois RN, Smalley WE (1996) Cyclooxygenase, NSAIDs, and colorectal cancer. *J Gastroenterol* 31 (6): 898–906

5 Burt RW (2000) Colon cancer screening. *Gastroenterology* 119: 837–853

6 Mandel JS, Church TR, Bond JH, Ederer, F, Geisser MS, Mongin SJ, Snover DC, Schuman LM (2000) The effect of fecal occult-blood screening in the incidence of colorectal cancer. *N Engl J Med* 343: 1603–1607

7 Anderson LM, May DS (1995) Has the use of cervical, breast and colorectal cancer screening increased in the United States? *Am J Public Health* 85: 840–842

8 Brown ML, Potosky AL, Thompson GB, Kessler LG (1990) The knowledge and use of

screening tests for colorectal and prostate cancer: data from the 1987 National Health Interview Survey. *Prev Med* 19: 562–574

9 Screening for colorectal cancer – United States (1997) *MMWR Morb Mortal Wkly Rep* (1999) 48: 116–121

10 Levin TR (2002) Flexible sigmoidoscopy for colorectal cancer screening: valid approach or short-sighted? *Gastroenterol Clin North Am* 31: 1015–1029

11 Sandler RS, Galanko JC, Murray SC, Helm JF, Woosley JT (1998) Aspirin and nonsteroidal anti-inflammatory agents and risk for colorectal adenoma. *Gastroenterology* 114: 441–447

12 Suh O, Mettlin C, Petrelli NJ (1993) Aspirin use, cancer, and polyps of the large bowel. *Cancer* 72: 1171–1177

13 Rosenberg L, Palmer JR, Zauber AG, Warshauer ME, Stolley PD, Shapiro S (1991) A hypothesis: nonsteroidal anti-inflammatory drugs reduce the incidence of large-bowel cancer. *J Natl Cancer Inst* 83: 355–358

14 Muscat JE, Stellman SD, Wynder EL (1994) Nonsteroidal antiinflammatory drugs and colorectal cancer. *Cancer* 74: 1847–1854

15 Steinbach G, Lynch PM, Phillips RKS, Wallace MH, Hawk E, Gordon GB, Wakabayashi N, Saunders B, Shen Y et al (2000) The effect of celecoxib, a cyclooxygenase-2-inhibitor, in familial adenomatous polyposis. *N Engl J Med* 342: 1946–1952

16 DuBois RN, Abramson SB, Crofford L, Gupta RA, Simon LS, Van De Putte LB, Lipsky PE (1998) Cyclooxygenase in biology and disease. *FASEB J* 12: 1063–1073

17 Abramson SR, Weissman G (1989) The mechanism of action of nonsteroidal anti-inflammatory drugs. *Arthritis Rheum* 32: 1–9

18 Smith WL, Garavito RM, DeWitt DL (1996) Prostaglandin endoperoxide H synthases (cyclooxygenases)-1 and -2. *J Biol Chem* 271: 33157–33160

19 Smith WL, DeWitt DL, Garavito RM (2000) Cyclooxygenases: structural, cellular, and molecular biology. *Ann Rev Biochem* 69: 145–182

20 Isakson P, Seibert K, Masferrer J, Salvemini D, Lee L, Needleman P (1995) Discovery of a better aspirin. *Adv Prostaglandin Thromboxane Leukotr Res* 23: 49–54

21 Simon LS, Weaver AL, Graham DY, Kivith AJ, Lipsky PE, Hubbard RC, Isakson PC, Verburg KM, Yu SS, Zhao WW, Geis GS (1999) Anti-inflammatory and upper gastrointestinal effects of celecoxib in rheumatoid arthritis. A randomised controlled trial. *JAMA* 282 (20): 1921–1928

22 DuBois RN, Awad J, Morrow J, Roberts II LJ, Bishop PR (1994) Regulation of eicasonoid production and mitogenesis in rat intestinal epithelial cells by transforming growth factor-alpha and phorbol ester. *J Clin Invest* 93: 493–498

23 Gabriel SE; Jaakkimainen L, Bombardier C (1991) Risk of serious gastrointestinal complications related to use of nonsteroidal anti-inflammatory drugs: a meta analysis. *Ann Intern Med* 115: 787–796

24 MacDonald TM, Morant SV, Robinson CC, Shield MJ, McGilchrist MM, Murray FE, McDevitt DG (1997) Association of upper gastrointestinal toxicity on non-steroidal anti-inflammatory drugs with continued exposure: cohort study. *BMJ* 315: 1333–1337

25 Henry D, Dobson A, Turner C (1993) Variability in the risk of major gastrointestinal from non-aspirin nonsteroidal anti-inflammatory drugs. *Gastroenterology* 105: 1078–1088
26 Griffin MR, Piper JM, Daugherty JR, Snowden M, Ray WA (1991) Nonsteroidal anti-inflammatory drug use and increased risk for peptic ulcer disease in elderly persons. *Ann Intern Med* 114: 257–263
27 Fu JY, Masferrer JL, Seibert K, Raz A, Needleman P (1990) The induction and suppression of prostaglandin H2 synthase (cyclooxygenase) in human monocytes. *J Biol Chem* 265: 12013–12017
28 Gierse JK, Hauser SD, Creely DP, Koboldt C, Rangmwala SH, Isakson PC, Seibert K (1995) Expression and selective inhibition of the constitutive and inducible forms of human cyclooxygenase. *Biochem J* 305: 479–484
29 Penning TD, Talley JJ, Bertenshaw SR, Carter JS, Collins PW, Docter S, Graneto MJ, Lee LF, Malecha JW, Miyashiro JM et al (1997) Synthesis and biological evaluation of the 1,5-diarylpyrazole class of cyclooxygenase-2 inhibitors: identification of 4-[5-(4-methylphenyl)-3-(trifluoromethyl)-1H-pyrazol-1-yl]benzenesulfonamide (SC-58635, celecoxib). *J Med Chem* 40: 1347–1365
30 Peipins LA, Sandler RS (1994) Epidemiology of colorectal adenomas. *Epidemiol Rev* 16: 273–297
31 Neugut AI, Jacobson JS, DeVivo I (1993) Epidemiology of colorectal adenomatous polyps. *Cancer Epidemiol Biomarkers Prev* 2: 159–176
32 Gupta RA, DuBois RN, Wallace MC (2002) New avenues for the prevention of colorectal cancer: targeting cyclooxygenase-2 activity. *Best Pract Res Clin Gastroenterol* 16: 945–956
33 Fearnhead NS, Wilding JL, Bodmer WF (2002) Genetics of colorectal cancer: hereditary aspects and overview of colorectal tumorigenesis. *Br Med Bull* 64: 27–43
34 Kinzler KW, Nilbert MC, Su LK, Vogelstein B, Bryan TM, Levy DB, Smith KJ, Preisinger AC, Hedge P, McKechnie D et al (1991) Identification of FAP locus genes from chromosome 5q21. *Science* 253: 661–665
35 Bisgaard ML, Fenger K, Bulow S, Niebuhr E, Mohr J (1994) Familial adenomatous polyposis (FAP): frequency, penetrance and mutation rate. *Hum Mutat* 3: 121–125
36 Debinski HS, Love S, Spigelmann AD, Phillips K (1996) Colorectal polyp counts and cancer risk in familial adenomatous polyposis. *Gastroenterology* 110: 1028–1030
37 Waddell WR, Gasner GF, Cerise EJ, Loughry RW (1989) Sulindac for polyposis of the colon. *Am J Surg* 157: 175–178
38 Giardiello FM, Hamilton SR, Krush AJ, Piantadosi S, Hylind LM, Celano P, Booker SV, Robinson CR, Offerhaus GJ (1993) Treatment of colonic and rectal adenomas with sulindac in familial adenomatous polyposis. *N Engl J Med* 328: 1313–1316
39 Rigas B, Goldman IS, Levine L (1993) Altered eicosanoid levels in human colon cancer. *J Lab Clin Med* 122: 518–523
40 Qiao L, Kozoni V, Tsioulias GJ, Koutsos MI, Hanif R, Shiff SJ, Rigas B (1995) Selected

eicosanoids increase the proliferation rat of human colon carcinoma cell lines and mouse colonocytes *in vivo*. *Biochem Biophys Acta* 1258: 215–223

41 Sano H, Kawahito Y, Wilder RL, Hashiramoto A, Mukai A, Asai S, Kimura S, Kato H, Kondo M, Hla T (1995) Expression of cyclooxygenase-1 and -2 in human colorectal cancer. *Cancer Res* 55: 3785–3789

42 Shiff SJ, Koutsos MI, Qiao L, Rigas B (1996) Nonsteroidal anti-inflammatory drugs inhibit the proliferation of colon adenocarcinoma cells: effects on cell cycle and apoptosis. *Exp Cell Res* 222(1): 179–188

43 Yao M, Kargmann S, Lam EC, Kelly CR, Zheng Y, Luk P, Kwong E, Evans JF, Wolfe MM (2003) Inhibition of cyclooxygenase-2 by rofecoxib attenuates the growth and metastatic potential of colorectal carcinoma in mice. *Cancer Res* 63: 586–592

44 Oshima M, Dinchuk JE, Kargman SL, Oshima H, Hancock B, Kwong E, Trzaskos JM, Evans JF, Taketo MM (1996) Suppression of intestinal polyposis in APC D716 mice by inhibition of cyclooxygenase (PGHS-2). *Cell* 87: 803–809

45 Sheng H, Shao J, Kirkland SC, Isakson P, Coffey RJ, Morrow J, Beauchamp RD, Dubois RN (1997) Inhibition of human colon cancer cell growth by selective inhibition of cyclooxygenase-2. *J Clin Invest* 99: 2254–2259

46 Reddy BS, Rao CV, Seibert K (1996) Evaluation of cyclooxygenase-2 inhibitor for potential chemopreventive properties in colon carcinogenesis. *Cancer Res* 56: 4566–4569

47 Pollard M, Luckert PH (1981) Effect of indomethacine on intestinal tumors induced in rats by the acetate derivative of dimethylnitrosamine. *Science* 214: 558–59

48 Moorghen M, Ince P, Finney KJ, Sunter JP, Watson AJ, Appleton DR (1990) The effect on of sulindac on colonic tumour formation in dimethylhydrazine-treated mice. *Acta Histochem* 39 (Suppl): 195–199

49 Skinner SA, Penney AG, O'Brien PE (1991) Sulindac inhibits the rate of growth and appearance of colon tumors in the rat. *Arch Surg* 126: 1094–1096

50 Reddy BS, Rao CV, Rivenson A, Kelloff G (1993) Inhibitory effect of aspirin on azoxymethane-induced colon carcinogenesis in F344 rats. *Carcinogenesis* 14: 1493–1497

51 Ross DS, Bitzer D, Roy T, Murphy JE (1988) Piroxicam inhibits the growth of an adenocarcinoma isograft in Fisher rats. *J Surg Res* 45: 249–253

52 Pollard M, Luckert P (1984) Effect of piroxicam on primary intestinal tumors induced in rats by N-methylnitrosourea. *Cancer Lett* 25: 117–121

53 Santini G, Sciulli MG, Marinacci R, Fusco O, Spoletini L, Pace A, Ricciardulli A, Natoli C, Procopio A, Maclouf J, Patrignani P (1999) Cyclooxygenase-independent induction of p21 WAF-1/cip1, apoptosis and differentiation by L-745,337, a selective PGH synthase-2 inhibitor, and salicylate in HT-29 cells. *Apoptosis* 4: 151–162

54 Williams C, Shattuck-Brandt RL, DuBois RN (1999) The role of COX-2 inhibitors in intestinal cancer. *Ann NY Acad Sci* 889: 72–83

55 Williams CS, Luongo D, Radhika A, Zhang T, Lamps LW, Nanney LB, Beauchamp RD, DuBois RN (1996) Elevated cyclooxygenase-2 levels in Min mouse adenomas. *Gastroentrology* 111: 1134–1140

56 DuBois RN, Radhika A, Reddy BS, Entingh AJ (1996) Increased cyclooxygenase-2 levels in carcinogen-induced rat colonic tumors. *Gastroenterology* 111: 1134–1140

57 Eberhard CE, Coffey RJ, Radhika A, Giardello FM, Ferrenbach S, DuBois RN (1994) Up-regulation of cyclooxygenase-2 gene expression in human colorectal adenomas and adenocarcinomas. *Gastroenterology* 107: 1183–1188

58 Kargman S, O'Neil G, Vickers P, Evans J, Mancini J, Jothy S (1995) Expression of prostaglandin G/H synthase-1 and -2 protein in human colon cancer. *Cancer Res* 55: 2556–2559

59 Beazar-Barclay Y, Levy DB, Moser AR, Dove WF, Hamilton SR, Vogelstein B, Kinzler KW(1996) Sulindac suppresses tumorigenesis in the Min mouse. *Carcinogenesis* 17: 1757–1760

60 Stack E, Dubois RN (2001) Role of cyclooxygenase inhibitors for the prevention of colorectal cancer. *Gastroenterol Clin North Am* 30(4): 1001–1010

61 Suleiman S, Rex DK, Sonnenberg A. (2002) Chemoprevention of colorectal cancer by aspirin: a cost-effectiveness analysis. *Gastroenterology* 122: 78–84

62 Sandler RS, Halabi S, Baron JA, Budinger S, Paskett E, Keresztes R, Petrelli N, Pipas M, Karp DD; Loprinzi CL et al (2003) A randomized trial of Aspirin to prevent colorectal adenomas in patients with previous colorectal cancer. *N Engl J Med* 348: 883–890

63 Derry S, Loke YK (2000) Risk of gastrointestinal haemorrhage with long term use of aspirin: meta-analysis. *BMJ* 321: 1183–1187

64 Hawkey CJ (2000) Nonsteroidal anti-inflammatory drug gastropathy. *Gastroenterology* 119: 521–535

65 Baron JA, Cole BF, Sandler RS, Haile RW, Ahnen D, Bresalier R, McKeown-Eyssen G, Summers RW, Rothstein R, Burke CA et al (2003) A randomized trial of aspirin to prevent colorectal adenomas. *N Engl J Med* 348: 891–899

66 Sample D, Wargovich M, Fischer SM, Inamdar N, Schwartz P, Wang X, Do KA, Sinicrope FA (2002) A dose-finding study of aspirin for chemoprevention utilizing rectal mucosal prostaglandin E(2) levels as a biomarker. *Cancer Epidemiol Biomarkers Prev* 11: 275–279

67 Ruffin MTIV, Krishnan K, Rock CL, Normolle D, Vaerten MA, Peters-Golden M, Crowell J, Kelloff G, Boland CR, Brenner DE (1997) Suppression of human colorectal mucosal prostaglandins: determining the lowest effective aspirin dose. *J Natl Cancer Inst* 89: 1152–1160

68 Smalley W, Ray WA, Daugherty J, Griffin MR (1999) Use of nonsteroidal anti-inflammatory drugs and the incidence of colorectal cancer: a population-based study. *Arch Intern Med* 159: 161–166

69 Rosenberg L, Louik C, Shapiro S (1998) Nonsteroidal antiinflammatory drug use and reduced risk of large bowel carcinoma. *Cancer* 82: 2326–2333

70 Provenzale D (2002) The cost-effectiveness of aspirin for chemoprevention of colorectal cancer. *Gastroenterology* 122: 230–233

71 Kune GA, Kune S, Watson LF (1988) Colorectal cancer risk, chronic illness, operations,

and medications: case control results from the Melbourne Colorectal Cancer Study. *Cancer Res* 48: 4399–4404

72 Rosenberg L, Palmer JR, Zauber AG et al (1991) A hypothesis: Nonsteroidal anti-inflammatory drugs reduce the incidence of large-bowel cancer. *J Natl Cancer Inst* 83: 355–358

73 Logan RF, Little J, Hawtin PG, Hardcastle JD (1993) Effect of aspirin and nonsteroidal anti-inflammatory drugs on colorectal adenomas: case-control study of subjects participating in the Nottingham faecal blood screening programme. *BMJ* 307: 285–289

74 Peleg II, Maibach HT, Brown SH, Wilcox CM (1994) Aspirin and nonsteroidal anti-inflammatory drug use and the risk of subsequent colorectal cancer. *Arch Intern Med* 154: 394–399

75 Rigau J, Pique JM, Rubio E, Olanas R, Tarrech JM, Bordas JM (1991) Effects of long-term sulindac therapy on colonic polyposis. *Ann Intern Med* 115: 952–954

76 Labayle D, Fischer D, Vielh P, Drouhin F, Pariente A, Bories C, Duhamel O, Trousset M, Attali P (1991) Sulindac causes regression of rectal polyps in familial adenomatous polyposis. *Gastroenterology* 101: 635–639

77 Ladenheim J, Garcia G, Titzer D, Herzenberg H, Lavori P, Edson R, Omary MB (1995) Effect of sulindac on sporadic colonic polyps. *Gastroenterology* 108: 1083–1087

78 Nugent KP, Farmer KC, Spigelmann AD, Williams CB, Phillips RK (1993) Randomized controlled trial of the effect of sulindac on duodenal and rectal polyposis and cell proliferation in patients with familial adenomatous polyposis. *Br J Surg* 80: 1618–1619

79 North GL (2001) Celecoxib as adjunctive therapy for treatment of colorectal cancer. *Ann Pharmacother* 35 (12): 1638–1643

80 Mann M, Sheng H, Shao J, William CS, Pisacane PI, Slixkokowski MX, Dubois RN (2001) Targeting cyclooxygenase 2 and HER-2/neu pathways inhibits colorectal carcinoma growth. *Gastroenterology* 120: 1713–1719

81 Ricchi P, Zarilli R, di Palma A, Acquaviva AM (2003) Nonsteroidal anti-inflammatory drugs in colorectal cancer: from prevention to therapy. *Br J Cancer* 88: 803–807

Inflammation, necrosis, and cancer

Michael T. Lotze

Translational Research, Molecular Medicine Institute, University of Pittsburgh School of Medicine, 300 Technology Drive, Pittsburgh, PA 15219, USA

Perspective

"Apophonia ... the spontaneous perception of connections and meaningfulness in unrelated things."

Pattern Recognition
William Gibson
Berkley Pub Group, 2004

William Gibson might have included cancer and inflammation as an example of "apophonia". The perception of this connection, however, has been anything but spontaneous. Cancer is generally thought of as disordered cell growth driven by the accumulation of genes that confer a growth advantage or prevent cellular senescence [1]. Inflammation is thought of primarily as a non-immune, acute host-defense process. When persistent, chronic inflammation and the associated immune response together play a role in several diseases including rheumatoid arthritis, asthma, and inflammatory bowel disease. The thoughtful clinician and scientist reflecting on the extraordinary advances in cancer biology and the search for causes of cancer are disappointed with how our premises have not yet translated into more effective therapy. Those studying diseases associated with inflammation raise a similar concern, with many of the therapeutic targets seemingly intractable. What are we missing? The editors of this volume have addressed the relatedness of these seemingly "unrelated" fields to reveal "meaningfulness" that is now more perceptible. This revelation could provide a synergistic base to allow the generation of new questions and to accelerate innovation in understanding and treatment of these diseases.

There is now a growing appreciation that cancer progression is facilitated by host mechanisms exploited by tumors to promote growth and dissemination. This includes inflammation. Indeed, thematic to this volume, cancers arise in the setting of chronic inflammation. We have recognized that interactions during chronic inflammation involve a cascade of cells and proinflammatory and proliferative factors interacting in a number of ways that ultimately drive epithelial and, to a lesser

Cancer and Inflammation, edited by Douglas W. Morgan, Ulf J. Forssmann and Marian T. Nakada

extent, stromal genomic instability [4–11]. This may be just the tip of the iceberg. Further elucidation of these interactions will challenge the existing paradigms that cancer is purely a genetic disorder and that chronic inflammation may be limited to only some of these chronic diseases. Crossover between these two fields will certainly benefit both. Recognition of the role of inflammation in cancer could lead to breakthroughs in new forms of therapies that alone, or in combination with more conventional cytotoxic agents or biologic therapies, could shift cancer from being a fatal disease to one that is chronic and manageable. Therapies for inflammatory diseases could benefit similarly. Already we know the value of crossover therapies using methotrexate and cyclooxygenase-2 inhibitors, addressed in some detail herein.

The processes occurring subsequent to inflammation (leukocyte infiltration, necrosis, angiogenesis, stromagenesis, and occasionally carcinogenesis) have been defined over the last quarter of a century. In contrast, the identification of inflammatory processes preceding the development of cancer has been slow to be recognized [12–31]. In virtually every tumor type that occurs in increased frequency with age, inflammation or hormonal cycling is an antecedent. During the cycles of cell growth and cell death characterizing most chronic inflammatory states, epigenetic changes proceed that are related to enhancing angiogenesis, inhibiting apoptotic death and, paradoxically, limiting thrombolysis (thereby promoting micro-necrosis). These cycles occur whether driven by bacteria, virus, toxins, smoke inhalation, solar irradiation, or hormonal cycling. Rounds of cellular proliferation and cell death are associated with hypermethylation of promoter regions within tumor-suppressor and proapoptotic genes, promoting cell survival. Following acquisition of genetic limitations in apoptotic pathways, increasing necrotic cell death leads to the release of cellular contents, including high-mobility-group box 1 protein (HMGB1) [32–35], ATP [36, 37], heat-shock protein 70 [9, 38–40], and uric acid [41] among others. These in turn recruit sentinel cells which diminish immune reactivity and promote tumor cell growth. Macrophages and other inflammatory cells produce a variety of factors, both pro-stromagenic and pro-angiogenic. In the absence of exogenous danger signals, they suppress immune reactivity. In my view, cancer is more a disease of abnormal cell death and associated inflammation than one solely of disordered cell growth.

Necrosis and cancer

In virtually every tumor type carefully examined, necrosis is a concomitant of poor prognosis. This includes breast cancer [42–44], renal cancer [45], colon cancer [46], sarcoma [2, 3, 45, 47, 48], and melanoma [49, 50]. Necrotic tumors, unlike apoptotic cells, release their cellular contents. Which factors are released has only become apparent over the last few years. These include uric acid [41], ATP [36, 37, 51, 52], heat-shock protein 70 [39, 40, 53], and HMGB1. HMGB1 is a highly conserved 30-kDa eukaryotic nuclear regulatory factor, released from other cells including activated macrophages [32, 54–59] and possibly natural killer cells. It stimulates tmor necrosis factor production and inflammation, promotes sickness behavior, is an endogenous pyrogen, enhances tumor growth, promotes endothelial activation, leukocyte recruitment and adhesion, and mediates death in sepsis [60]. HMGB1 is a biologically potent costimulus of inflammation promoting interferon γ release in the presence of interkeukin-1, -2, and -12. It is elevated to extraordinary levels in the serum of patients with metastatic melanoma, suggesting its potential utility as an important new target for patients with unscheduled necrotic cell death and cancer. We have assessed detection in the serum of cancer patients and shown it to be elevated in patients with pancreatic cancer and melanoma. High levels of HMGB1 were found in all melanoma sera (30–2719 ng/ml) compared with 25.2 ng/ml in recovered and 83.7 ng/ml in dying septic patients (normal undetectable). The application of antibodies to HMGB1 is supported by the available data in cancer and other chronic inflammatory states [58]. Clearly HMGB1 could be one of the common links involving both of these disorders.

Immunity and cancer

As tumors progress, it is commonplace to observe immune deficits not only in cells within the tumor microenvironment but frequently in the systemic circulation as well [61–66]. This has alarmed the tumor immunologist and limited the biologic therapist's ability to "initiate" an immune response. In many instances, as noted above, immune infiltrates can indeed be observed in adult tumors and shown to correlate with improved survival. As tumors progress, they diminish their infiltrate and appear to have more substantial immune changes, the origins of which are still obscure. We would suggest that these changes are the consequence of global and specific downregulation of immune reactivity mediated by immune sentinels including plasmacytoid dendritic cells [67–69] and the consumption of tryptophan [70] or other factors necessary for lymphoid cell survival and function, as a consequence of diminished toll-like receptor (TLR) signaling and persistent necrotic cell death. If these notions are accurate, means to modify the inflammatory response with new anti-inflammatory agents in the clinic will generate a new class of cancer therapeutics.

References

1 Ben-Porath I, Weinberg RA (2004) When cells get stressed: an integrative view of cellular senescence. *J Clin Invest* 113: 8–13

2 Gustafson P, Akerman M, Alvegard TA, Coindre JM, Fletcher CD, Rydholm A, Willen H (2003) Prognostic information in soft tissue sarcoma using tumour size, vascular invasion and microscopic tumour necrosis-the SIN-system. *Eur J Cancer* 39: 1568–1576

3 Hasegawa T, Yamamoto S, Yokoyama R, Umeda T, Matsuno Y, Hirohashi S (2002) Prognostic significance of grading and staging systems using MIB-1 score in adult patients with soft tissue sarcoma of the extremities and trunk. *Cancer* 95: 843–851

4 Herzog CR, Bodon N, Pittman B, Maronpot RR, Massey TE, Anderson MW, You M, Devereux TR (2004) Carcinogen-specific targeting of chromosome 12 for loss of heterozygosity in mouse lung adenocarcinomas: implications for chromosome instability and tumor progression. *Oncogene* 23: 3033–3039

5 Duensing S, Munger K (2004) Mechanisms of genomic instability in human cancer: Insights from studies with human papillomavirus oncoproteins. *Int J Cancer* 109: 157–162

6 Tang R, Changchien CR, Wu MC, Fan CW, Liu KW, Chen JS, Chien HT, Hsieh LL (2004) Colorectal cancer without high microsatellite instability and chromosomal instability – an alternative genetic pathway to human colorectal cancer. *Carcinogenesis* 25: 841–846

7 Nassif NT, Lobo GP, Wu X, Henderson CJ, Morrison CD, Eng C, Jalaludin B, Segelov E (2004) PTEN mutations are common in sporadic microsatellite stable colorectal cancer. *Oncogene* 23: 617–628

8 Richardson C, Stark JM, Ommundsen M, Jasin M (2004) Rad51 overexpression promotes alternative double-strand break repair pathways and genome instability. *Oncogene* 23: 546–553

9 Hunt CR, Dix DJ, Sharma GG, Pandita RK, Gupta A, Funk M, Pandita TK (2004) Genomic instability and enhanced radiosensitivity in Hsp70.1- and Hsp70.3-deficient mice. *Mol Cell Biol* 24: 899–911

10 Liu G, Parant JM, Lang G, Chau P, Chavez-Reyes A, El-Naggar AK, Multani A, Chang S, Lozano G (2004) Chromosome stability, in the absence of apoptosis, is critical for suppression of tumorigenesis in Trp53 mutant mice. *Nat Genet* 36: 63–68

11 Stergiou L, Hengartner MO (2004) Death and more: DNA damage response pathways in the nematode C. elegans. *Cell Death Differ* 11: 21–28

12 Templeton A (1980) Pre-existing, non-malignant disorders associated with increased cancer risk. *J Environ Pathol Toxicol* 3: 387–397

13 Lotze MT (1997) Future directions for recombinant interleukin-2 in cancer: a chronic inflammatory disorder. *Cancer J Sci Am* 3: S106–S108

14 Jankowski JA, Harrison RF, Perry I, Balkwill F, Tselepis C (2000) Barrett's metaplasia. *Lancet* 356: 2079–2085

15 Balkwill F, Mantovani A (2001) Inflammation and cancer: back to Virchow? *Lancet* 357: 539–545

16 Fitzpatrick FA (2001) Inflammation, carcinogenesis and cancer. *Int Immunopharmacol* 1: 1651–1667

17 Ishitsuka T, Kashiwagi H, Konishi F (2001) Microsatellite instability in inflamed and neoplastic epithelium in ulcerative colitis. *J Clin Pathol* 54: 526–532
18 O'Byrne KJ, Dalgleish AG (2001) Chronic immune activation and inflammation as the cause of malignancy. *Br J Cancer* 85: 473–483
19 O'Byrne KJ, Dalgleish AG (2002) Infection and cancer. *Lancet* 358: 156
20 Brigati C, Noonan DM, Albini A, Benelli R (2002) Tumors and inflammatory infiltrates: friends or foes? *Clin Exp Metastasis* 19: 247–258
21 Chang YT, Wu MS, Shun CT, Lin MT, Chang MC, Lin JT (2002) Association of polymorphisms of interleukin-1 beta gene and Helicobacter pylori infection with the risk of gastric ulcer. *Hepatogastroenterology* 49: 1474–1476
22 Coussens LM, Werb Z (2002) Inflammation and cancer. *Nature* 420: 860–867
23 Fitzgerald RC, Abdalla S, Onwuegbusi BA, Sirieix P, Saffed IT, Burnham WR, Farthing MJ (2002) Inflammatory gradient in Barrett's oesophagus: implications for disease complications. *Gut* 51: 316–322
24 Howell WM, Calder PC, Grimble RF (2002) Gene polymorphisms, inflammatory diseases and cancer. *Proc Nutr Soc* 61: 447–456
25 Offersen BV, Knap MM, Marcussen N, Horsman MR, Hamilton-Dutoit S, Overgaard J (2002) Intense inflammation in bladder carcinoma is associated with angiogenesis and indicates good prognosis. *Br J Cancer* 87: 1422–1430
26 Shacter E, Weitzman SA (2002) Chronic inflammation and cancer. *Oncology (Huntingt)* 16: 217–226, 229; discussion 230–232
27 Guo HH, Loeb LA (2003) Tumbling down a different pathway to genetic instability. *J Clin Invest* 112: 1793–1795
28 Rao M, Yang W, Seifalian AM, Winslet MC (2003) Role of cyclooxygenase-2 in the angiogenesis of colorectal cancer. *Int J Colorectal Dis* 19: 1–11
29 Slaviero KA, Clarke SJ, Rivory LP (2003) Inflammatory response: an unrecognised source of variability in the pharmacokinetics and pharmacodynamics of cancer chemotherapy. *Lancet Oncol* 4: 224–232
30 Lucia MS, Torkko KC (2004) Inflammation as a target for prostate cancer chemoprevention: pathological and laboratory rationale. *J Urol* 171: S30–S35
31 Solakidi S, Dessypris A, Stathopoulos GP, Androulakis G, Sekeris CE (2004) Tumour-associated trypsin inhibitor, carcinoembryonic antigen and acute-phase reactant proteins CRP and alpha1-antitrypsin in patients with gastrointestinal malignancies. *Clin Biochem* 37: 56–60
32 Scaffidi P, Misteli T, Bianchi ME (2002) Release of chromatin protein HMGB1 by necrotic cells triggers inflammation. *Nature* 418: 191–195
33 O'Connor KA, Hansen MK, Rachal Pugh C, Deak MM, Biedenkapp JC, Milligan ED, Johnson JD, Wang H, Maier SF, Tracey KJ et al (2003) Further characterization of high mobility group box 1 (HMGB1) as a proinflammatory cytokine: central nervous system effects. *Cytokine* 24: 254–265
34 Andersson U, Erlandsson-Harris H, Yang H, Tracey KJ (2002) HMGB1 as a DNA-binding cytokine. *J Leukoc Biol* 72: 1084–1091

35 Czura CJ, Wang H, Tracey KJ (2001) Dual roles for HMGB1: DNA binding and cytokine. *J Endotoxin Res* 7: 315–321
36 Schmidt A, Ortaldo JR, Herberman RB (1984) Inhibition of human natural killer cell reactivity by exogenous adenosine 5'-triphosphate. *J Immunol* 132: 146–150
37 Schnurr M, Toy T, Stoitzner P, Cameron P, Shin A, Beecroft T, Davis ID, Cebon J, Maraskovsky E (2003) ATP gradients inhibit the migratory capacity of specific human dendritic cell types: implications for P2Y11 receptor signaling. *Blood* 102: 613–620
38 Buttiglieri S, Galetto A, Forno S, De Andrea M, Matera L (2003) Influence of drug-induced apoptotic death on processing and presentation of tumor antigens by dendritic cells. *Int J Cancer* 106: 516–520
39 Millar DG, Garza KM, Odermatt B, Elford AR, Ono N, Li Z, Ohashi PS (2003) Hsp70 promotes antigen-presenting cell function and converts T-cell tolerance to autoimmunity *in vivo*. *Nat Med* 9: 1469–1476
40 Noessner E, Gastpar R, Milani V, Brandl A, Hutzler PJ, Kuppner MC, Roos M, Kremmer E, Asea A, Calderwood SK et al (2002) Tumor-derived heat shock protein 70 peptide complexes are cross-presented by human dendritic cells. *J Immunol* 169: 5424–5432
41 Shi Y, Evans JE, Rock KL (2003) Molecular identification of a danger signal that alerts the immune system to dying cells. *Nature* 425: 516–521
42 Gilchrist KW, Gray R, Fowble B, Tormey DC, Taylor SGt (1993) Tumor necrosis is a prognostic predictor for early recurrence and death in lymph node-positive breast cancer: a 10-year follow-up study of 728 Eastern Cooperative Oncology Group patients. *J Clin Oncol* 11: 1929–1935
43 Kato T, Kameoka S, Kimura T, Tanaka S, Nishikawa T, Kobayashi M (2002) p53, mitosis, apoptosis and necrosis as prognostic indicators of long-term survival in breast cancer. *Anticancer Res* 22: 1105–1112
44 Kato T, Kameoka S, Kimura T, Nishikawa T, Kobayashi M (2003) The combination of angiogenesis and blood vessel invasion as a prognostic indicator in primary breast cancer. *Br J Cancer* 88: 1900–1908
45 Frank I, Blute ML, Cheville JC, Lohse CM, Weaver AL, Zincke H (2002) An outcome prediction model for patients with clear cell renal cell carcinoma treated with radical nephrectomy based on tumor stage, size, grade and necrosis: the SSIGN score. *J Urol* 168: 2395–2400
46 Hunter GJ, Willson SA, Chapman M (1983) Necrotic carcinoma of the colon. *Clin Radiol* 34: 297–299
47 Miyajima K, Oda Y, Oshiro Y, Tamiya S, Kinukawa N, Masuda K, Tsuneyoshi M (2002) Clinicopathological prognostic factors in soft tissue leiomyosarcoma: a multivariate analysis. *Histopathology* 40: 353–359
48 Cheville JC, Blute ML, Zincke H, Lohse CM, Weaver AL (2001) Stage pT1 conventional (clear cell) renal cell carcinmoa: pathological features associated with cancer specific survival. *J Urol* 166: 453–456
49 Cole DJ, Taubenberger JK, Pockaj BA, Yannelli JR, Carter C, Carrasquillo J, Leitman S,

Steinberg SM, Rosenberg SA, Yang YC (1994) Histopathological analysis of metastatic melanoma deposits in patients receiving adoptive immunotherapy with tumor-infiltrating lymphocytes. *Cancer Immunol Immunother* 38: 299–303

50 Scheffer SR, Nave H, Korangy F, Schlote K, Pabst R, Jaffee EM, Manns MP, Greten TF (2003) Apoptotic, but not necrotic, tumor cell vaccines induce a potent immune response *in vivo*. *Int J Cancer* 103: 205–211

51 Agteresch HJ, Rietveld T, Kerkhofs LGM, van den Berg JWO, Wilson JHP, Dagnelie PC (2002) Beneficial effects of adenosine triphosphate on nutritional status in advanced lung cancer patients: a randomized clinical trial. *J Clin Oncol* 20: 371–378

52 Yaglom JA, Ekhterae D, Gabai VL, Sherman MY (2003) Regulation of necrosis of H9c2 myogenic cells upon transient energy deprivation: rapid deenergization of mitochondria precedes necrosis and is controlled by reactive oxygen species, stress kinase JNK, HSP72, and ARC. *J Biol Chem* 278: 50483–50496

53 Di YP, Repasky EA, Subjeck JR (1997) Distribution of HSP70, protein kinase C, and spectrin is altered in lymphocytes during a fever-like hyperthermia exposure. *J Cell Physiol* 172: 44–54

54 Scaffidi P, Misteli T, Bianchi ME (2002) Release of chromatin protein HMGB1 by necrotic cells triggers inflammation. *Nature* 418: 191–195

55 Bustin M (2002) At the crossroads of necrosis and apoptosis: signaling to multiple cellular targets by HMGB1. *Sci STKE* 151: PE39

56 Bonaldi T, Talamo F, Scaffidi P, Ferrera D, Porto A, Bachi A, Rubartelli A, Agresti A, Bianchi ME (2003) Monocytic cells hyperacetylate chromatin protein HMGB1 to redirect it towards secretion. *EMBO J* 22: 5551–5560

57 Gardella S, Andrei C, Ferrera D, Lotti LV, Torrisi MR, Bianchi ME, Rubartelli A (2002) The nuclear protein HMGB1 is secreted by monocytes via a non-classical, vesicle-mediated secretory pathway. *EMBO Rep* 3: 995–1001

58 Lotze MT, DeMarco RA (2003) Dealing with death: HMGB1 as a novel target for cancer therapy. *Curr Opin Invest Drugs* 4 (12): 1405–1409

59 Park JS, Svetkauskaite D, He Q, Kim JY, Strassheim D, Ishizaka A, Abraham E (2003) Involvement of TLR 2 and TLR 4 in cellular activation by high mobility group box 1 protein (HMGB1). *J Biol Chem* 279: 7370–7377

60 Yang H, Ochani M, Li J, Qiang X, Tanovic M, Harris HE, Susarla SM, Ulloa L, Wang H, Di Raimo R et al (2004) Reversing established sepsis with antagonists of endogenous high-mobility group box 1. *Proc Natl Acad Sci USA* 101: 296–301

61 Takagi S, Chen K, Schwarz R, Iwatsuki S, Herberman RB, Whiteside TL (1989) Functional and phenotypic analysis of tumor-infiltrating lymphocytes isolated from human primary and metastatic liver tumors and cultured in recombinant interleukin-2. *Cancer* 63: 102–111

62 Sedlmayr P, Rabinowich H, Elder EM, Ernstoff MS, Kirkwood JM, Herberman RB, Whiteside TL (1991) Depressed ability of patients with melanoma or renal cell carcinoma to generate adherent lymphokine-activated killer cells. *J Immunother* 10: 336–346

63 Saito T, Dworacki G, Gooding W, Lotze MT, Whiteside TL (2000) Spontaneous apop-

tosis of CD8+ T lymphocytes in peripheral blood of patients with advanced melanoma. *Clin Cancer Res* 6: 1351–1364

64 Dworacki G, Meidenbauer N, Kuss I, Hoffmann TK, Gooding W, Lotze M, Whiteside TL (2001) Decreased zeta chain expression and apoptosis in CD3+ peripheral blood T lymphocytes of patients with melanoma. *Clin Cancer Res* 7: 947s–957s

65 Hoffmann TK, Muller-Berghaus J, Ferris RL, Johnson JT, Storkus WJ, Whiteside TL (2002) Alterations in the frequency of dendritic cell subsets in the peripheral circulation of patients with squamous cell carcinomas of the head and neck. *Clin Cancer Res* 8: 1787–1793

66 Beckebaum S, Cicinnati VR, Dworacki G, Muller-Berghaus J, Stolz D, Harnaha J, Whiteside TL, Thomson AW, Lu L, Fung JJ, Bonham CA (2002) Reduction in the circulating pDC1/pDC2 ratio and impaired function of *ex vivo*-generated DC1 in chronic hepatitis B infection. *Clin Immunol* 104: 138–150

67 Vermi W, Bonecchi R, Facchetti F, Bianchi D, Sozzani S, Festa S, Berenzi A, Cella M, Colonna M (2003) Recruitment of immature plasmacytoid dendritic cells (plasmacytoid monocytes) and myeloid dendritic cells in primary cutaneous melanomas. *J Pathol* 200: 255–268

68 Gomez J, Borras FE, Singh R, Rajananthanan P, English M, Knight SC, Navarrete CV (2004) Differential up-regulation of HLA-DM, invariant chain, and CD83 on myeloid and plasmacytoid dendritic cells from peripheral blood. *Tissue Antigens* 63: 149–157

69 Hartmann E, Wollenberg B, Rothenfusser S, Wagner M, Wellisch D, Mack B, Giese T, Gires O, Endres S, Hartmann G (2003) Identification and functional analysis of tumor-infiltrating plasmacytoid dendritic cells in head and neck cancer. *Cancer Res* 63: 6478–6487

70 Munn DH, Mellor AL (2004) IDO and tolerance to tumors. *Trends Mol Med* 10: 15–28

Index

acquired immune system 75
activation-induced cell death (AICD) 129
active MMP 74
adenocarcinoma 2, 8, 153, 180
adenoma 180
adenoma-carcinoma sequence 178
adhesion molecule 101, 102, 109
angiogenesis 21, 58, 62, 80, 82, 108, 160
angiogenic support 21
angiogenic switch 82
angiogenin 108
anti-inflammatory drug 81
apophonia 189
apoptosis 24, 32, 123–136, 160
apoptosome 124
apoptotic resistance 126, 130, 131
arachidonic acid 148, 177
arsenic 22
asbestos 22
asbestosis 11
ascite formation 55
aspirin 81
ATP 25, 190
AU-rich sequence 151
Avastin (an anti-VEGF monoclonal antibody) 12

B lymphocyte 75
bacille Calmette-Guérin (BCG) 30
Barrett's esophagus (BE) 8, 154
basement membrane 78
basic fibroblast growth factor (bFGF) 100, 106
batimastat 83
Bcl 123, 126, 134
Bcl-2 126, 134
bladder cancer 2, 10
blood surrogate 34
breast cancer 190
breast tissue 22
Bretscher and Cohn model 25
broad-spectrum MPI 83

carcinogenic, COX-2 activity 159
catalytic domain, MMP 71
CCR7 58
celecoxib 111
cell-adhesion molecule 110
chemokine 53, 54, 61, 63, 77, 78, 101, 102, 105, 107, 108
chemokine receptor 53, 54
chemokine receptor antagonist 61, 63
chemoprotection 157
chemoradiotherapy 162
chemotactic mediator 76
chemotaxis 77
chemotherapeutic agents 162
chronic gastritis 2
chronic inflammation 81, 131, 148
chronic pancreatitis 9, 155
chymase 77
clinical trials, with MPIs 83
colitis-associated cancer 156
colon cancer 156, 190
colorectal cancer (CRC) 6, 177, 182

colorectal cancer, prevention 182
Corynebacterium parvum 30
COX-independent anti-cancer effect 161
COX-1 150, 153
COX-2 111, 150, 159, 178, 180
COX-2 inhibitor 177, 182
COX-2 pathway 180
Crohn's disease 157
CSF-1 26, 102, 103
CTLA4 30
CXCR4 58
cysteine switch 73
cytochrome C 124
cytokine 101, 103, 105, 107
cytoprotective role, COX-1 expression 153
cytotoxic T lymphocyte 130

de novo cancer 80
dendritic cell (DC) 21, 29, 32, 78, 103
double-stranded RNA 27
dysplasia, precancerous 153

E1A (viral oncogenic protein) 125
eicosanoid 148
endogenous MMP inhibitor 74
endogenous pyrogen 191
endopeptidase 77
endothelial activation 191
endothelial cell 109
eosinophil 81
epithelial metaplasia 132
Epstein-Barr virus 22
E-selectin 110
esophageal adenocarcinoma (EAC) 8, 153
esophageal squamous cell carcinoma (ESCC) 153
expression of matrix metalloproteinase (MMP) 73
extracellular matrix (ECM) 75, 99, 109
extracellular matrix metalloproteinase inducer (EMMPRIN) 74
extracellular matrix remodeling 75
extravasation 78

Fas ligand (FasL) 32, 123, 126, 133
FLIP 129
furin-susceptible insert 74

gastric adenocarcinoma 2
gastritis 2
gastro-esophageal reflux disease (GERD) 8, 154
G-CSF 26
genetic instability 159
genomic instability 21
glioblastoma cell 58
glioma 55
GM-CSF 26, 28
granzyme 32
growth factor 103, 105

head and neck squamous cell cancer (HNSCC) 153
heat-shock protein 25, 191
Helicobacter pylori 2–4, 22, 81, 131, 154
hepatic cirrhosis 156
hepatitis B virus 22
hepatitis C 4, 22, 156
hepatitis C virus 22
hepatocellular carcinoma (HCC) 2, 4, 156
high-mobility-group box 1 protein (HMGB1) 190, 191
HMGB-1 25
Hodgkin's disease 22, 55
host response 85
Hsp70 25
human carcinoma of the breast and cervix 55
human papillomavirus 22

IFNs α, β and γ 26
IL-1 26, 106, 107
IL-1α 28, 29
IL-1β 28, 29
IL-2 26
IL-3 26
IL-4 26, 107
IL-6 25, 102, 107

IL-7 25
IL-8 107
IL-10 25, 27
IL-11 25
IL-12 26, 28, 30
IL-18 26, 28, 30
IL-1F5 29
IL-1F7 29
IL-1F9 29
IL-1RA 29
IL-2 receptor-α (IL-2Rα) 78
immunity 25, 26, 75, 77
immunity, signals 25, 26
immunologic "ignorance" 22
immunologic quiescence 33, 34
infiltrating leukocyte 55, 57
inflammatory bowel disease (IBD) 2, 6, 130, 131, 134
inflammatory cell 76–79, 81, 82
inflammatory cell-derived MMP 76, 82
inhibitor of apoptosis (IAP) 128
innate immune system 75
iNOS 132
integrin 110
intercellular adhesion molecule-1 (ICAM-1) 110
interferon γ (IFNγ) 22
intestinal cancer growth 180
intestinal metaplasia 154
intestinal tumor 80
intraductal papillary-mucinous tumor (IPMT) 155
invasion 79
isomerase 150

JAK/STAT 26

Kaposi's sarcoma 57
K-*ras* 155

Langerhans cell 78
latent matrix metalloproteinase 73
leukocyte 55, 57, 99, 101, 105, 191
leukocyte infiltrate 54-57
leukocyte recruitment 101, 191
leukotriene 148
lipopolysaccharide (LPS) 31
lipoxygenase 150
lymphocyte 75, 78, 105
lymphokine-activated killer cell (LAK) 30

α2-macroglobulin 74
macrophage 75, 76, 81, 82, 102, 103, 108
macrophage colony-stimulating factor (M-CSF or CSF-1) 26, 102, 103
malignancy 80
malignant melanoma 58
mast cell 75, 76, 81, 82, 103
matrix metalloproteinase (MMP) 57, 71–86, 101
matrix metalloproteinase and inflammation 75
matrix metalloproteinase and neoplastic progression 79
matrix metalloproteinase family members 71–73
matrix metalloproteinase inhibitor (MPI) 74, 80, 82
matrix metalloproteinase localization 74
matrix metalloproteinase mRNA expression 73
matrix metalloproteinase promotor region 73
M-CSF 26, 102, 103
melanoma 25, 58, 190
membrane-type matrix metalloproteinase (MT-MMP) 71
mesothelioma 11
metaplasia 132, 154
metastase 58, 79, 80, 82, 83
MHC class I chain-like genes A and B (MICA/B) 22
microenvironment 81
micro-necrosis 190
migration 78
mitogen-activated protein kinase (MAPK) 151
MMP-9 80, 82
monocyte 76, 77, 102–108

monocyte chemoattractant protein (MCP) 77
monocyte chemotactic protein-1 (MCP-1) 100, 102, 103, 108
multiple myeloma 58

natural killer (NK) cell 21, 29, 75
necrotic cell death 24, 32
neoplastic cell 79
neoplastic progression 80, 81
neuroendocrine tumor 155
neutrophil 75, 76, 81, 104
NF-κB 63, 128, 134
nitric oxide 25
NK cell 21, 29, 75
non-steroidal anti-inflammatory drug (NSAID) 99, 111, 157, 178, 182
nuclear factor κB (NF-κB) 63, 128, 134

ovarian cancer 55, 58

p53 125, 132
pancreatic cancer 9
pancreatic ductal carcinoma (PDC) 155
pancreatic intraepithelial neoplasia 155
pancreatic islet cell cancer 82
pancreatic islet cell carcinogenesis 80
pancreatitis 9, 155
PD-ECGF 106
PGHS-2 synthase 151
phospholipase A2 (PLA2) 149
plasmacytoid dendritic cell 191
plasminogen activator receptor 100
platelet-derived growth factor (PDGF) 100
polymorphonuclear neutrophil (PMN) 104
precancerous dysplasia 153
pre-clinical animal model 83
proliferation 160
pro-MMP 76
propeptide domain 71
prostaglandin 148, 178
prostaglandin H2 178
prostanoid 25
proteinase 71–86, 103, 109
proteolytic processing 75

reactive oxygen species 103
recruitment 77, 85
recruitment pathway 85
remodeling 75
renal cancer 190
resistance to apoptosis 125, 133
reversion-inducing-cysteine-rich protein with Kazal motifs (RECK) 74

sarcoma 55, 190
Schistosomiasis 2, 10
sickness behavior 191
signals in immunity0 25, 26
single-nucleotide polymorphism (SNP) 73
single-stranded DNA 27
skin carcinogenesis 82
smoking 22
squamous carcinogenesis 80
squamous cell carcinoma 55, 153
stroma 81
stromagenic support 21
stromal fibroblast 79
suppressor of cytokine signaling 1 (SOC1) 26
suppressor of cytokine signaling 3 (SOC3) 26
survivin 135
synthetic MPI 82

T-lymphocyte 75
Th2 cell 57
thalidomide 111
therapeutic efficacy 83
thrombolysis 190
thromboxane 148
tissue inhibitor of matrix metalloproteinases (TIMP) 71, 74, 80
tissue remodeling 21
TNF-related apoptosis-inducing ligand (TRAIL) 32, 135
TP53 126, 136

transforming growth factor β (TGFβ) 25, 57, 100
tryptase 77
tryptopan 191
tumor growth 79, 80, 191
tumor microenvironment 82
tumor necrosis factor α (TNFα) 22, 56, 100, 111
tumor progression 80
tumor-associated leukocyte infiltrate by chemokines 54
tumor-associated macrophage (TAM) 102
tumor-associated MMP 81
tumor-infiltrating lymphocyte 78

ulcerative colitis 157
uric acid 25, 190
urokinase plasminogen activator receptor (uPAR) 100
uterine tissue 22

vascular cell 79
vascular cell adhesion molecule-1 (VCAM-1) 110
vascular endothelial growth factor (VEGF) 100, 102, 103, 105

xenograft 158

The PIR-Series
Progress in Inflammation Research

Homepage: http://www.birkhauser.ch

Up-to-date information on the latest developments in the pathology, mechanisms and therapy of inflammatory disease are provided in this monograph series. Areas covered include vascular responses, skin inflammation, pain, neuroinflammation, arthritis cartilage and bone, airways inflammation and asthma, allergy, cytokines and inflammatory mediators, cell signalling, and recent advances in drug therapy. Each volume is edited by acknowledged experts providing succinct overviews on specific topics intended to inform and explain. The series is of interest to academic and industrial biomedical researchers, drug development personnel and rheumatologists, allergists, pathologists, dermatologists and other clinicians requiring regular scientific updates.

Immunology and Drug Therapy of Atopic Skin Diseases,
C.A.F. Bruijnzeel-Komen, E.F. Knol (Editors), 2000
Novel Cytokine Inhibitors, G.A. Higgs, B. Henderson (Editors), 2000
Inflammatory Processes. Molecular Mechanisms and Therapeutic Opportunities,
L.G. Letts, D.W. Morgan (Editors), 2000*Cellular Mechanisms in Airways Inflammation*,
C. Page, K. Banner, D. Spina (Editors), 2000
Inflammatory and Infectious Basis of Atherosclerosis, J.L. Mehta (Editor), 2001
Muscarinic Receptors in Airways Diseases, J. Zaagsma, H. Meurs, A.F. Roffel (Editors), 2001
TGF-β and Related Cytokines in Inflammation, S.N. Breit, S. Wahl (Editors), 2001
Nitric Oxide and Inflammation, D. Salvemini, T.R. Billiar, Y. Vodovotz (Editors), 2001
Neuroinflammatory Mechanisms in Alzheimer's Disease. Basic and Clinical Research,
J. Rogers (Editor), 2001
Disease-modifying Therapy in Vasculitides,
C.G.M. Kallenberg, J.W. Cohen Tervaert (Editors), 2001
Inflammation and Stroke, G.Z. Feuerstein (Editor), 2001
NMDA Antagonists as Potential Analgesic Drugs,
D.J.S. Sirinathsinghji, R.G. Hill (Editors), 2002
Migraine: A Neuroinflammatory Disease? E.L.H. Spierings, M. Sanchez del Rio (Editors), 2002
Mechanisms and Mediators of Neuropathic pain, A.B. Malmberg, S.R. Chaplan (Editors), 2002
Bone Morphogenetic Proteins. From Laboratory to Clinical Practice,
S. Vukicevic, K.T. Sampath (Editors), 2002
The Hereditary Basis of Allergic Diseases, J. Holloway, S. Holgate (Editors), 2002
Inflammation and Cardiac Diseases, G.Z. Feuerstein, P. Libby, D.L. Mann (Editors), 2003
Mind over Matter – Regulation of Peripheral Inflammation by the CNS,
M. Schäfer, C. Stein (Editors), 2003
Heat Shock Proteins and Inflammation, W. van Eden (Editor), 2003
Pharmacotherapy of Gastrointestinal Inflammation, A. Guglietta (Editor), 2004
Arachidonate Remodeling and Inflammation, A.N. Fonteh, R.L. Wykle (Editors), 2004
Recent Advances in Pathophysiology of COPD, P.J. Barnes, T.T. Hansel (Editors), 2004
Cytokines and Joint Injury, W.B. van den Berg, P. Miossec (Editors), 2004

GPSR Compliance

The European Union's (EU) General Product Safety Regulation (GPSR) is a set of rules that requires consumer products to be safe and our obligations to ensure this.

If you have any concerns about our products, you can contact us on ProductSafety@springernature.com

In case Publisher is established outside the EU, the EU authorized representative is:

Springer Nature Customer Service Center GmbH
Europaplatz 3
69115 Heidelberg, Germany

Batch number: 10577884

Printed by Printforce, the Netherlands